THE PSYCHIATRY RESIDENT HANDBOOK

HOW TO THRIVE IN TRAINING

THE PSYCHIATRY RESIDENT HANDBOOK

HOW TO THRIVE IN TRAINING

Edited by

Sallie G. De Golia, M.D., M.P.H.

Raziya S. Wang, M.D.

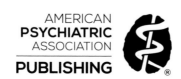

AMERICAN
PSYCHIATRIC
ASSOCIATION
PUBLISHING

Copyright © 2023 American Psychiatric Association Publishing

ALL RIGHTS RESERVED

First Edition

Manufactured in the United States of America on acid-free paper
27 26 25 24 23   5 4 3 2 1

American Psychiatric Association Publishing
800 Maine Avenue SW, Suite 900
Washington, DC 20024-2812
www.appi.org

Library of Congress Cataloging-in-Publication Data
A CIP record is available from the Library of Congress.
ISBN 9781615374113 (paperback), 9781615374120 (ebook)

British Library Cataloguing in Publication Data
A CIP record is available from the British Library.

CONTENTS

PART 3
Approaching Clinical Work

PART 5

Developing a Career

Preface

Psychiatry residency training can be a meaningful and life-changing experience, especially with the guidance of wise mentors. The authors of this book endeavor to formalize wise guidance from experienced residency faculty as well as current residents-in-training from across the United States. In each chapter, the authors provide useful explanations and tips for residents and make explicit what residents otherwise often learn implicitly. Our hope is that this guide will help residents anticipate challenges and thrive during this phase in their psychiatry careers.

Contributors

Rashi Aggarwal, M.D.
Professor and Director, Residency Training, Department of Psychiatry, Rutgers New Jersey Medical School, Newark, New Jersey

Neal D. Amin, M.D., Ph.D.
Clinical Assistant Professor, Stanford University, Stanford, California

Nientara Anderson, M.D., M.H.S.
Resident Psychiatrist, Yale University School of Medicine, New Haven, Connecticut

Timothy Ando, M.D.
Psychiatrist, Baywell Psychiatry Group, San Francisco, California

Melissa R. Arbuckle, M.D., Ph.D.
Professor of Psychiatry, Director of Adult Psychiatry Residency Training, and Vice Chair for Education, Columbia University Irving Medical Center and New York State Psychiatric Institute, New York, New York

Cybèle Arsan, M.D.
Psychiatrist, Kaiser Permanente Oakland Medical Center, Oakland, California

Janet Baek, M.D.
Child and Adolescent Psychiatry Fellow, Stanford University School of Medicine, Stanford, California

Clayton A. Barnes, M.D., M.P.H.
Medical Director of the Alcohol and Drug Abuse Prevention and Treatment Program, Joint Base Elmendorf-Richardson Hospital, JBER, Richardson, Alaska

Sara Baumann, M.D.
Assistant Clinical Professor of Psychiatry, University of California, Davis, Sacramento, California

Antoine Beayno, M.D.
Resident, Department of Psychiatry, Icahn School of Medicine at Mount Sinai Morningside/West, New York, New York

Iverson Bell, M.D., DLFAPA
Director of Residency Training and Associate Professor, Department of Psychiatry, University of Tennessee Health Science Center, Memphis, Tennessee

Jeana Benton, M.D.
Assistant Professor, University of Nebraska Medical Center, Omaha, Nebraska

Laurel J. Bessey, M.D.
Assistant Professor of Psychiatry and Associate Residency Training Director, University of Wisconsin School of Medicine and Public Health, Madison, Wisconsin

Seamus Bhatt-Mackin, M.D., FAPA, CGP, AGPA-F
Director, Program for Clinical Group Work, VA Mid-Atlantic Mental Illness Research, Education and Clinical Center (MIRECC), Durham, North Carolina

Adam Brenner, M.D.
Director of Adult Psychiatry Residency Training and Vice Chair for Education in Psychiatry, University of Texas Southwestern Medical Center, Dallas, Texas

Deborah L. Cabaniss, M.D.
Professor of Clinical Psychiatry and Associate Director of Adult Psychiatry Residency Training, Columbia University/New York State Psychiatric Institute, New York, New York

Hugh Caldwell, M.D.
PGY-4 Resident, Department of Psychiatry, University of Tennessee Health Science Center, Memphis, Tennessee

Jorien Campbell, M.D.
Forensic Child and Adolescent Psychiatrist, Forensic Psychiatric Associates, Irvine, California

Enrico G. Castillo, M.D., M.S.H.P.M.
Assistant Professor and Associate Vice Chair for Justice, Equity, Diversity, and Inclusion, Jane and Terry Semel Institute for Neuroscience and Human Behavior at UCLA, Department of Psychiatry and Biobehavioral Sciences, UCLA David Geffen School of Medicine, Los Angeles, California

Metin Cayirolgu, M.D.
Attending Psychiatrist, Department of Psychiatry, Northwell Health, New York, New York

Joanna Chambers, M.D.
Associate Professor of Clinical Psychiatry and OB/GYN, Indiana University School of Medicine, Indianapolis, Indiana

Sarah C. Collica, M.D.
Chief Resident, Department of Psychiatry and Behavioral Sciences, Johns Hopkins Medical Institutions, Baltimore, Maryland

Rachel Conrad, M.D.
Instructor in Psychiatry, Brigham and Women's Hospital, Boston, Massachusetts

Takesha Cooper, M.D., M.S.
Associate Professor and Program Director, Psychiatry Residency Training Program; Vice-Chair of Education, UCR Department of Psychiatry and Neurosciences; Equity Advisor and Chair of Medical School Admissions Committee, UC Riverside School of Medicine, Riverside, California

Ann Crawford-Roberts, M.D., M.P.H.
Psychiatrist, San Ysidro Health, San Diego, California

Erin M. Crocker, M.D.
Clinical Associate Professor, Department of Psychiatry, University of Iowa, Iowa City, Iowa

E. Ann Cunningham, D.O.
Psychiatry Residency Program Director at Community Health Network, Community Health Network, Indianapolis, Indiana

Sallie G. De Golia, M.D., M.P.H.
Clinical Professor and Co-Residency Director, Department of Psychiatry and Behavioral Sciences, Stanford University School of Medicine, Stanford, California

Michael DeGroot, M.D.
Assistant Professor, Department of Psychiatry and Behavioral Sciences, University of Minnesota Medical School, Minneapolis, Minnesota

Vanessa de la Cruz, M.D.
Louisiana State Medical Director, Eleanor Health, New Orleans, Louisiana

Matthew L. Edwards, M.D.
Assistant Professor and Assistant Director of Residency Training, Department of Psychiatry and Behavioral Sciences, Stanford University School of Medicine, Stanford, California

Laura Erickson-Schroth, M.D.
Chief Medical Officer, The Jed Foundation; Psychiatrist, Hetrick-Martin Institute for LGBTQ Youth; Assistant Professor, Columbia University Medical Center, New York, New York

Carrie Ernst, M.D.
Associate Professor of Psychiatry and Medical Education, Icahn School of Medicine at Mount Sinai, Mount Sinai Hospital, New York, New York

Ambarin Faizi, D.O.
Adult and Forensic Psychiatrist, Forensic Psychiatric Associates, Irvine, California

Aaron Feiger, M.D.
Medical Instructor, Department of Psychiatry and Behavioral Sciences, Duke University, Durham, North Carolina

Christine T. Finn, M.D.
Vice Chair for Clinical Services and Associate Professor, Dartmouth Hitchcock Medical Center, Lebanon, New Hampshire

Laura Flores, Ph.D.
M.D.-Ph.D. scholar, University of Nebraska Medical Center, College of Medicine, Omaha, Nebraska

Allison Ford, M.D.
Assistant Professor, Department of Psychiatry, University of Tennessee Health Science Center, Memphis, Tennessee

Amy Gallop, M.D.
Resident, Department of Psychiatry, St. Louis University, St. Louis, Missouri

Daniel E. Gih, M.D.
Associate Professor, University of Nebraska Medical Center, Omaha, Nebraska

Teddy G. Goetz, M.D., M.S.
PGY-2 Psychiatry Resident, Department of Psychiatry, University of Pennsylvania, Philadelphia, Pennsylvania

Nichole Goodsmith, M.D., Ph.D.
Assistant Professor, VA Greater Los Angeles Healthcare System and Jane and Terry Semel Institute for Neuroscience and Human Behavior at UCLA, Department of Psychiatry and Biobehavioral Sciences, UCLA David Geffen School of Medicine, Los Angeles, California

Tracey M. Guthrie, M.D.
Professor, Clinician Educator, Vice Chair for Clinical Faculty Affairs, Assistant Dean for Diversity in the Division of Biology and Medicine, and Program Director, Adult Psychiatry Residency Training Program, Department of Psychiatry and Human Behavior, Warren Alpert Medical School of Brown University, Providence, Rhode Island

Nekisa Haghighat, M.D., M.P.H.
Resident Physician, Department of Psychiatry and Neurosciences, UC Riverside School of Medicine, Riverside, California

Elizabeth E. Hathaway, M.D.
Psychiatry Resident, Indiana University School of Medicine, Indianapolis, Indiana

Paul Hill, M.D.
Associate Director of Residency Training and Assistant Professor, Department of Psychiatry, University of Tennessee Health Science Center, Memphis, Tennessee

Erick Hung, M.D.
Professor of Clinical Psychiatry, University of California, San Francisco School of Medicine, San Francisco, California

Jeffrey Hunt, M.D.
Professor (Teacher Scholar Track), Department of Psychiatry and Human Behavior, Alpert Medical School of Brown University, Providence, Rhode Island

Jessica Isom, M.D., M.P.H.
Clinical Instructor, Department of Psychiatry, Yale University, New Haven, Connecticut

Oluwole Jegede, M.D., M.P.H.
Assistant Professor of Psychiatry, Yale University School of Medicine, New Haven, Connecticut

James Kahn, M.D.
Professor of Medicine, Stanford University School of Medicine, Palo Alto, California

Michael Kelly, M.D.
Chief of Forensics, Department of State Hospitals—Coalinga, Coalinga, California

Anna Kerlek, M.D.
Child and Adolescent Psychiatry Program Training Director, Nationwide Children's Hospital and The Ohio State University College of Medicine, Columbus, Ohio

Manal Khan, M.D.
Assistant Clinical Professor of Psychiatry, Division of Child and Adolescent Psychiatry; UCLA Semel Institute for Neuroscience and Behavior, David Geffen School of Medicine at UCLA, Los Angeles, California

Murad M. Khan, M.D.
PGY-4 Psychiatry Resident, Department of Psychiatry, Yale School of Medicine, New Haven, Connecticut

You Na P. Kheir, M.D.
Child and Adolescent Psychiatry Fellow, Indiana University School of Medicine, Indianapolis, Indiana

Kristen Kim, M.D.
Child and Adolescent Psychiatry Fellow, Department of Psychiatry, University of California San Diego, San Diego, California

Grace Lee, M.D.
Clinical Assistant Professor, Department of Psychiatry and Behavioral Sciences, Stanford University School of Medicine, Stanford, California

Zachary Lenane, M.D., M.P.H.
Attending Psychiatrist, Whiting Forensic Hospital, Connecticut Department of Mental Health and Addiction Services, Middletown, Connecticut

Melissa M. Ley-Thomson, M.D.
Resident in Psychiatry, Dartmouth Hitchcock Medical Center, Lebanon, New Hampshire

Karen Li, M.D.
Child and Adolescent Psychiatry Fellow, Stanford University, Palo Alto, California

Csilla N. Lippert, M.D., Ph.D.
Staff Psychiatrist, VA Palo Alto Health Care System, Palo Alto, California

Juan David Lopez, M.D.
Clinical Assistant Professor, Department of Psychiatry and Behavioral Sciences, Stanford University School of Medicine, Stanford, California

Vishal Madaan, M.D.
Chief of Education and Deputy Medical Director, American Psychiatric Association, Washington, D.C.

Aekta Malhotra, M.D., M.S.
Medical Director, Apollo Psychiatry, Plano, Texas

Jennifer E. Manegold, M.D., M.S.
Fellow in Child and Adolescent Psychiatry, Jane and Terry Semel Institute for Neuroscience and Human Behavior at UCLA, Department of Psychiatry and Biobehavioral Sciences, UCLA David Geffen School of Medicine, Los Angeles, California

Tessa L. Manning, M.D.
Assistant Professor, Department of Psychiatry, University of Oklahoma School of Community Medicine, Tulsa, Oklahoma

Natalie Maples, Dr.P.H.
Assistant Professor, UT Health San Antonio, San Antonio, Texas Email address for complimentary book ordering information:

Melissa Martinez, M.D.
Professor, UT Health San Antonio, San Antonio, Texas

Phelan E. Maruca-Sullivan, M.D.
Assistant Professor, Department of Psychiatry, Yale University, New Haven, Connecticut

Alka Mathur, M.D.
Clinical Assistant Professor (Affiliate), Stanford School of Medicine; Medical Director, Virtual Behavioral Health Services, Veterans Affairs Palo Alto Healthcare System, Palo Alto, California

Jessica L. W. Mayer, M.D.
Pediatrics/Psychiatry/Child Psychiatry Resident, Indiana University School of Medicine, Indianapolis, Indiana

Patrick McGuire, D.O.
Core Faculty for Community Health Network, Indianapolis, Indiana

Michael O. Mensah, M.D., M.P.H.
Postdoctoral scholar and Psychiatrist, Yale University School of Medicine, New Haven, Connecticut

Isabella Morton, M.D., M.P.H.
Clinical Instructor, VA Greater Los Angeles Healthcare System and Jane and Terry Semel Institute for Neuroscience and Human Behavior at UCLA, Department of Psychiatry and Biobehavioral Sciences, UCLA David Geffen School of Medicine, Los Angeles, California

Katharine J. Nelson, M.D.
Associate Professor, Department of Psychiatry and Behavioral Sciences, University of Minnesota Medical School, Minneapolis, Minnesota

William Newman, M.D.
Professor of Psychiatry, St. Louis University, St. Louis, Missouri

Tram Nguyen, M.D.
Staff Physician, Bay Area Clinical Associates, San Jose, California

Aaron Owen, M.D.
Clinical Assistant Professor of Psychiatry, University of Wisconsin School of Medicine and Public Health, Madison, Wisconsin

Daniella Palermo, M.D.
Clinical Assistant Professor of Psychiatry and Human Behavior and Curriculum Director, General Adult Psychiatry Residency Program, Warren Alpert Medical School of Brown University, Providence, Rhode Island

Amit Parikh, M.D.
Child and Adolescent Psychiatrist, Sports Psychiatrist, Los Angeles, California

Michael Polignano, M.D.
Clinical Assistant Professor and Associate Program Director, Stanford Addiction Medicine Fellowship, Department of Psychiatry and Behavioral Sciences, Stanford University School of Medicine, Stanford, California

Zheala Qayyum, M.D., M.M.Sc.
Assistant Professor of Psychiatry, Boston Children's Hospital, Harvard Medical School, Cambridge, Massachusetts

Harika Reddy, M.D.
Resident Physician, Department of Psychiatry and Neurosciences, UC Riverside School of Medicine, Riverside, California

Rebecca Rendleman, M.D.
Associate Professor of Clinical Psychiatry, Weill Cornell Medicine, New York, New York

James I. Rim, J.D., M.D.
Assistant Clinical Professor of Psychiatry, Columbia University Irving Medical Center and New York State Psychiatric Institute, New York, New York

Robert Rohrbaugh, M.D.
Professor, Department of Psychiatry, Yale University, New Haven, Connecticut

Anne E. Ruble, M.D., M.P.H.
Director of Psychotherapy Training and Associate Director for Residency Education, Department of Psychiatry and Behavioral Sciences, Johns Hopkins Medical Institutions, Baltimore, Maryland

Mohona Sadhu, M.D.
Assistant Professor, Department of Psychiatry, University of Texas Southwestern Medical Center, Dallas, Texas

Bronwyn Lane Scott, M.D.
Resident, Psychiatry, Mayo Clinic, Rochester, Minnesota
Email address for complimentary book ordering information: Bronwyn Lane Scott, scott.bronwyn@mayo.edu

Sourav Sengupta, M.D., M.P.H.
Associate Professor, Psychiatry and Pediatrics, Departments of Psychiatry and Pediatrics, Jacobs School of Medicine and Biomedical Sciences, University at Buffalo, Buffalo, New York

Jon Sole, M.D.
Resident, Psychiatry, Stanford University, Palo Alto, California

Gillian L. Sowden, M.D.
Residency Program Director and Assistant Professor, Dartmouth Hitchcock Medical Center, Lebanon, New Hampshire

Vinod H. Srihari, M.D.
Professor, Department of Psychiatry, Yale University, New Haven, Connecticut

Kristoffer Strauss, M.D., M.B.A.
Child and Adolescent Psychiatry Fellow, Stanford University School of Medicine, Stanford, California

Oliver M. Stroeh, M.D.
Clarice Kestenbaum, M.D., Associate Professor of Education and Training in the Division of Child and Adolescent Psychiatry, Columbia University Vagelos College of Physicians and Surgeons, New York, New York

Rajesh R. Tampi, M.D., M.S., DFAPA, DFAAGP
Chairman, Department of Psychiatry and Behavioral Sciences, Cleveland Clinic, Cleveland, Ohio

Lia Thomas, M.D.
Professor, Department of Psychiatry, University of Texas Southwestern Medical Center, Dallas, Texas

Jonathan Tsang, M.D.
Psychiatrist, Santa Clara Valley Medical Center—Emergency Psychiatric Services, San Jose, California

Sanya Virani, M.D., M.P.H.
Assistant Professor, Department of Psychiatry; Associate Program Director, Addiction Psychiatry Fellowship, University of Massachusetts Chan Medical School; Director of Addiction Services, Worcester Recovery Center and Hospital, Worcester, Massachusetts

Phuong Vo, M.D., M.S.
Resident Physician, Department of Psychiatry and Neurosciences, UC Riverside School of Medicine, Riverside, California

Ashley E. Walker, M.D.
Associate Professor, Department of Psychiatry, University of Oklahoma School of Community Medicine, Tulsa, Oklahoma

Raziya S. Wang, M.D.
Former Designated Institutional Official and Program Director, San Mateo Psychiatry Residency Training Program, San Mateo, California; Clinical Assistant Professor (Affiliated), Department of Psychiatry and Behavioral Sciences, Stanford University School of Medicine, Stanford, California

Diana Willard, M.D.
Clinical Assistant Professor, Department of Psychiatry and Behavioral Sciences, Stanford University School of Medicine, Stanford, California

J. Corey Williams, M.D., M.A.
Assistant Professor of Psychiatry, Medstar-Georgetown University Hospital, Washington, D.C.

Matthew G. Yung, M.D.
Psychiatry Resident, University of Texas Southwestern Medical Center, Dallas, Texas

DISCLOSURES

The following contributors to this book have indicated a financial interest in or other affiliation with a commercial supporter, a manufacturer of a commercial product, a provider of a commercial service, a nongovernmental organization, and/or a government agency, as listed below:

Adam Brenner, M.D., receives royalties from Wolters-Kluwer.

Carrie Ernst, M.D., receives royalties from American Psychiatric Association Publishing.

Jeffrey Hunt, M.D., is senior editor for a monthly psychopharmacology newsletter for John Wiley and receives grant support from NIMH.

Vishal Madaan, M.D., receives research support from Supernus, Allergan, Boehringer Ingelheim, Pfizer, Purdue Pharma, and NICHD and honoraria from American Psychiatric Association and American College of Psychiatrists.

Melissa Martinez, M.D., has conducted research supported by Otsuka Pharmaceuticals and is the ownder of Curbpsych.

Katharine J. Nelson, M.D., receives royalties from UpToDate and Oxford University Press, honoraria from grand round presentations, and a research grant from the American Board of Psychiatry and Neurology.

The following contributors have indicated that they have no financial interests or other affiliations that represent or could appear to represent a competing interest with their contributions to this book:

Rashi Aggarwal, M.D.; Neal D. Amin, M.D., Ph.D.; Nientara Anderson, M.D., M.H.S.; Timothy Ando, M.D.; Melissa R. Arbuckle, M.D. Ph.D.; Janet Baek, M.D.; Clayton A. Barnes, M.D., M.P.H.; Sara Baumann, M.D.; Antoine Beayno, M.D.; Iverson Bell, M.D., DLFAPA; Jeana Benton, M.D.; Laurel J. Bessey, M.D.; Seamus Bhatt-Mackin, M.D., FAPA, CGP, AGPA-F; Deborah L. Cabaniss, M.D.; Hugh Caldwell, M.D.; Jorien Campbell, M.D.; Enrico G. Castillo, M.D., M.S.H.P.M.; Metin Cayirolgu, M.D.; Joanna Chambers, M.D.; Rachel Conrad, M.D.; Takesha Cooper, M.D., M.S.; Ann Crawford-Roberts, M.D., M.P.H.; E. Ann Cunningham, D.O.; Sallie G. De Golia, M.D., M.P.H.; Michael DeGroot, M.D.; Vanessa de la Cruz, M.D.; Matthew L. Edwards, M.D.; Laura Erickson-Schroth, M.D.; Ambarin Faizi, D.O.; Aaron Feiger, M.D.; Christine T. Finn, M.D.; Laura Flores, Ph.D.; Allison Ford, M.D.; Amy Gallop, M.D.; Daniel E. Gih, M.D.; Teddy G. Goetz, M.D., M.S.; Nichole Goodsmith, M.D., Ph.D.; Tracey M. Guthrie, M.D.; Nekisa Haghighat, M.D., M.P.H.; Elizabeth E. Hathaway, M.D.; Paul Hill, M.D.; Erick Hung, M.D.; Jessica Isom, M.D., M.P.H.; Oluwole Jegede, M.D., M.P.H.; James Kahn, M.D.; Michael Kelly, M.D.; Anna Kerlek, M.D.; Manal Khan, M.D.; Murad M. Khan, M.D.; You Na P. Kheir, M.D.; Kristen Kim, M.D.; Zachary Lenane, M.D., M.P.H.; Grace Lee, M.D.; Melissa M. Ley-Thomson, M.D.; Karen Li, M.D.; Csilla N. Lippert, M.D., Ph.D.; Juan David Lopez, M.D.; Aekta Malhotra, M.D., M.S.; Jennifer E. Manegold, M.D., M.S.; Tessa L. Manning, M.D.; Natalie Maples, Dr.P.H.; Phelan E. Maruca-Sullivan, M.D.; Alka Mather, M.D.; Jessica L. W. Mayer, M.D.; Patrick McGuire, D.O.; Michael O. Mensah, M.D., M.P.H.; Isabella Morton, M.D., M.P.H.; William Newman, M.D.; Tram Nguyen, M.D.; Aaron Owen, M.D.; Daniella Palermo, M.D.; Amit Parikh, M.D.; Michael Polignano, M.D.; Harika Reddy, M.D.; Rebecca Rendleman, M.D.; James I. Rim, J.D., M.D.; Robert Rohrbaugh, M.D.; Anne Ruble, M.D., M.P.H.; Mohona Sadhu, M.D.; Bronwyn Lane Scott, M.D.; Sourav Sengupta, M.D., M.P.H.; Jon Sole, M.D.; Vinod H. Srihari, M.D.; Kristoffer Strauss, M.D., M.B.A.; Oliver M. Stroeh, M.D.; Rajesh R. Tampi, M.D., M.S., DFAPA, DFAAGP; Lia Thomas, M.D.; Jonathan Tsang, M.D.; Sanya Virani, M.D., M.P.H.; Phuong Vo, M.D., M.S.; Raziya S. Wang, M.D.; Diana Willard, M.D.; J. Corey Williams, M.D., M.A.; Matthew G. Yung, M.D.

PART I

Understanding Residency

CHAPTER 1

Framing the Residency Experience

Sallie G. De Golia, M.D., M.P.H.
Raziya S. Wang, M.D.

Welcome to psychiatry residency! You are embarking on a comprehensive training to equip you to help your patients live healthier and more fulfilling lives. Your training will include seemingly disparate areas of focus, from neuroscience, psychotherapy, quality improvement, and teaching to navigating cultural differences and social advocacy, yet all are core aspects of the psychiatric experience. While striving to integrate an intensive training experience, you will be navigating a formative period in your personal life, bridging possibly your last "training" experience and your first unsupervised job as a psychiatrist. Our hope is to help make your journey as smooth and meaningful as possible by making explicit that which is often left implicit during training, leading to confusion, frustration, and/or missed opportunities. This book, written by psychiatry educators and often coauthored by psychiatry residents in training, provides important pearls and tips to engaging meaningfully in residency while also maintaining a fulfilling life.

KEY POINTS

- Psychiatry residents bring a variety of intersectional identities and personal experiences that enrich the field of psychiatry.

- The transition from medical student to psychiatry resident is significant, and new residents may benefit from support systems to promote the professional and personal growth that makes training an enriching experience.

- Having a training "road map" may help psychiatry residents focus on the most relevant stage of professional development while also keeping the big picture in mind.

WHO WE ARE

According to the National Resident Matching Program, psychiatry programs filled 2,030 incoming postgraduate year 1 (PGY-1) positions in the 2022 Match. Of the matched applicants, 1,298 were M.D.s, 411 were D.O.s, 188 were U.S. international medical graduates (IMGs), and 133 were non-U.S. IMGs. This represented an overall 24% increase in the number of matched applicants to psychiatry since 2018. In addition, 10 positions were filled in psychiatry–family medicine programs, and 3 were filled in psychiatry-neurology (National Resident Matching Program 2022).

Data gathered from the 2020–2021 academic year by the Accreditation Council for Graduate Medical Education (ACGME) showed that 49.1% of all active psychiatry residents identified as female and 49.8% identified as male, with no residents identifying as nonbinary and 76 declining to report. With regard to race and ethnicity, of 6,976 active residents in 2020–2021, 48.4% identified as white, 25.3% identified as Asian; 5.5% identified as Hispanic, Latino, or of Spanish origin; 6.8% identified as Black or African American; 0.2% identified as American Indian or Alaska Native; 0.03% identified as Native Hawaiian or Pacific Islander; 8.4% identified as multiple race/ethnicity; 2.4% identified as "other"; and 3% were "unknown" (Accreditation Council for Graduate Medical Education 2021). In addition to these reported demographic factors, psychiatry residents bring rich individual life experiences to the training environment. Residents' personal experiences, intersectional identities, and diverse interests nourish the field of psychiatry and help advance care for patients.

THE BIG TRANSITION

As a group of trainees, psychiatry residents enter medicine for a variety of reasons—to be clinicians, researchers, inventors, educators, administrators, advocates, and more—but with the same overarching goal of helping others. Up to now, you have mastered the skill of getting high marks on tests and doing well in clerkships, but that focus is about to change.

Transitioning from a highly dependent learner role in medical school to being a far more directly responsible member of the health care team in residency has been described as the most stressful transition during medical training (Teunissen and Westerman 2011). Most of you are leaving the role of full-time student to become a full-time employee with the astonishing charge to care for someone's health and well-being. Of course, your role as a student is not officially over (nor will it ever be), but now the content learning occurs on your "own time" and with a different focus: how to provide the most appropriate care for individuals whose treatment has been entrusted to you. With this change, you will be immersed in a world of new rules to be navigated while acquiring new skills and knowledge, expanding your attitudes and allowing them to evolve, and developing a professional manner in a variety of contexts. Your identity as a psychiatrist will start to develop and consolidate over time. You are also transitioning from a culture where you may have experienced a certain level of recognition—chair of a psychiatry interest group, class representative in your school of medicine, or teaching assistant for histology—to one where you have been "demoted," yet again, to the lowest rung: intern. However, you are resilient! Indeed, West et al. (2020) found that physicians showed higher levels of resilience than the general U.S. working population. You would not have made it through medical school otherwise.

Despite this resilience, burnout occurs in individuals in medical training more often than in age-matched nonmedical peers (Dyrbye et al. 2014). Compared with these nonmedical peers, you must manage a variety of systemic factors, including inefficient electronic health records and cumbersome clinical processes. You may already have felt as if life is "on hold" because you may have delayed important milestones such as establishing a romantic relationship, having children, or buying a house.

As a psychiatry trainee, you also will witness the ravages of depression and psychosis and the unspeakable traumas your patients have experienced. You may lose a patient to suicide, experience sleepless nights, or feel insurmountable uncertainty while trying to manage some difficult patients or deal with challenging colleagues and staff. We hope this book helps you recognize that you are not alone. There are strategies to help you harness your resilience and also advocate for change in our systems of care. Although the challenges are complex, with careful planning and intention, you can find a meaningful balance between your residency demands and your life outside. In addition, while pursuing such a laudable path as psychiatry, you are apt to experience tremendous personal and professional growth in ways you cannot yet anticipate.

As you progress through the years of psychiatry training, you will encounter different challenges and tasks in your professional and personal development. Having a "road map" may help you focus your energies on the most relevant learning for your stage of training while also keeping the big picture in mind. Table 1–1 provides an outline of psychiatry training and professional development across the years.

PGY-I

Your experience in residency will transform you over time and have a significant impact on your professional identity development. The internship year can be exhilarating yet frightening. You may have just moved to a completely new geographic location or may have matched at a residency program where you have to establish a new social network for yourself and, possibly, your significant other. You may experience a completely different and unfamiliar sociocultural context, not only within your institution but also within the community where you have chosen to live. If you are a non-U.S. IMG, you may further have to manage acculturation to the United States. You may have to master new institutional or rotation cultures, procedures, and knowledge. You may have to adjust to new patient populations, staff and attending personalities, and expectations.

In the clinical setting, you can no longer "hide" behind your resident or attending physician. You will be expected to evaluate patients on your own and make decisions while also learning new protocols and managing relationships in a new multidisciplinary setting. On-call attending physicians will rely on your interviews, description of data, preliminary impressions of what is going on with your patients, and thoughts on how to proceed. Remember, learning when to ask for help is a key skill that will guide your training and patient care.

As your patients look to you as the all-knowing expert, your identity as an impostor may loom large. In contrast, your attendings and super-

TABLE 1–1. Stages of development

PGY year	Clinical rotations	Professional and identity development tasks
PGY-1	• Often primarily hospital-based psychiatry and required medicine and neurology months • Some programs introduce night float for the first time	• Transition into a new program and/or new geographic location • Learn new institutional culture • Increase clinical independence and clinical decision-making • Manage relationships in a multidisciplinary setting • Develop a self-directed approach to content learning • Learn to ask for help
PGY-2	• Often primarily hospital-based psychiatry, including consultation-liaison and subspecialty rotations • Some programs introduce outpatient psychiatry • Some programs introduce scholarly time • Some programs introduce psychotherapy training	• Shift identity away from medical and toward psychiatric physician • Realize that even small incremental changes in patient clinical status may represent significant improvements in their health • Build skills in teaching and mentorship of early learners • Develop interprofessional communication and team collaboration skills • Develop health advocacy skills
PGY-3	• Often the first opportunity to practice outpatient psychiatry • Continue subspecialty rotations • Some programs offer scholarly time • Start or continue psychotherapy training	• Transition to outpatient practice • Build leadership, scholarship, teaching, or advocacy skills • Consider fast track to child and adolescent psychiatry fellowship • Start to integrate identity as psychotherapist

TABLE 1–1. Stages of development *(continued)*

PGY year	Clinical rotations	Professional and identity development tasks
PGY-4	• Many programs offer elective time, leadership roles (e.g., chief resident), and scholarly time • Many programs offer preattending opportunities	• Integrate roles as a more experienced practitioner, including teacher, scholar, advocate, and clinical team leader • Consider postgraduate employment or further training in fellowship • Consider posttraining role as supervisor

visors will seem powerful and valuable (Fann et al. 2003). In the first year, it often can feel that you are directly responsible for your patients and should be able to make them better. This sense of significant responsibility while feeling inexperienced can lead to feelings of ambivalence, self-doubt, and frustration (Fann et al. 2003). You also may start to recognize that your abilities and those of other providers, as well as the therapeutics used, are more limited than you anticipated. Rest assured that you will learn to manage these challenges as you continue to hone your skills and gain experience through your training.

Before you know it, you will be preparing handoffs to your colleagues and moving on to a different and unfamiliar location in the hospital or another care setting. These rapid shifts in rotation sites have been associated with resident stress, negative coping strategies, and perceived negative impact on patient care (Bernabeo et al. 2011). Embracing the discomfort, staying cognitively flexible, being clear about expectations, and asking for and integrating real-time feedback will help you cope more effectively (Bone and Flaxman 2006; Houser et al. 2018; Lloyd et al. 2013).

And just as you develop surer footing in your clinical skills and knowledge as a medical physician, you face the transition of letting go of medicine to welcome in your emerging identity as a psychiatrist. Even though you intentionally selected this specialty, the transition is not always smooth; letting go of the dominant culture in which you have been marinating for almost 4 years can be difficult for some.

Yet in spite of all these challenges, PGY-1 can also be a year of fulfillment and meaning-making. You are finally in a position to play a significant role in helping your patients. Your already-honed skills in active listening will continue to lead you toward that goal. In addition, your coresidents, and many psychiatrists before you, have navigated similar challenges and joys. They will now be part of your professional community going forward, providing the foundation for a meaningful future career in psychiatry.

PGY-2

By the time you are a PGY-2 resident, you are probably far more comfortable with the systems within which you work and have developed confidence in your ability to care for hospital patients and engage with colleagues. However, it also may become confusing and frustrating to notice that there are competing forces pulling you in different directions depending on your supervisor and/or role model. Expectations can vary around such activities as prerounding, presentation styles, interventions, and documentation, as well as autonomy. Your increased capacity to tolerate uncertainty and your growing skills in communication and self-directed learning will ease your path through these challenges.

At this stage, you may begin to idealize your supervisors less and perceive them as less valuable and therefore may feel less dependent on them as you develop your confidence (Fann et al. 2003). With more confidence, a decreased sense of vulnerability, and deepened identity as a psychiatrist, you may be able to start focusing more on teaching medical students and seeking leadership positions such as running team meetings, initiating consultations, or becoming involved in the school of medicine or residency program activities. This is also the year you may be eligible for a number of national fellowships, including those through the American Psychiatric Association and other national psychiatric associations. These are terrific ways to broaden your scope of psychiatry, receive external mentorship, and start to network with peers and leaders committed to the field of psychiatry. By the end of PGY-2, you may have developed a more realistic view of psychiatry and its impact on patients while starting to view your supervisors and role models as having both important strengths and limitations.

PGY-3

If you are not already immersed in outpatient care, your PGY-3 year will be the start of yet another significant inflection point: moving into the outpatient realm. Your increasing sense of confidence may be derailed momentarily as you again become the newbie on the block, trying to figure out the new systems and culture of the outpatient settings. Yearning for the safety of the protected inpatient unit with 24/7 monitoring and safety checks, you are now faced with increased uncertainty because you are not directly privy to much of your patients' daily lives and have limited impact on their follow-through. You *will* learn to manage your uncertainty or anxiety about this. As you progress, you will gain comfort in your outpatient risk evaluations and will participate in the more long-term goals of this model of care. Whereas your inpatient goals might have been to stabilize acute symptoms and connect your patient to resources, your outpatient experience includes an opportunity to partner with your patients in building goals that include their recovery and quality of life.

Your developing professional identity will morph as you take on this new role as an outpatient therapist, psychopharmacologist, and/or interventionalist. You also might be exposed to scholarly pursuits, including quality improvement, research, or curricular development. You also may consider leading projects, getting involved in committees or advocacy work, or teaching in new venues within the medical school or community or at the national level. Finally, you may have a bit more space to reflect on your growth, better identify specific knowledge gaps, and develop strategies on how to fill those gaps. You may continue to reflect more deeply on the forces that have shaped you up to this point in your training and how they align with your personal and professional values as you continue the process of differentiating yourself within the field. You also may start to seriously consider life after residency as you begin to integrate both inpatient and outpatient experiences. If child and adolescent psychiatry (CAP) has been on your mind, this is a time to determine whether you will want to apply for fast-tracking into a CAP fellowship program or stay to complete your fourth year before starting fellowship.

PGY-4

Finally, you will arrive at your final year of residency training, PGY-4, when putting plans together for postresidency life will dominate. You may consider whether you will apply for a fellowship or faculty position or consider industry, private or group practice, or an administrative or community position. You may also start to feel as though you are more able to balance clinical responsibilities with personal obligations and choices. It is during this year that you may start to see yourself as equally valuable and powerful as your supervisors (Fann et al. 2003). You may open yourself more to broader perspectives in order to consolidate your professional identity as a psychiatrist. During this year, you also may start developing supervisory skills as you begin to contemplate becoming a supervisor yourself.

For many, PGY-4 comes rather abruptly as you realize your training is nearly completed, yet there is so much more to master. Some feel an urgency to take as many didactics as possible and expose themselves to a variety of clinical situations they have yet to experience. Others may find importance in consolidating a lifelong learning plan. As you leave the security of a training program, you will need to find ways to stay abreast of the literature and expand your knowledge and skills. Training does *not* stop after residency or fellowship but extends throughout your lifetime through reading, social media, professional conferences, grand rounds, specialty training experiences, consultations, mentorship, and/or journal clubs or peer learning groups. Our field continues to evolve, and residency training ultimately is only the initial stepping-stone to a career of lifelong learning and service and your own contributions to our field.

TIPS FOR USING THIS RESOURCE

As you move through your training, we recommend using this book intermittently. As you reach a certain stage in residency, review the chapters that are most relevant to your experiences.

Chapter 2, "The U.S. Mental Health Care Landscape," provides a lay of the land—an overview of mental health care in the United States. Many of us starting out in psychiatry had little perspective on how the field developed, its vast richness, or a sense of where our field of psychiatry was headed. We hope this chapter provides some grounding as you start your adventure in the diverse and expansive field of psychiatry.

Part 2, "Centering Our Identities," highlights our diverse identities, provides context for your own experiences, and offers helpful strategies to better navigate residency training.

We explore various clinical venues in Part 3, "Approaching Clinical Work," with the aim of providing helpful perspectives and advice on how to get the most out of your clinical experiences, while recognizing that your emotional experience may be shared among many residents.

Many of you will seek a career as a clinician, educator, mentor, scholar, leader, and/or writer. Part 4, "Building Skills," focuses on the important skills beyond clinical expertise needed for a career in psychiatry. In addition to these competencies, being able to tolerate the inherent uncertainty that is pervasive in our field is also an important skill that you can develop over time.

As you move through your 4 years, you will start to direct more attention to your career goals. These goals are covered in Part 5, "Developing a Career." Some of you will be focused on career development from day one of residency, whereas others will take in experiences over time and try to make sense of them near the beginning or middle of the fourth year. However you approach career planning, these chapters will provide you with a framework for considering future endeavors.

Finally, the ever-present challenge in residency and beyond is how to balance and integrate a career with your personal life. We explore these topics in Part 6, "Maintaining a Professional and Personal Life."

We hope you will find this book to be a valuable resource over the course of your residency training, and we look forward to being a part of your journey.

SPECIFIC CHALLENGES AND STRATEGIES

⌘ **In medical school, there were quizzes, tests, and grades to help me assess my mastery of material. Now that I'm a resident, I'm not sure if I'm learning everything I need to know.** The transition from medical student to psychiatry resident is a big one. Make sure to give yourself the time and space to navigate this adjustment and keep in mind that your growth as a psychiatrist will not be confined to the 4 years designated to residency training. Psychiatry practice involves lifelong learning that will extend throughout your career. In the meantime, familiarize yourself with the goals and objectives of your clinical rotations and academic assignments. These objectives will help you orient yourself to what you need to know and will help you put feedback from attending physicians in context. The ACGME Milestones for Psychiatry can also provide a map of the expected progress of psychiatry residents through training. A link to the helpful *Milestones Guidebook for Residents and Fellows* is provided in the "Resources" section.

⌘ **Because I'm just a trainee, I feel like I'm doing my patients a disservice by not providing the experienced, comprehensive care that they could get from an attending.** Although it is true that you are learning the practice of psychiatry, your patients can still receive high-quality care in the teaching setting. It is important to always inform your patients that you are a trainee and to give the name of your designated attending supervisor. Obtaining this informed consent allows you and your patient to navigate access to appropriate care in the training setting together. Working closely with your attending and asking for feedback will help you identify the aspects of clinical care you have built up proficiency to practice more independently and the aspects for which you should seek supervision and assistance. In addition, keep in mind that as a trainee, you may have more time to spend building a therapeutic alliance and listening to your patient than to your attending. This connection can be the key to developing the trust that will lead to a successful treatment plan and may be an advantage for the patient who sees a psychiatry resident for care.

SELF-REFLECTIVE QUESTIONS

1. What challenges or stressors am I encountering at my current stage of training? What resources are available to assist me?
2. What are my personal training goals and how can I meet them? Is there a mentor or more advanced resident who can guide me?

RESOURCES

Accreditation Council for Graduate Medical Education: Psychiatry milestones. Chicago, IL, Accreditation Council for Graduate Medical Education, 2020. Available at: www.acgme.org/globalassets/pdfs/milestones/psychiatrymilestones.pdf. Accessed April 27, 2022.

Eno C, Correa R, Stewart NH, et al: Milestones guidebook for residents and fellows. Chicago, IL, Accreditation Council for Graduate Medical Education, 2020. Available at: www.acgme.org/globalassets/pdfs/milestones/milestonesguidebookforresidentsfellows.pdf. Accessed April 27, 2022.

REFERENCES

Accreditation Council for Graduate Medical Education: Data resource book academic year 2020–2021. Chicago, IL, Accreditation Council for Graduate Medical Education, 2021. Available at: www.acgme.org/globalassets/pfassets/publicationsbooks/2020-2021_acgme_databook_document.pdf. Accessed April 12, 2022.

Bernabeo EC, Holtman MC, Ginsburg S, et al: Lost in transition: the experience and impact of frequent changes in the inpatient learning environment. Acad Med 86(5):591–598, 2011 21436668

Bone FW, Flaxman PE: The ability of psychological flexibility and job control to predict learning, job performance, and mental health. Journal of Organ Behavioral Management 26(1–2):113–130, 2006

Dyrbye LN, West CP, Satele D, et al: Burnout among U.S. medical students, residents, and early career physicians relative to the general U.S. population. Acad Med 89(3):443–451, 2014 24448053

Fann JR, Hunt DD, Schaad D: A sociological calendar of transitional stages during psychiatry residency training. Acad Psychiatry 27(1):31–38, 2003 12824119

Houser MM, Worzella G, Burchsted S, et al: Wellness skills for medical learners and teachers: perspective taking and cognitive flexibility. MedEdPORTAL 14:10674, 2018 30800874

Lloyd J, Bond FW, Flaxman P: The value of psychological flexibility: examining psychological mechanisms underpinning a cognitive behavioural therapy intervention for burnout. Work Stress 27(2):181–199, 2013

National Resident Matching Program: Advance data tables: 2022 main residency match. National Resident Matching Program, 2022. Available at: www.nrmp.org/wp-content/uploads/2022/03/Advance-Data-Tables-2022-FINAL.pdf. Accessed April 12, 2022.

Teunissen PW, Westerman M: Opportunity or threat: the ambiguity of the consequences of transitions in medical education. Med Educ 45(1):51–59, 2011 21155868

West CP, Dyrbye LN, Sinsky C, et al: Resilience and burnout among physicians and the general US working population. JAMA Netw Open 3(7):e209385, 2020 32614425

CHAPTER 2

The U.S. Mental Health Care Landscape

Aaron Owen, M.D.

Laurel J. Bessey, M.D.

You are entering psychiatry at an exciting time in the field. Understanding of neuroscience is growing exponentially, but the clinical application of this knowledge remains limited. Although treatment options are increasing, psychiatry is still waiting for the era of the genome to supplant the era of the syndrome. Psychiatrists must develop lifelong learning skills to keep up with this ever-growing knowledge base. To examine what current psychiatric practice looks like, in this chapter we review how psychiatry developed as a medical specialty, discuss the current practice settings and treatment modalities, and predict what the future of psychiatry holds. We end by discussing some challenges to the field and proposed solutions.

KEY POINTS

- The field of psychiatry has a rich history that shapes the way we practice today.

- Psychiatrists practice in a variety of settings and with multidisciplinary teams.

- Psychiatric patients face health care inequities and mental illness stigma.

- Psychiatrists must advocate for patients legislatively and in health care systems.

- The future of psychiatry includes opportunities and challenges.

LANDSCAPE OF THE PAST

Imagine becoming a psychiatrist at the beginning of the twentieth century. The field had already existed for 100 years, and the number of people in state-run asylums in the United States was soaring (Shorter 1997). Far from expecting to cure your patients, you could offer primarily mere confinement. Similar to today, you would work in a system marred by racist ideologies and incomplete science. Neurologist Sigmund Freud was developing theories about the unconscious roots of "neurotic" disorders (work that would contribute to the original psychodynamically oriented *Diagnostic and Statistical Manual of Mental Disorders* [DSM]; American Psychiatric Association 1952). At the same time, psychiatrist Emil Kraepelin was researching the biological origin of psychiatric disease and developing a classification system based on syndromes. Thus, you would participate in a lifelong debate about how much of mental illness is socially and psychologically constructed versus the result of a biological brain abnormality.

Given this lack of clear understanding of etiology, you and your colleagues would rely largely on serendipity in developing treatments. Fast forward to the mid-1900s, and your practice would be informed by some pivotal advancements. Elemental lithium was isolated in 1821, became the first medicine demonstrated to be effective in the treatment of a mental disorder in 1948, and was made available in the United States in 1970. The year of the original DSM publication, 1952, was also the year the first clinical trial of an antipsychotic, chlorpromazine, was published, and the first monoamine oxidase inhibitor, the tuberculosis drug iproniazid, was reconceived as an antidepressant. Electroconvulsive therapy (ECT) gained widespread clinical use in the United States as early as the 1940s but remains one of the most controversial treatments in medicine (largely because of its portrayal as cruel and punitive, but also stemming from the legitimate drawbacks of early administration without anesthesia). On the other hand, shortly after its introduction in 1988, the selective serotonin reuptake inhibitor fluoxetine became wildly popular as the first antidepressant not lethal in overdose.

One of the largest policy initiatives in mental health was deinstitutionalization in the 1960s (vis-à-vis the Community Mental Health Act of 1963, P.L. 88-164). Deinstitutionalization appealed to policy makers at the time who found that with this shift they were able to make budget cuts at various levels of government. The idea of reintegrating asylum patients into the community gained further traction with the introduction of antipsychotic drugs and the notion that people with severe mental illness could be readily treated as outpatients. Proponents of the burgeoning antipsychiatry movement (with vocal adherents, including Scientologists) made moralistic arguments in favor of integrating patients into society at large. In reality, large volumes of patients were discharged to homelessness or incarceration when promised funding for community psychiatry never materialized. In many cases, stigma toward patients actually worsened, and grassroots peer advocacy groups and community treatment programs were formed. The result is our current system of public mental health, which is plagued by underfunding and fragmentation (see Chapter 21, "Public Mental Health").

Stigma against the field of psychiatry itself dates back to the earliest days of the profession. This includes stigma around psychiatry as a pseudoscience as well as the perception that psychiatrists are nefarious or "functionaries of the oppressive state" (Sartorius et al. 2010). Indeed, many psychiatrists were involved in the eugenics movement and perpetuating racist policies by supporting such ideas as drapetomania to target individuals fleeing slavery and "protest psychosis" to delegitimize Black Americans advocating for civil rights (Metzl 2009). Psychiatric theories pathologizing homosexuality contributed to antigay stigma well into the 1970s. Social activism around that time led to a major advancement in LGBTQ+ rights with the removal of homosexuality as a DSM diagnosis in DSM-III (American Psychiatric Association 1980).

Partly in response to this general climate of mistrust of psychiatry, the 1980 publication of DSM-III marked a shift toward empiricism and embracing of the biological understanding of mental illness (Sanders 2011). DSM-III also initiated an axial diagnostic structure that delineated major psychiatric ailments from personality disorders and general medical conditions and added context for sociocultural factors (allowing biologically and psychoanalytically oriented psychiatrists to share a common framework). Thus, there was a simultaneous movement toward the biopsychosocial formulation and a greater social consciousness. Introduction of managed care in the 1980s also profoundly altered the practice of psychiatry, for the first time limiting visits, choice of medications, and length of hospitalizations. Although outpatient psychiatrists were predominantly psychotherapists throughout most of the twentieth century, by the early 2000s, as few as 1 in 10 practiced psychotherapy extensively after residency (Mojtabai and Olfson 2008).

CURRENT LANDSCAPE

Psychiatry is the medical specialty focused on diagnosing and treating mental illness. Psychiatrists have remained perennially hopeful that research would be able to unlock the neurobiological basis for mental illness, but by the advent of DSM-5 (American Psychiatric Association 2013) and DSM-5-TR (American Psychiatric Association 2022), the overall categories remain descriptive in nature. In general, psychiatrists practice in conjunction with multiple professions to provide comprehensive mental health care (see Chapter 14, "Working in a Multidisciplinary Team") and often serve as team leaders (see Chapter 29, "Leadership"). Both psychiatrists (M.D., D.O.) and psychologists (Ph.D., Psy.D.) possess doctorate-level degrees. Psychiatrists, psychologists, and licensed psychotherapists (e.g., L.C.S.W., M.S.W., L.P.C., M.F.T.) are all trained to accurately diagnose mental illness and recommend psychological treatment. However, of these mental health professionals, only psychiatrists are trained to provide both medical and psychological interventions. Medical treatments for less complex mental illness may also be offered by primary care physicians, nurse practitioners, and physician assistants, depending on resources in your area of practice.

As with other medical conditions, a large portion of mental illness treatment occurs in the primary care doctor's office. One study showed that between the study periods 1995–1998 and 2007–2010, a statistically significant increase occurred in primary care visits involving psychotropic medications, from 11.08% to 26.74% of visits (OR=3.43; 95% CI 2.16–2.71) (Olfson et al. 2014). Primary care doctors are usually a first stop for patients seeking care for mental health concerns, and they are able to manage a variety of conditions depending on the resources and standard of care in their region of practice. For example, in many rural areas, psychiatrists are scarce, so primary care doctors treat the whole spectrum of mental illness (Abed Faghri et al. 2010). Likewise, psychiatrists who do practice in rural areas often function as generalists. In urban areas or academic settings, psychiatrists are more readily available and may subspecialize in treatment of patients within narrow symptomatology (e.g., forensic psychiatry, addiction, pain, sleep) or age range (e.g., child and adolescent, geriatric). Therefore, in these settings, primary care doctors usually treat straightforward cases and refer patients with more complex cases or treatment-refractory illness to psychiatrists.

Many psychiatrists find that they transition between practice settings as their career progresses. Although customarily assigned to inpatient work at the beginning of residency, graduating psychiatrists will practice in a range of settings, from inpatient to outpatient (including small-group practice, large institutions, psychiatry emergency departments [EDs], and collaborative care in primary care doctors' offices). Psychiatry also retains one of the highest rates of private practice among medical specialties (about 50%), but this is a declining trend (Hawkins 2018). Inpatient psychiatrists operate similarly to the hospitalists of internal medicine, running psychiatric units in larger general hospitals, dedicated psychiatric hospitals, and residential facilities. Psychiatrists also cover consultation-liaison roles within hospitals. Depending on the system in which you practice, the facility may either have dedicated psychiatric EDs or rely on consultations called to assess psychiatric concerns among patients presenting to the general ED. In either case, you will need to familiarize yourself with the laws in your state that govern involuntary commitment of the mentally ill (see Chapter 19, "Legal Issues").

During residency, you will be expected to become an adept psychopharmacologist, and a majority of your patient interactions are likely to involve management of medication regimens. Common practice categorizes medication by class (e.g., antidepressants, mood stabilizers), although the mechanisms of action may vary within a class. Many psychiatric medications were not developed with psychiatric disorders in mind and are used in off-label ways with varying degrees of evidence. It is imperative that you follow the principle of "do no harm" by monitoring for side effects of treatment as well as discontinuing medications that are not effective for your individual patient.

Nonpharmacological somatic therapies remain reserved primarily for treatment-resistant psychiatric disorders. For example, transcranial magnetic stimulation has been adopted in widespread clinical practice but may not be readily available to underserved populations. ECT has a long track record and robust data for efficacy in refractory cases such as severe depression and catatonia. In these instances, ECT can be lifesaving, but its adverse cognitive effects and stigma limit use. The most invasive intervention, psychosurgery, has been the most marred by a history of misuse. Although the idea of treating mental illness with surgery still evokes images of "ice pick lobotomies," this has not completely undermined progress. Current surgeries involve implanting devices for deep brain and vagus nerve stimulation, and only infrequently does surgery involve severing the brain tissue itself (e.g., cingulotomy for intractable obsessive-compulsive disorder).

It is helpful to think of treatment modalities not as gold standard interventions but as trends that fluctuate over time, are heavily influenced by reimbursement and pharmaceutical marketing, and inherently are bound to the prevailing scientific understanding and societal views of mental illness (Scull 2019). Studies looking at comparative effectiveness of medical versus psychological treatments for psychiatric disorders reveal that the combination is often superior (Cuijpers et al. 2014; Kamenov et al. 2017). Although trained in psychological treatments, most psychiatrists refer their psychotherapy cases to other professionals (Mojtabai and Olfson 2008). The way we define our roles can also change (as evidenced by the fact that most psychiatrists are no longer "asylum superintendents"), and you will have to determine your own interests and impact (see Chapters 33–36 in Part 5, "Developing a Career"). Regardless of whether you perform formal psychotherapy in your career, the core skills you acquire from psychotherapy training can imbue every patient interaction with a therapeutic element. In fact, multiple studies show that an enhanced doctor-patient relationship improves clinical outcome for both psychotherapy and psychopharmacological treatments of mental illness (Blatt and Zuroff 2005; Krupnick et al. 1996).

CHALLENGES IN PSYCHIATRY

Although modern psychiatry offers many tools for treatment and exciting advances, it is not without challenges. A few of these challenges center on stigma, efforts of nonpsychiatry providers to expand their scope of practice, and psychiatry's ability to address health inequities.

Stigma

The first of these challenges includes the stigma of mental illness and the field of psychiatry itself. Although a science with increasing evidence, psychiatry is still challenged by the antipsychiatry movement, most vocally by the Church of Scientology. This group was founded in the early 1950s in Los Angeles, California, and has sought to stop psychiatric practice and replace it with its own techniques (Kent and Manca 2014). Scientology has inspired multiple subgroups, including the Citizens Commission on Human Rights (CCHR). CCHR portrays itself as a champion of rights for psychiatric patients and, at times, has identified individual instances of questionable psychiatric practices. However, CCHR more commonly fuels online conspiracy theories (Kent and Manca 2014).

In addition to the stigma raised by overt antipsychiatry movements, being diagnosed with mental illness holds broader, more subtle stigma.

This stigma stems partly from false beliefs that mental disorders are personally controllable and that people with mental illness are frightening and unpredictable. Stigma makes seeking treatment very difficult for some of our patients and may even lead them to potentially harmful treatments offered by antipsychiatry groups. It is our role to provide our patients with factual medical information and evidence-based treatments. We must also advocate for our profession both legislatively and through public awareness groups such as the National Alliance on Mental Illness. In recent years, stigma has decreased because of education efforts and improved public recognition of mental illness as treatable. Recent movements include the push to integrate mental health specialists with other first responders and the adaptation of a national crisis line number, 988. The overall result is that mental illness has been brought out of the shadows and today is something as likely to be discussed by adolescents as acne and trending pop stars.

Other Professions Seeking to Extend Scope of Practice

As a field, psychiatry is also faced with the challenge of other professions seeking to expand their scope of practice. Controversially, nurse practitioners (NPs) and physician assistants (PAs) are seeking, through legislative efforts, to practice without physician supervision. This would, it is argued, improve access to care (on the basis of the premise that training in these fields is shorter but adequate for NPs and PAs to practice independently). Additionally, psychologists are seeking to expand their practice to include prescribing and have gained this privilege in some states. Psychology lobbies argue similarly to increase access, contending that with the addition of a psychopharmacology course, psychologists have enough training to safely prescribe psychotropic medications. Psychiatrist organizations, including the American Psychiatric Association, argue that NPs and PAs do not have the same level of extensive training as psychiatrists. They argue that without supervision, independent practice of these providers could lead to lower quality of care for patients. Further, psychiatry lobbies argue that patients need to understand the level of training their provider has undergone, which is often not readily apparent by one's credentials. To address this challenge, we as psychiatrists need to advocate for our patients and profession individually and as part of local and national medical organizations (see Chapter 32, "Advocacy"). We can also educate our patients in clinic about the training and qualifications of each type of mental health care provider.

Health Care Inequities

Finally, a major challenge is that health care inequities remain evident in psychiatry today. Although mental health care insurance coverage parity has become standard in the past decade, patients with mental illness still face barriers to receiving care, including lack of health insurance or underinsurance and mental illness stigma. As a result, only an estimated 43% of people with mental illness receive treatment (American Psychiatric Association 2017). People with severe mental illness have higher mortality rates than the general population, usually due to increased burden of physical illness and unequal quality of health care (Lawrence and Kisely 2010). Additionally, racial/ethnic minority groups with mental health concerns are not treated equitably. For example, racial/ethnic minority youth with mental health issues more often end up in the juvenile justice system than do white youth with mental health issues (American Psychiatric Association 2017). This racial inequity is further propagated by the lack of diversity among psychiatrists. From 1987 to 2016, underrepresented minorities had less representation in psychiatry at all levels of training compared with the demographics of the U.S. population (10.4% of practicing psychiatrists vs. 32.6% of the U.S. population) (Wyse et al. 2020). Mental health care inequities in diverse populations are addressed in more detail in Chapter 8, "Working With Historically Oppressed Patient Populations."

LANDSCAPE OF THE FUTURE

Our field will continue to experience growth as we face challenges that arise. We are hopeful that progress will be made in reducing the stigma of mental illness through efforts outlined in this chapter. With this progress, more patients will seek care, leading to more timely access to psychiatrists. To address the resulting workforce shortage, we will need to change the way we practice. Namely, psychiatrists will increasingly take on roles collaborating in nontraditional mental health settings. We will continue to see an increase in integrated and collaborative care. As psychiatrists, we will need to become adept leaders of multidisciplinary teams and nimble practice managers, with more stable patients being referred back to primary care. Telepsychiatry has undergone a rapid expansion (most notably during the COVID-19 pandemic) and is likely here to stay, helping patients in rural or other underserved areas gain access to mental health services (see Chapter 18, "Telehealth Services").

Additionally, we need to address structural inequities in the care provided to patients and racism at the individual, organizational, and societal levels. We also need to address these inequities through work-force expansion of diverse providers to reflect the demographics of the population we treat. Efforts toward this end include increasing the pipe-line of diverse individuals, starting with high school–age or college-age students and using more holistic review of applications to medical school and residency and in hiring staff and faculty.

We will continue to face the challenges and uncertainty of current mental health crises as they evolve. From 1999 to 2018, the United States has seen a 35% increase in the suicide rate (Hedegaard et al. 2020). This statistic is likely to increase further as our world faces the mental health fallout from the pandemic. This increase in the suicide rate will require more study and the development of innovative approaches to suicide prevention. Additionally, we continue to face the multitudes of people affected by the opioid epidemic. Psychiatrists will continue to be leaders in addressing this epidemic, given our expertise in treating addiction. Over time, most psychiatrists will likely be adept at prescribing medi-cation-assisted treatment for opioid use disorder. We also face a rapidly aging population. We will need to find avenues to allow patients access to mental health care in long-term care facilities and account for a loom-ing wave of provider retirements.

The future also brings opportunity. Our knowledge of neuroscience will grow, leading to a more personalized approach to the care of psy-chiatric illness using genetics, epigenetics, biomarkers, and imaging. This may also allow for novel interventional psychiatry modalities. We have already seen early success with ketamine treatment for depression, and, as research continues, we may see emergence of novel treatments such as psychedelic-assisted therapy. Increased acknowledgment of structural inequities and racism during the COVID-19 pandemic has also fueled education and advocacy to address these issues and close health disparities.

Psychiatry remains a field where there is continued humanity. Bear-ing witness to our patients' suffering and offering support through psy-chotherapy and systemic advocacy will continue to be paramount. Even the greatest technology cannot supplant human connection.

Specific Challenges and Strategies

⌘ **My patient is requesting a medication regimen that their thera-pist recommended.** Collaborative (split) treatment with a separate therapist can be challenging. You will benefit from communicating openly and directly so as to not perpetuate conflict. Obtain a release of information form to talk to the therapist, and then have a collegial conversation with them. The therapist is generally trying to be helpful and will be happy to know they can contact you directly with concerns. Your prescribing license is on the line, so take the therapist's insights as a useful data point and ultimately make your own decision with the aid of your clinical supervisor. Also, remember that patients often interpret what various providers tell them and may be communicating their own desires indirectly.

⌘ **My patient is a single parent and lost his job (and insurance coverage). What can I do to help him access care?** Job loss can be a detriment to a person's sense of efficacy and meaning, and the resulting social isolation can contribute to depression, substance use, and other mental health crises that require direct intervention. Lack of access is a frequent contributor to poor care and disparities. This issue includes too few psychiatrists; inpatient psychiatric bed shortages; and social determinants of health such as lack of transportation, low socioeconomic status, and unemployment. This patient is likely eligible for a special enrollment period for Marketplace insurance and may qualify for a subsidy or Medicaid to cover costs. Issues like this one must be addressed on individual and systemic levels. Legislative advocacy on behalf of patients is needed to support programs to expand mental health care access.

⌘ **My patient's family encourages her to stop taking medications when she feels better, saying it is a moral weakness to depend on pills.** Mental illness stigma exists in individuals and also our social structure. In the media, mentally ill people are often depicted as violent, and symptoms of severe mental illness are viewed as character flaws. That said, both medication adherence and familial support may be intimately linked to a patient's outcome. In this case, it is necessary to explore cultural factors around the role of family in decision-making and possibly include support people in future appointments.

SELF-REFLECTIVE QUESTIONS

1. How has my personal narrative shaped my view of psychiatry?
2. How does the history of psychiatry guide my view of the field, and how might it impact my patients' or the public's perceptions? How might I relate to patients who are skeptical of or hesitant about treatment?
3. What do I know about how mental health care is approached in other countries and cultures? What similarities and differences exist?
4. Where do I see psychiatry as a field 10 years from now? Fifty years?

RESOURCES

For diagnostic reference: American Psychiatric Association: Diagnostic and Statistical Manual of Mental Disorders, 5th Edition, Text Revision. Washington, DC, American Psychiatric Association, 2022

For an overview of psychiatry: Sadock BJ, Sadock VA, Ruiz P: Kaplan and Sadock's Synopsis of Psychiatry: Behavioral Sciences/Clinical Psychiatry, 11th Edition. Philadelphia, PA, Wolters Kluwer, 2015

For historical perspective: Shorter E: A History of Psychiatry: From the Era of the Asylum to the Age of Prozac. Chichester, UK, John Wiley, 1997

For sociological critique: Scull A: Psychiatry and Its Discontents. Berkeley, University of California Press, 2019

For in-depth pharmacology: Schatzberg AF, Nemeroff CB (eds): The American Psychiatric Association Publishing Textbook of Psychopharmacology, 5th Edition. Arlington, VA, American Psychiatric Association Publishing, 2017

For a quick prescriber guide: Stahl SM: Stahl's Essential Psychopharmacology: Prescriber's Guide, 5th Edition. New York, Cambridge University Press, 2014

For clinical interviewing: Shea SC: Psychiatric Interviewing: The Art of Understanding: A Practical Guide for Psychiatrists, Psychologists, Counselors, Social Workers, Nurses, and Other Mental Health Professionals, 3rd Edition. Edinburgh, UK, Elsevier, 2017

For neurology: Kaufman DM, Geyer HL, Milstein MJ: Kaufman's Clinical Neurology for Psychiatrists, 8th Edition. New York, Elsevier, 2016

For advocacy: Shim RS, Vinson SY (eds): Social (In)justice and Mental Health. Washington, DC, American Psychiatric Association Publishing, 2021

REFERENCES

Abed Faghri NM, Boisvert CM, Faghri S: Understanding the expanding role of primary care physicians (PCPs) to primary psychiatric care physicians (PPCPs): enhancing the assessment and treatment of psychiatric conditions. Ment Health Fam Med 7(1):17–25, 2010 22477919

American Psychiatric Association: Diagnostic and Statistical Manual of Mental Disorders. Washington, DC, American Psychiatric Association, 1952

American Psychiatric Association: Diagnostic and Statistical Manual of Mental Disorders, 3rd Edition. Washington, DC, American Psychiatric Association, 1980

American Psychiatric Association: Diagnostic and Statistical Manual of Mental Disorders, 5th Edition. Arlington, VA, American Psychiatric Association, 2013

American Psychiatric Association: Diagnostic and Statistical Manual of Mental Disorders, 5th Edition, Text Revision. Washington, DC, American Psychiatric Association, 2022

American Psychiatric Association: Mental health disparities: diverse populations. December 19, 2017. Available at: www.psychiatry.org/psychiatrists/cultural-competency/education/mental-health-facts. Accessed October 24, 2020.

Blatt SJ, Zuroff DC: Empirical evaluation of the assumptions in identifying evidence based treatments in mental health. Clin Psychol Rev 25(4):459–486, 2005 15893862

Cuijpers P, Sijbrandij M, Koole SL, et al: Adding psychotherapy to antidepressant medication in depression and anxiety disorders: a meta-analysis. World Psychiatry 13(1):56–67, 2014 24497254

Hawkins M: The silent shortage: a white paper examining supply, demand and recruitment trends in psychiatry. Dallas, TX, Merritt Hawkins, February 22, 2018. Available at: www.merritthawkins.com/uploadedFiles/merritthawkins_whitepaper_psychiatry_2018.pdf. Accessed January 30, 2021.

Hedegaard H, Curtin SC, Warner M: Increase in suicide mortality in the United States, 1999–2018 (NCHS Data Brief No 362). Hyattsville, MD, National Center for Health Statistics, 2020

Kamenov K, Twomey C, Cabello M, et al: The efficacy of psychotherapy, pharmacotherapy and their combination on functioning and quality of life in depression: a meta-analysis. Psychol Med 47(3):414–425, 2017 27780478

Kent SA, Manca TA: A war over mental health professionalism: scientology versus psychiatry. Ment Health Relig Cult 17(1):1–23, 2014 24348087

Krupnick JL, Sotsky SM, Simmens S, et al: The role of the therapeutic alliance in psychotherapy and pharmacotherapy outcome: findings in the National Institute of Mental Health Treatment of Depression Collaborative Research Program. J Consult Clin Psychol 64(3):532–539, 1996 8698947

Lawrence D, Kisely S: Inequalities in healthcare provision for people with severe mental illness. J Psychopharmacol 24(4)(suppl):61–68, 2010 20923921

Metzl JM: The Protest Psychosis: How Schizophrenia Became a Black Disease. Boston, MA, Beacon Press, 2009

Mojtabai R, Olfson M: National trends in psychotherapy by office-based psychiatrists. Arch Gen Psychiatry 65(8):962–970, 2008 18678801

Olfson M, Kroenke K, Wang S, et al: Trends in office-based mental health care provided by psychiatrists and primary care physicians. J Clin Psychiatry 75(3):247–253, 2014 24717378

Sanders JL: A distinct language and a historic pendulum: the evolution of the Diagnostic and Statistical Manual of Mental Disorders. Arch Psychiatr Nurs 25(6):394–403, 2011 22114794

Sartorius N, Gaebel W, Cleveland HR, et al: WPA guidance on how to combat stigmatization of psychiatry and psychiatrists. World Psychiatry 9(3):131–144, 2010 20975855

Scull A: Psychiatry and Its Discontents. Berkeley, University of California Press, 2019

Shorter E: A History of Psychiatry: From the Era of the Asylum to the Age of
Prozac. Chichester, UK, John Wiley, 1997

Wyse R, Hwang WT, Ahmed AA, et al: Diversity by race, ethnicity, and sex
within the US psychiatry physician workforce. Acad Psychiatry 44(5):523–
530, 2020 32705570

PART 2

Centering Our Identities

CHAPTER 3

Centering Our Identities

Matthew L. Edwards, M.D.
Michael Polignano, M.D.

You may be coming to psychiatry as someone who is older; a parent; from an economically disadvantaged background; transitioning from another career or changing paths in medicine; or living with chronic illness, disability, or a learning difference. You may be someone whose faith or culture is of profound and central importance to your life and self-understanding. You may identify with a racial or ethnic minority group or as underrepresented in medicine (UiM) (see Chapter 4, "The Underrepresented in Medicine Experience"). You may identify as a gender or sexual minority (see Chapter 5, "Gender and Sexual Identity"). You may have completed your medical training outside the United States (see Chapter 6, "Professional and Personal Life"). As you approach residency, you may wonder two things: 1) whether you have the attributes needed to succeed in a residency and as a practicing psychiatrist and 2) whether you really want to "belong" to the culture of medicine and psychiatry—whether you want to identify with the beliefs, attitudes, and practices that constitute psychiatric training and being a psychiatrist in the United States (Weurlander et al. 2019).

These beliefs, attitudes, and practices—the norms of residency and professional practice—are often implicit, not explicit. They are embedded, for example, in the policies, practices, and curriculum of a training program; in the ways that faculty model interactions with patients, trainees, and each other; and in the qualities of the built environment that allow certain kinds of physical access but not others.

Such norms may be centered in part on a background understanding of "who" a psychiatrist-in-training "should be"—perhaps someone who is a younger single white cisgender male; without illness (*especially* mental illness) or disability; without any visible signs of identification with a particular faith or culture; unencumbered by financial concerns, a family, or other responsibilities outside psychiatric training; and who completed medical school in the United States. In other words, they are centered on an idea of someone whose life experience and identity are perhaps very different from yours.

In this chapter we discuss navigating the difference between who you are and the hidden standard of normalcy around which the practices of residency programs and professional psychiatry have historically been constructed.

KEY POINTS

- Your "differences" are strengths that are key to being a good psychiatrist.

- Remembering your larger purpose can help you navigate circumstances that challenge your identity.

- You can address isolation and a sense of "otherness" by seeking community and mentorship.

VALUE YOUR DIFFERENCES AS SOURCES OF STRENGTH

Your history and identity are not limiting "differences" that must be overcome in order for you to belong and succeed. Just the opposite! Your history and identity are sources of strength and skill that will support you through residency and make you a better psychiatrist.

You May Have a Deepened Capacity for Empathy

If you are living with illness, disability, or a learning difference, your experience has very likely deepened your capacity for providing empathic, compassionate care to your patients. This may be especially true if you have been living with health problems during medical training

(Roberts et al. 2011). Likewise, if you are a parent, or caring for a family member, you have had to develop the capacity for "tuning in" to the unexpressed emotional states of others, and thus your experience of providing care to others may have also enriched your capacity for empathy.

You May Understand the Importance of Relational, Sociocultural, and Spiritual Factors in Health

Raising a family may have led you to consider the role of the family and community in healthy development. Similarly, if you are living with strong faith or a strong cultural identity, you might better understand the importance of community in supporting your patients' well-being and how living with strong faith can provide a moral compass and sense of purpose. If you have chosen medicine after a previous career, you understand how work has shaped your sense of self. Because of these experiences, you will be able to approach your patients not as isolated individuals defined by a diagnosis but as the whole people they are, people whose family and community relationships, whose cultural and religious identities, whose professional and personal roles all profoundly affect their mental health.

You May Have Learned to Balance Competing Demands on Your Time

As someone who had another career; is raising a family; is living with the need for daily self-care because of illness, disability, or a learning difference; or has had to balance work with schooling, you will have had to learn how to balance competing demands on your time in ways that your peers may not have.

You Can Assume a "Decentered" Perspective

If you have had a nontraditional path to psychiatry or you identify with a minoritized or underrepresented group, you may have learned to hold multiple perspectives on yourself without reflexively overidentifying with any single perspective. For example, if you are living with a disability, you may have heard messages that you "can't" accomplish certain things that others do, or if you identify with a minoritized group, you may have faced barriers to advancement while also hearing and acting on messages about your ability to succeed. In other words, you already have some practice with *decentering* from stories that do not tell your truth. This is an essential skill for a psychiatrist—to simultaneously bear in mind the stories we tell about ourselves and our patients, listening to all of them without getting lost in any of them.

REMEMBER YOUR LARGER PURPOSE

During your training, you may get subtle and not-so-subtle messages that some aspect of your identity is "incompatible" with being a physician or psychiatrist. Perhaps you get the message that parents cannot be "team players" in residency because of other demands on their time, or that overt signs of cultural identity are incompatible with a "neutral" professional presentation, or that physicians should be immune from illness or disability (McKevitt and Morgan 1997). You may encounter frank hostility or an ever-accumulating, exhausting series of microaggressions related to your race, ethnicity, or gender.

The messages of incompatibility may also manifest in practices that prevent you from fully participating in either residency or some important part of your life outside residency. For example, rounding practices and the built environment may limit full participation by residents living with illness or disability; call schedules and other work expectations may take time away from necessary self-care or family obligations; and limitations on moonlighting may increase financial challenges for those coming from economically disadvantaged backgrounds.

In these circumstances, you might imagine that you must either disavow some vitally important part of your life or identity in order to be a physician or else abandon being a physician to be true to yourself and your needs. However, there is a third option that starts with remembering the larger purpose that led you to a psychiatry residency. As someone who has traveled a nonprescribed path, you almost certainly have been thoughtful and deliberate in choosing to enter medical school and residency. Why did you choose to become a psychiatrist? What do you hope to accomplish as a psychiatrist? Can your residency program, however inhospitable it may currently seem, help you to achieve your goals? Keeping the answers to these questions in mind will help you to endure during moments of crisis and to forge an identity as a psychiatrist that is centered on your values.

FIND COMMUNITY AND MENTORS

You may feel socially isolated because your past experience has brought you perspectives, interests, and priorities different from those of your peers or because you have different demands on your time outside residency (Chur-Hansen 2003). This may worsen the experience of feeling different, marginal, or other. To address social isolation, you can look for peer support or affinity groups at your institution—for example, support groups for parents, for residents and medical staff living with disability, for people of a particular faith or culture, or for those who are UiM. You can also look outside your institution for groups at other institutions or in the community. Developing connections with colleagues by joining your program's process group for residents may be helpful. Your participation within the broader residency group helps to decenter the implicit understanding of who a psychiatrist is.

When building community, you may at first seek support of others who are like you in some identifiable way (e.g., with respect to race or ethnicity, gender, religion or culture, illness or disability, or social class). Whereas these *strong ties* with similar-seeming others provide important support, so-called *weak ties*, often formed through relationships with individuals less similar to ourselves, are more likely to be influential in fostering community and effecting institutional change. Such weak ties may form in groups organized around a shared professional interest (e.g., your residency cohort or a group interested in public psychiatry). Although you may not share characteristics such as race, gender, or socioeconomic or geographic background with other members of such groups, your common interest allows for an affinity that can further your personal and professional development. Because such groups are often tied to institutions (e.g., your residency program or the American Psychiatric Association), the collective membership of such groups bound by "weak" ties can be a powerful voice for change. As one leading expert on social networks stated, weak ties "are…indispensable to individuals' opportunities and to their integration into communities." Without weak ties, "strong ties, breeding local cohesion, lead to overall fragmentation" (Granovetter 1973, p. 1378). As you search for and begin to build new communities, consider the factors that lead you to form connections with various people, groups, and ideas and consider including affiliations joined by weak ties as well as strong ones.

Finding a mentor can also be important as you develop your identity. Consider seeking a mentor who is someone you identify with, whose practice of psychiatry you admire, and whose presence challenges the implicit norm of "who" a psychiatrist should be. Mentors can provide practical guidance and explicit emotional support, but their greatest value may be to signal by their presence that they (and therefore you) belong in your setting (Schwarz and Zetkulic 2019). You may find mentors in fellow trainees who are further along than you, in faculty or staff at your institution, or in people at other institutions who are visible and accessible to you. Just as your mentor's presence can signal to you that you belong, so your presence can signal to others who identify with you that *they* belong, thus beginning a *positive feedback loop* that loosens the grip of invisible norms dictating who belongs in medicine (Schwarz and Zetkulic 2019) (see Chapter 33, "Mentorship and Sponsorship").

TAKE ACTION

At some point, you may want to push to change practices at your institution to reform the institutional and systemic defaults that prevent full participation by historically excluded groups. You may want, for example, to reform the moonlighting policy to allow those from economically disadvantaged backgrounds more opportunity for financial security. When you set out to advocate for change, we suggest that you work in a way that feels appropriate to you. Some people seek allies—community—to take collective action; others may wish to engage with institutions through individuals who have a formal position of power, such as house staff leadership. Some may organize within their residency program; others may organize around concerns shared across departments (see Chapter 32, "Advocacy").

You may not want or feel empowered to organize for change in these ways. That's OK. Change occurs simply through your presence in your program; your presence makes a place in the world of medicine for yourself and others who may identify with you. Your presence thus embodies change, and in so doing offers hope to patients and others who can see someone like themselves at work in medicine.

SPECIFIC CHALLENGES AND STRATEGIES

⌘ **I can't support myself and my family on a resident's salary.** Residents from socioeconomically disadvantaged backgrounds remain UiM. Recent data from the American Association of Medical Colleges show that more than 75% of medical school students came from families with incomes in the top two quintiles (American Association of Medical Colleges 2018). Only 5% of matriculants came from families in the lowest quintile, compared with 24% of matriculants from the highest quintile. This disparity, combined with rising debt (averaging more than $200,000) among American medical graduates, creates financial constraints for many residents from socioeconomically disadvantaged backgrounds. You also may experience financial stress if you are coming to medicine later in life or from another career and thus are losing income during peak earning years. If you have a family, you may have to support your partner, children, or other family members (Chur-Hansen 2003). If you are living with chronic illness or disability, you may have medical expenses that increase financial stress. Although your resident salary may be a welcome relief from years of accruing debt in college and medical school, it typically will not be sufficient to change your overall financial picture. Although it may be difficult to reverse the downstream effects of socioeconomic disadvantage and its impact on financial well-being, there are ways you can mitigate the financial burden of medical training.

To reduce your chances of incurring further debt, make and live within a budget that considers regional costs of living, known expenses, and unexpected situations. Assess your eligibility for loan deferment, forbearance, and consolidation opportunities; loan forgiveness programs; and income-based repayment. Investigate opportunities and program policies for moonlighting to supplement your resident income. If your program does not allow moonlighting, consider pointing out that this policy disproportionately affects residents from economically disadvantaged backgrounds. Learn about your program's meal and travel reimbursements, relocation and housing assistance, and institutional discounts (e.g., for transportation, fitness, insurance). Meet with a financial adviser to discuss your short- and long-term financial goals. Access financial literacy tools from the Association of American Medical Colleges, the U.S. Department of Education, and other organizations (see also Chapter 41, "Practical Finances").

⌘ **I want to get support for my disability without jeopardizing my medical career.** Although increasing numbers of medical trainees are reporting disabilities, particularly those related to mental health (Meeks et al. 2019), rates of reporting of mental health disability nevertheless remain very low compared with the estimated prevalence (Meeks et al. 2020a). Indeed, reporting disabilities, particularly those related to mental health, may come with risks. A recent survey of residency program directors suggested that applicants who disclosed a diagnosis of depression were likely to be ranked lower than applicants who did not, all other factors being equal (Pheister et al. 2020). These risks may be due to the cultural norm in medicine that physicians should not be ill or disabled (McKevitt and Morgan 1997).

Despite the risks, there are clearly benefits to some form of disclosure, including the possibility of accessing institutional support, obtaining accommodations, and taking medical leave when necessary. This points to a dilemma faced by trainees with learning differences, chronic illness, or disabilities, particularly mental health–related disabilities: Do the benefits of disclosing a disability and requesting help outweigh the risks related to stigma and discrimination? Is there a way to get support without jeopardizing one's medical career?

When approaching this issue, keep in mind that your acceptance into residency, your training, and your employment as a resident are all subject to protections afforded by the Americans with Disabilities Act. Learn about your program's and your institution's disability policies by contacting some or all of the following: the office of accessible education (if your program is associated with an academic institution), the office of graduate medical education (GME), or the human resources department at your medical center (because residents are employees as well as trainees). Some questions to ask yourself and your institution: Does your program or GME office clearly specify a disability policy and clearly specify procedures for requesting accommodations? (Many GME programs do not specify a disability policy or procedures for requesting accommodations; Meeks et al. 2020b.) Can you request accommodations confidentially, without having to disclose the nature of your disability to your program directors, who may also be evaluating you? Does your program include people with disabilities in its statement of diversity? Find out if there are any groups for residents and medical staff living with disability. Talk with other residents who are living with learning differences or disabilities to find out their experience with disclosure and requesting accommodations.

SELF-REFLECTIVE QUESTIONS

1. Has my identity as a psychiatrist-in-training been supported or challenged by *other* identities I may have?
2. Has my identity been affected by identities that others ascribe to me?
3. How does my life experience or identity allow me to better help my patients?
4. Have I been part of a group where I felt unwelcome or that I didn't belong? How did I navigate that experience?
5. What is the most important reason I am training to be a psychiatrist? How can my awareness of this reason sustain me during difficult times?

RESOURCES

Coalition for Disability Access in Health Science Education: www.hsmcoalition.org

Brenner AM, Balon R, Guerrero APS, et al: Training as a psychiatrist when having a psychiatric illness. Academic Psychiatry 42(5):592–597, 2018 30105576

Hochschild A, Machung A: The Second Shift: Working Families and the Revolution at Home. New York, Penguin, 2012

Society for Physicians with Disabilities, www.physicianswithdisabilities.org

REFERENCES

American Association of Medical Colleges: An updated look at the economic diversity of U.S. medical students. Washington, DC, American Association of Medical Colleges, 2018. Available at: www.aamc.org/data-reports/analysis-brief/report/updated-look-economic-diversity-us-medical-students. Accessed June 6, 2022.

Chur-Hansen A: Mature-aged medical students: a qualitative study. Learning in Health and Social Care 2(3):159–168, 2003

Granovetter MS: The strength of weak ties. Am J Sociol 78(6):1360–1380, 1973

McKevitt C, Morgan M: Illness doesn't belong to us. J R Soc Med 90(9):491–495, 1997 9370984

Meeks LM, Case B, Herzer K, et al: Change in prevalence of disabilities and accommodation practices among US medical schools, 2016 vs 2019. JAMA 322(20):2022–2024, 2019 31769816

Meeks LM, Plegue M, Case B, et al: Assessment of disclosure of psychological disability among US medical students. JAMA Netw Open 3(7):e2011165–e2011165, 2020a 32701156

Meeks LM, Taylor N, Case B, et al: The unexamined diversity: disability policies and practices in US graduate medical education programs. J Grad Med Educ 12(5):615–619, 2020b 33149832

Pheister M, Peters RM, Wrzosek MI: The impact of mental illness disclosure in applying for residency. Acad Psychiatry 44(5):554–561, 2020 32415458

Roberts LW, Warner TD, Moutier C, et al: Are doctors who have been ill more compassionate? Attitudes of resident physicians regarding personal health issues and the expression of compassion in clinical care. Psychosomatics 52(4):367–374, 2011 21777720

Schwarz CM, Zetkulic M: You belong in the room: addressing the underrepresentation of physicians with physical disabilities. Acad Med 94(1):17–19, 2019 30157092

Weurlander M, Lönn A, Seeberger A, et al: Emotional challenges of medical students generate feelings of uncertainty. Med Educ 53(10):1037–1048, 2019 31509285

CHAPTER 4

The Underrepresented in Medicine Experience

Daniella Palermo, M.D.
Tracey M. Guthrie, M.D.

We find ourselves in the midst of a racial reckoning in America, a period of divisiveness perhaps most comparable to the civil rights movement of the 1950s and 1960s. The dehumanization and murder of Black and Brown bodies at the hands of police remind us that racism is embedded in the DNA of this country. The emboldening of white supremacy groups by a sitting U.S. president reminds us that the oppression of Black and Brown bodies continues to benefit the white majority. The adoption of immigration policies intended to criminalize and brutalize those seeking opportunity and refuge within our borders reminds us that people of color are not welcome. The disproportionate morbidity and mortality associated with COVID-19 infection within Black and Latinx communities remind us that the health care system remains undeserving of our trust. The lack of representation of Black and Brown voices within the house of medicine reminds us that this is still an unsafe space for people of color.

In this chapter you will find perspectives and insights into the manifestations of the historically, and often intentionally, deficient pipeline for people of color into the field of medicine and guidance on how to navigate the current experience of being underrepresented in medicine

(UiM). We write this chapter from the perspective of a Black, cisgender, gay woman of West Indian descent who completed residency in the Northeast in the late 1990s and an Indigenous Afro-Latina who is the proud daughter of immigrants, a first-generation college graduate who completed her residency at a predominantly white institution in the Northeast in 2018. We write this chapter with the hope of doing more than recapitulating the structural and systemic injustices that have established and perpetuated the underrepresentation of physicians of color in medicine. We write this chapter because we want to be seen for all that we are and all that others like us must overcome for the privilege of the white coat. We hope that in speaking truth to the experience of the UiM, you, as a trainee, will find validation of your own experience as well as opportunities to overcome the barriers we face. If you do not identify as a UiM trainee, we hope that this chapter highlights opportunities to progress from acting as an ally to acting as a co-conspirator against inequities.

KEY POINTS

- Structural racism is embedded within the institution of medicine, resulting in a long history of exclusion and oppression of minoritized individuals.

- Historical racism within medicine must be taught, validated, and understood in order to enact changes that will promote equity and inclusivity for UiM trainees.

- UiM trainees face a unique set of challenges with respect to professional identity development, access to mentorship and sponsorship opportunities, obtaining clinical supervision that acknowledges racial identity and promotes integration with the professional self, and navigating experiences of interpersonal racism.

- Community building, mentorship, and social supports are critical to the UiM trainee's well-being, professional development, and success as they navigate the white-dominant culture of medicine.

- For non-UiM trainees, solidarity must extend beyond allyship. As co-conspirators, they must ask and listen to how they can show up, using their privilege while committing resources to promoting equity.

PIPELINE AND HISTORICAL RACISM

Historically *underrepresented minorities in medicine* is a term initially used by the Association of American Medical Colleges (AAMC), consisting of Blacks, Mexican Americans, Native Americans, and mainland Puerto Ricans. In 2003, the AAMC adopted the more flexible term *underrepresented in medicine*. As of 2018, only 5.8% of the physician workforce identified as Hispanic/Latinx, 5.0% as Black/African American, and 0.3% as American Indian or Alaska Native (Association of American Medical Colleges 2019). In psychiatry, UiMs are underrepresented at the trainee level, comprising 16.2% of resident physicians. Although representation among practicing psychiatrists is difficult to ascertain, current data suggest that only 10.4% of practicing physicians and 8.7% of faculty belong to a historically underrepresented group (Wyse et al. 2020). With a U.S. population that is 33.8% minority (13.6% Black, 18.9% Hispanic/Latinx, and 1.3% American Indian or Alaska Native), psychiatry, like all other medical specialties, fails to reflect the already existing diversity of our country (U.S. Census Bureau 2021). When looking into the future, the U.S. Census Bureau projects that half of all Americans will belong to a minority group by the year 2044 (Colby and Ortman 2015). This shift toward a *majority minority* demographic will have implications across all sectors of U.S. life, including health care. In order to adequately meet the health needs of the increasingly diverse nation, we will need to fundamentally disrupt the power structures and institutional policies that currently maintain the status quo.

When we fail to recognize that the field of medicine is not immune to the deleterious effects of structural and interpersonal racism, we remain complicit in the continued exclusion and oppression of minoritized individuals. From a historical standpoint, this practice of exclusion was operationalized well over a century ago through the Flexner Report. This report, published in 1910, is credited with the elevation and standardization of American medical education. Its high-quality training and professional standards established the United States' reputation of medical excellence, but its recommendations also led to the closing of 72% of predominantly Black medical schools, introduced admissions standards that excluded most Blacks from enrolling in medical school, and promoted the marginalization of Black physicians as "hygienists and sanitarians," segregated to Black communities (Sullivan and Suez Mittman 2010). In the decades that followed, the field of medicine remained a white-dominant space. When combined with discriminatory policies denying Blacks access to education, loans, and property ownership, these admissions standards made a career in medicine practically inaccessible to Blacks on the basis of race. It was not until the 1960s that U.S. medical schools began to actively recruit Blacks, with admission to all medical schools being delayed until 1966 (Pinder-Amaker and Leary 2019). Despite this change, discriminatory practices and policies persist, excluding UiMs from matriculation in and graduation from medical schools (Serchen et al. 2021).

Beyond the deliberate exclusion from medical education, the medical establishment, particularly psychiatry, has earned the mistrust of the Black community by bringing legitimacy to racial stratification and racism. Negative impacts on the mental health of Blacks in the United States date as far back as the 1600s, with the dehumanization of Black bodies through enslavement. Historically, medical terminology was used to validate the inferiority of blackness, with one example being the concept of "negritude" introduced by Benjamin Rush, M.D., often referred to as the "Father of Psychiatry," which equated blackness with a mild form of leprosy that could be cured only by becoming white (Jackson 2002). Psychiatry also has a history of legitimizing slavery, with Samuel Cartwright, M.D., coining the mental health disorder known as drapetomania, which pathologized the desire for freedom among the enslaved and called for whipping as its treatment (Willoughby 2018). To support the claims of the 1840 U.S. Census, which declared that enslaved Blacks were free of mental illness but became prey to mental disturbances when set free, psychiatric professionals manufactured data suggesting that "insanity" rates were directly correlated with proximity to the North (Suite et al. 2007). These oppressive theories continued to emerge into the 1890s, with physicians such as James Woods Babcock and T.O. Powell attributing the increased rates of insanity to emancipation (Medlock et al. 2019). Additionally, the eugenics movement of the early 1900s promoted the "breeding out" of undesirable traits of Blacks and other minority groups with efforts that brought about immigration restrictions, interracial marriage bans, and forced sterilization (Dowbiggin 1997). In later years, the fight for equality during the civil rights era was similarly pathologized, as described in Jonathan Metzl's book *Protest Psychosis* (Metzl 2009).

With some of the most heinous acts of medical abuse against minoritized communities being perpetrated by government entities and the medical establishment (e.g., the Tuskegee syphilis experiment; Brandt 1978), one can understand how minoritized individuals developed mistrust in the medical establishment, deterring them from seeking and engaging in both health care and medical research. We have been reminded of this recently in the context of the COVID-19 pandemic, with the emergence of a vaccine and the skepticism toward it that has been identified among Black and Brown communities. Black, Latinx, and Indigenous communities are among the groups hardest hit by the coronavirus pandemic, enduring infection rates that are 1.4, 1.7, and 1.8 times higher, respectively, than that of their white/non-Hispanic counterparts. When it comes to mortality, Black, Latinx, and Indigenous communities also suffer disproportionately, being 1.7, 1.8, and 2.1 times more likely to experience death as a result of COVID-19 infection when compared with whites (Centers for Disease Control and Prevention 2022). However, Blacks, Indigenous people, and other persons of color remain among the most reluctant to roll up their sleeves—a problem that lies not in the individual but in a medical system that has historically dehumanized them.

THE UiM RESIDENT: PROFESSIONAL IDENTITY FORMATION

For Black and Brown physicians, the sociohistorical context of racism and discrimination of this country is foundational to our experiences of *otherness*. We are taxed with having to consciously monitor and manage the negative attributes ascribed to our racial identities, forcing us to censor and/or conceal our true selves in an attempt to assimilate (Osseo-Asare et al. 2018). We find ourselves in a constant state of negotiation as we navigate spaces that either define us by our minoritized identity or remain oblivious to it. This experience reinforces a duality that becomes almost insurmountable in the absence of an environment that promotes integration, not just within the medical community but, more importantly, among minoritized physicians themselves.

Although extant research in professional identity formation has aimed to define how medical education teaches us to think, feel, and act as physicians, it has done so in the context of a white-dominant culture. In doing so, it has failed to integrate the experiences of people who have been historically underrepresented and systematically oppressed. For us, the experience of becoming involves both learning and unlearning as we aim to reconcile newly acquired privilege with the parts of ourselves that remain continuously disadvantaged. As society continues to struggle to see us for who we are, we are deprived of the opportunity to exist as both our true cultural selves and as physicians, furthering the divide between our personal and professional identities, which is otherwise known as *double consciousness* (Wyatt et al. 2020).

For many people of color, the quest for integration leads us to seek out opportunities to connect with Black and Brown communities like our own. Beyond the desire to "give back," we also find that it is in these spaces that we feel safe, accepted, and celebrated for who we are. Whether it be a racially concordant clinical encounter or mentoring a student from a minoritized group, we are granted the privilege of existing within our role as a physician without sacrificing aspects of our racial identity.

What is most critical for you to be aware of as a trainee is your positionality within medicine and academia. To better understand positionality within these spaces is to understand the self, the historical context by which you have existed, and how the institution presently embraces and values you. Understanding the self is to understand who you are and what you represent. To understand your historical positionality is to understand how you have been either overrepresented or underrepresented in academic medicine. And finally, it is critical to be aware of the institution's commitment to promoting diversity, equity, and inclusion while empowering yourself and others to question, push back, and demand meaningful change.

As the embodiment of change, you belong. It will be a struggle at times to accept this, but it is true. When you have doubts about it, seek support from friends, colleagues, and former classmates who helped you navigate medical school. You are not the only one who has this feeling. We all had it and still do. Rail against internalizing this feeling. Talk about it with others. Do not be silent about it. Seek help, support, therapy, whatever you may need to cope. You are not less than. We need you here.

MENTORSHIP

First and foremost as a UiM trainee, seek mentorship. In addition to providing emotional support, mentors can demystify the experience of navigating the many challenges of becoming a physician without compromising other aspects of your identity. Access to mentorship also serves to empower the first-generation physician while expanding on existing support networks. Although the process of finding a mentor can be difficult in itself, UiMs are up against a unique set of challenges due to lack of representation, which then limits opportunities for race-concordant mentorship. In seeking mentorship, we aim to identify individuals who share in our experience in an effort to promote the merger between our racial and professional identities. However, barriers with respect to the recruitment, retention, and advancement of UiM physicians in academic settings have deprived UiMs of the opportunity to see themselves in positions of power and privilege, perpetuating the experience of otherness. Here are some steps UiMs can take to address these challenges:

- Join organizations at your institution that support UiM residents. In academic institutions, this may entail connecting with the diversity office or physician groups. If they do not exist, explore regional and national organizations that can provide a sense of connectedness and belonging.
- Find your people. Seek out the minority house staff association at your institution. If it does not exist, consider the benefits of establishing a supportive space for trainees to build community. If there is a diversity group, seek it out.
- Seek out community supports. These may include houses of worship and social organizations that you identify with, including sports and outdoor groups.
- Use your family and friends as support. Spend your vacation time with them, visit often, and let them remind you why you are on this journey.

It is important to recognize the importance of trust as essential to successful mentorship. Non-UiM mentors, specifically, must acknowledge the historical events in the field of medicine that fostered a level of mistrust among underrepresented and disadvantaged communities while also recognizing the ways in which mistrust can manifest in the context of mentorship. In doing so, non-UiM mentors should recognize that trust must be earned before expecting their mentee to freely accept their guidance. By genuinely investing in the sponsorship of UiM trainees, non-UiM mentors can also begin to reshape the narrative of historical exclusion and suppression by the white majority.

SUPERVISION

Supervision is the cornerstone of training for psychiatry residents. When we fail to acknowledge and discuss the identities of trainees or supervisors, we are limiting the development of our professional identities (Cook 1994). In her 1994 article "Racial Identity in Supervision," Cook reminded us that the goal of supervision is to help integrate our personal and professional identities. Without a discussion of identity, biases against patients will remain unexplored, patients will not have the opportunity to understand fundamental parts of themselves, trainees will not know how to process intense feelings they have about themselves and/or patients, and for UiM trainees, they will be unseen and ignored once again (Cook 1994).

While recognizing that power differentials exist in the supervision dyad, we would like to empower all residents to bring discussions regarding race into the room if and when a supervisor fails to do so. Whether it be dialogue regarding your own racial identity, experiences as a physician as a result of your identity, or observations regarding the physician-patient dyad as it relates to racial concordance or nonconcordance, this is the space to process how your identities shape who you are as a physician and how you relate to patients. Without such discussion, it is hard to envision how trainees will develop the skills needed to navigate race-based dialogues with their future patients. Some suggestions on how to approach this situation include the following:

- *Advocate.* It may not be obvious to program leadership that assigning you to a supervisor with a similar identity as your own may be beneficial to your development. Inquire about this as an option during your residency training.
- *Inquire.* If there are other UiM residents in your program, inquire if they found certain supervisors open, helpful, and supportive. Seek out those supervisors during your training.
- *Speak up.* Inform your supervisor if supervision is not addressing the issues that you would like to discuss. Raise topics that you are interested in learning about. Advocate for yourself within your supervision. Supervisors may be open to finding their own mentorship, guidance, and support to help you on your educational journey.
- *Use the Cultural Formulation Interview.* Conducting the DSM-5-TR Cultural Formulation Interview (American Psychiatric Association 2022) with your patient can be an avenue through which you can bring about discussions relating to race and culture in the context of supervision.

Although representation remains limited, it is imperative that institutions establish clear and intentional strategic plans to recruit, support, retain, and promote UiM students, trainees, physicians, and researchers. Institutions, in particular, should take a vested interest in understanding why UiM physicians too infrequently climb the ranks to senior leadership and too often leave academic medicine entirely. Many have spoken of the "leaky" pipeline that results from senior leadership expressing support for diversity without investing in educational initiatives or promoting change to the discriminatory policies that are barriers to promotion and advancement, thus perpetuating inequity and exclusion.

DIFFICULT CONVERSATIONS AND EXPERIENCES

As UiM physicians, we are burdened by the difficult conversations that result from the experience of practicing medicine in a society that does not naturally see us as competent, trustworthy physicians. We encounter patients who cannot conceive, or simply refuse to accept, that someone who looks like us could be their doctor. Ongoing sociopolitical polarization (e.g., anti-immigrant sentiments, anti-Blackness) can manifest as biased patient behaviors that range from microaggressions to outright refusal of care. These experiences themselves bring about a significant psychological tax on us, and we also find ourselves feeling increasingly isolated as we question how and with whom to process these experiences.

Although hospitals and academic institutions have policies protecting against workplace discrimination at the hands of supervisors and colleagues, such policies do not exist against racism or biased behavior from patients. During a time in which some Americans feel emboldened to speak and act in bigoted ways, institutional policies addressing racially biased patient encounters are necessary in order to mitigate the repeated victimization of UiMs at both the trainee level and faculty level. For trainees specifically, race-based discrimination has been found to be the most prevalent type of mistreatment and discrimination, at approximately 19% (Whitgob et al. 2016). Recognizing the psychological tax of this experience and the likely reality that this is an underestimation of the prevalence of such discriminatory acts, continued silence is not an option. For the trainee, it is important to have an understanding of how the institution responds, which is something that should be explored as early as the residency application process. Trainees should have a clear understanding of what resources are available, both for reporting (e.g., Title IX office, human resources, program leadership), including anonymous ways to do so, and supports for the UiM (e.g., mentorship, peer support groups, therapy). (See Chapter 39, "Handling Mistreatment and Discrimination.")

The UiM physician's experience of racism brings about a conflict within ourselves and the identities we hold. First, our duty to the patient and the clinical acuity of the situation may require us to cast aside our humanity in order to fulfill a professional role. In the event of a medical emergency and/or the unavailability of a colleague or supervisor to step in, we may find ourselves unable to respond in a way that would preserve the other aspects of our identity. In some situations, we may find ourselves able to cultivate a therapeutic alliance following an incident of discrimination, encouraging the patient to challenge prejudicial beliefs and creating the space for learning. However, we must acknowledge that not everyone has the capacity for this, nor should the UiM physician have to take on this additional duty. For that reason, it is important for program directors, hospital leadership, and clinical supervisors to respect and empower UiM trainees and faculty to establish boundaries, which may include removing ourselves from the situation entirely.

The hierarchical nature of medicine and academia brings about an additional set of challenges for the UiM trainee. When experiencing discrimination from patients, you may find yourself in the presence of faculty and/or clinical supervisors who fail to acknowledge and/or address it, invalidating your experience. In doing so, they miss the opportunity to support your growth and success as a minoritized individual and physician. Additionally, having a supervisor who elects to remain a silent bystander can lead you to question how you should feel and whether or not you should respond to racism, eliciting feelings of isolation and otherness, only adding to the initial insult.

ALLIES AND CO-CONSPIRATORS

For non-UiM trainees, it is important to understand what it means to be an ally versus a co-conspirator. Allyship should be considered a starting point, while recognizing that our times call for much more. Allyship has great intentions, but true solidarity must extend beyond the theoretical support for equity through reading, watching, and learning about the experiences of minoritized individuals. Co-conspirators, on the other hand, offer meaningful support while showing up with, not for, the communities they support. They ask and listen to how they can show up, using their privilege while committing resources and putting themselves on the line. In order to move along the continuum from allyship to co-conspirator, you must anticipate mistakes. Acknowledge them, apologize, and do better. Some strategies for allies include the following:

- *Educate yourself.* This is where the work must start. However, it cannot end here. Approach this lifelong process with openness and humility. You cannot do the work without having an understanding of the historical and present-day forces that created and maintain systems of oppression. There are numerous lists of recommended resources for self-directed learning that you can access (see the "Resources" section at the end of this chapter).

- *Recognize your privilege.* It is important to understand that growing up oblivious to systems of oppression is part of the problem. The privilege and power of being white, if not used to disrupt existing structures, actually maintain the shackles that remain in place for people of color. Beyond recognizing your privilege, you must also acknowledge the pain and trauma this has caused for us as people of color. Be willing to sit with this pain as we move toward healing.

- *Acknowledge when you are taking up too much space.* Stand with us or behind us, not in front of us. Take your advocacy cues from your UiM colleagues.

- *Demand change.* Your voice is inherently valued. Given the hierarchical nature of medicine and academia, many trainees may struggle to perceive themselves as being positioned to make demands. However, we want to empower you to find your voice and speak out against bias and discrimination. Whether it is holding your institution accountable with respect to recruitment, retention, and inclusion efforts; antiracist curriculum development; and/or "teach-up" programs that would allow for faculty to learn from trainees, be the force that brings about change.

SPECIFIC CHALLENGES AND STRATEGIES

Case Vignette 1: The Semiannual

As a high-achieving Haitian-American postgraduate year 2 (PGY-2) psychiatry resident, you value your education above all. However, training in a predominantly white residency program has presented some challenges. When your program director reviews your evaluations with you, he notes that two evaluations (from the same attending physician) are below those of your peers. Comments on your evaluations have a consistent theme of you being disengaged, being unreliable with patient follow-up, and having a lower psychopharmacology knowledge base compared with your peers. Your program director does not make note of the fact that these comments are in sharp contrast to your first year and your second year to date. He is disappointed in you and simply asks how you are going to correct this problem. During your meeting, you feel angry, blindsided, and attacked. You do not agree with any of these assessments and feel that you are being judged incorrectly. You feel overwhelmed, not sure what to say or how to say it. You leave the semiannual evaluation meeting as soon as possible feeling upset and angry.

✤ Unclear expectations, inconsistent feedback, and harsher evaluations are unfortunately common experiences that you may have as a UiM resident (Liebschutz et al. 2006) or that you may see your colleagues experience in training. Here again you will need support to not internalize these feelings. Discuss the issue with your colleagues, allies, mentors, and family. Do not simply accept the evaluation as a deficit without interrogating it further. Repeatedly having to use your time and energy to protect yourself against racism and bias is exhausting. Find time during your training to rejuvenate. Get out into nature, exercise, play music, cook, be with family and friends, read, whatever you do to reset and refill yourself. You need to do more of it during training, not less. It may not be possible at the moment for you to challenge the program director's assessment, but you should do so eventually. The fact that this feedback is based on only one evaluation when the many others have the opposite view needs to be stated. Biases need to be called out to be seen and to be changed.

Case Vignette 2: Patient Racism

You are a PGY-1 resident who self-identifies as a Latinx, cisgender, heterosexual male. While on an inpatient service, a patient refuses to see you, stating that he does not want to meet with a "foreign doctor" and wants an "American-trained physician that speaks without an accent." Your attending tells you that she will see the patient without you, and there is no further discussion about the incident. The attending physician contributes to your feeling as if you have failed in some way and/or as if you are incapable.

✤ Inaction on the part of the attending physician makes her complicit with the racist remark. Until she states otherwise, her actions indicate that she agrees with the patient's comments. At first, you may be in shock or stunned and not know how you feel. Allow yourself time to sort out your feelings. When you are ready to talk about the incident, discussing it with someone can prevent you from internalizing the racist views that were projected onto you. Find a coresident, friend, attending physician, supervisor, program director, or ally to talk to about this incident. Coping with racism during training can be overwhelming and emotionally exhausting. Part of your self-care may need to include individual therapy and support with a culturally competent therapist.

✤ If you are a coresident, mentor, or supervisor for this resident, acknowledge what just happened to them and allow them to talk about it if they are ready to do so. If you witness the racial event, you too may be overwhelmed and unable to respond appropriately. Know that it is never too late to validate the resident's feelings and provide support.

✤ We want to support you in your desire to give feedback to the attending physician about how she made you feel. We also want to acknowledge that the power differential between you and the attending is real and may give you pause about giving this feedback. You should feel comfortable exploring your options and seeking mentorship. You may want to do this alone with the attending or with the support of the chief resident, the program director, or a mentor. You may want to wait until your rotation with this attending is over to provide this feedback, or you may choose to give it immediately. Decide what you want to say and role-play the conversation with an ally or colleague if that is helpful to you. The correct course of action is the one that works best for you. Whatever you decide to do, your experience is valid and important.

⌘ This case describes the actions of one attending, but systemic issues play a role in why she thought this was an appropriate response. We must educate the academic community on how to respond appropriately to racist comments by patients. This is everyone's responsibility. Providing feedback to the program and/or hospital system may help change how attendings manage the issue of patient racism. Education to all supervisors on how to appropriately manage these situations will create an environment of support for you and all trainees who come after you. Use your residency committees (e.g., education, curriculum), program director meetings, and residency retreats as places to raise these concerns within your program.

SELF-REFLECTIVE QUESTIONS

1. What am I doing for my own self-care?
2. Do I know who my allies are within my residency program or institution?
3. How is my program or institution supporting UiM trainees in their professional development and advancement?
4. What am I doing to educate myself and my colleagues about how to be antiracist?
5. How am I educating myself about health care disparities? Am I aware of my own biases?
6. How am I using my voice within my department to advocate for change?

RESOURCES

National Organizations Offering Community, Mentorship, and Fellowship Opportunities

American Association of Directors of Psychiatry Residency Training fellowships: www.aadprt.org/annual-meeting/awards-fellowships/award-detail?awardsid=69

Association of LGBTQ+ Psychiatrists: www.aglp.org

Association of Black Women Physicians: www.blackwomenphysicians.org

American Psychiatric Association Fellowships: www.psychiatry.org/residents-medical-students/residents/fellowships

Black Psychiatrists of America: www.blackpsychiatrists.org

Latino Medical Student Association: https://national.lmsa.net

National Hispanic Medical Association: www.nhmamd.org

National Medical Association: www.nmanet.org

Student National Medical Association: https://snma.org

Creating Inclusive Curricula

Alpert Medical School of Brown University: Creating inclusive curricula: considerations for review of curricular materials for inclusivity, diversity, and bias-free instruction. Program in Educational Faculty Development, Alpert Medical School of Brown University. Available at: facultydev.med.brown.edu/sites/g/files/dprerj596/files/CREATING%20INCLUSIVE%20CURRICULA.AMS_.pdf. Accessed September 19, 2021.

REFERENCES

American Psychiatric Association: Core Cultural Formulation Interview, in Diagnostic and Statistical Manual of Mental Disorders, Fifth Edition, Text Revision. Washington, DC, American Psychiatric Association, 2022, pp 864–867

Association of American Medical Colleges: Figure 18: Percentage of all active physicians by race/ethnicity, 2018, in Diversity in Medicine: Facts and Figures. Washington, DC, Association of American Medical Colleges, 2019. Available at: www.aamc.org/data-reports/workforce/interactive-data/figure-18-percentage-all-active-physicians-race/ethnicity-2018#:~:text=Figure%2018%20shows%20the%20percentage,as%20Black%20or%20African%20American. Accessed November 2, 2022.

Brandt AM: Racism and research: the case of the Tuskegee Syphilis Study. Hastings Cent Rep 8(6):21–29, 1978 721302

Centers for Disease Control and Prevention: COVID-19 hospitalization, and death by race/ethnicity. Atlanta, GA, Centers for Disease Control and Prevention, September 15, 2022. Available at: www.cdc.gov/coronavirus/2019-ncov/covid-data/investigations-discovery/hospitalization-death-by-race-ethnicity.html. Accessed October 8, 2022.

Colby S, Ortman JM: Projections of the size and composition of the U.S. population: 2014 to 2060: current population reports. Suitland, MD, U.S. Census Bureau, March 2015. Available at: www.census.gov/content/dam/Census/library/publications/2015/demo/p25-1143.pdf. Accessed December 19, 2020.

Cook DA: Racial identity in supervision. Counselor Education and Supervision 34(2):132–141, 1994

Dowbiggin IR: Keeping America Sane: Psychiatry and Eugenics in the United States and Canada, 1880–1940. Ithaca, NY, Cornell University Press, 1997

Jackson V: In our own voice: African-American stories of oppression, survival and recovery in mental health systems. Off Our Backs 33(7/8):19–21, 2002

Liebschutz JM, Darko GO, Finley EP, et al: In the minority: Black physicians in residency and their experiences. J Natl Med Assoc 98(9):1441–1448, 2006 17019911

Medlock MM, Shtasel D, Trinh N, et al (eds): Racism and Psychiatry: Contemporary Issues and Interventions. Cham, Switzerland, Humana Press, 2019, pp 3–17

Metzl JM: The Protest Psychosis: How Schizophrenia Became a Black Disease. Boston, MA, Beacon Press, 2009

Osseo-Asare A, Balasuriya L, Huot SJ, et al: Minority resident physicians' views on the role of race/ethnicity in their training experiences in the workplace. JAMA Netw Open 1(5):e182723, 2018 30646179

Pinder-Amaker S, Leary K: Changing institutional values and diversifying the behavioral health workforce, in Racism and Psychiatry: Contemporary Issues and Interventions. Edited by Medlock MM, Shtasel D, Trinh, NT, Williams DR. Cham, Switzerland, Humana Press, 2019, pp 181–203

Serchen J, Doherty R, Hewett-Abbott G, et al: Understanding and Addressing Disparities and Discrimination in Education and in the Physician Workforce: A Position Paper of the American College of Physicians. Philadelphia, PA, American College of Physicians, 2021

Suite DH, La Bril R, Primm A, Harrison-Ross P: Beyond misdiagnosis, misunderstanding and mistrust: relevance of the historical perspective in the medical and mental health treatment of people of color. J Natl Med Assoc 99(8):879–885, 2007 17722664

Sullivan LW, Suez Mittman I: The state of diversity in the health professions a century after Flexner. Acad Med 85(2):246–253, 2010 20107349

U.S. Census Bureau: QuickFacts: population estimates, July 1, 2021. Suitland, MD, U.S. Census Bureau, 2021. Available at: www.census.gov/quickfacts/fact/table/US/PST045221. Accessed October 8, 2022.

Willoughby CDE: Running away from drapetomania: Samuel A. Cartwright, medicine, and race in the antebellum South. J South Hist 84(3):579–614, 2018

Whitgob EE, Blankenburg RL, Bogetz AL: The discriminatory patient and family: strategies to address discrimination towards trainees. Acad Med 91(11):S64–S69, 2016 27779512

Wyatt TR, Rockich-Winston N, Taylor TR, et al: What does context have to do with anything? A study of professional identity formation in physician-trainees considered underrepresented in medicine. Acad Med 95(10):1587–1593, 2020 32079956

Wyse R, Hwang WT, Ahmed AA, et al: Diversity by race, ethnicity, and sex within the US psychiatry physician workforce. Acad Psychiatry 44(5):523–530, 2020 32705570

CHAPTER 5

Gender and Sexual Identity

Murad M. Khan, M.D.
Teddy G. Goetz, M.D., M.S.
Laura Erickson-Schroth, M.D.

Psychiatry residency has the potential to be an intensely reward-ing experience for many people because it provides multiple avenues for career growth as well as internal growth. However, if you are an LGBTQ+ resident, you may encounter challenges in several ways that make their learning environments more difficult to navigate. To date,

---

Positionality statements: Murad M. Khan (he/they) is a Pakistani, South Asian/Brown, Muslim, gay/queer, cisgender male PGY-4 psychiatry resident. Teddy G. Goetz (they/he) is a white, Jewish, queer, nonbinary transmasc PGY-2 psychiatry resident with chronic ill-ness. Laura Erickson-Schroth (she/they) is a white, queer, nonbinary psychiatrist who su-pervises residents in the psychiatric emergency room.

there has been a paucity of studies exploring sexual and gender minority health–related training during psychiatry residency. Missing from the literature are the voices of residents and their lived experiences within medical training. In response, we provide quotations from psychiatry residents about their own unique intersectional experiences (collected through an informal, voluntary convenience sample survey, disseminated anonymously via Google Forms through professional networks). Although these examples are not representative of *all* LGBTQ+ psychiatry residents, they may offer insights into different relevant challenges faced by individuals.

This chapter serves as a resource for LGBTQ+ and allied psychiatry residents as well as LGBTQ+ medical students interested in psychiatry. Although the chapter references *residents*, it may prove useful to fellows as well. Ultimately, structural solutions from program leadership are necessary: investing resources into creating rigorous and equitable curricula, recruiting and retaining LGBTQ+ faculty and faculty with expertise in LGBTQ+ mental health, and taking ownership of creating environments that allow all of their trainees to thrive. Therefore, this chapter also may be useful to program directors and other residency administrators hoping to improve educational and work environments for residents.

KEY POINTS

- LGBTQ+ psychiatry residents experience multiple challenges in the realms of training, career guidance, mentorship, health care, and safety.

- Resources that have been developed by LGBTQ+ residents and faculty often can mitigate some of the harm inflicted by training.

- Finding community with LGBTQ+ and allied psychiatry residents and faculty is essential for wellness, education, and organizing for change.

RESIDENCY TRAINING

Health disparities between LGBTQ+ and non-LGBTQ+ people are extensively documented and reflected in the training that residents receive (Hirschtritt et al. 2019; Nowaskie 2020). Many LGBTQ+ residents are deeply passionate about caring for patients who share one or more identities with them, some choosing to pursue psychiatry primarily for this reason. However, it is rare for residents to feel prepared to do so adequately, regardless of how they identify. Reasons it may be important for LGBTQ+ residents to be aware of these realities include the following:

- Realistic expectations can prepare residents to access resources for their professional development.
- Preparation can mitigate the deleterious impact of training-related distress.
- Acknowledgment of these experiences can reduce distress in climates where resistance and gaslighting are widespread.
- Information can empower residents to ask for curriculum reform in mainstream content, bolster LGBTQ+-specific content, and address concerns in the clinical environment.

Residency Didactics

Mainstream psychiatry curricula often miss multiple opportunities to address LGBTQ+ concerns. It is common to discuss prevalence of mental disorders by gender, but these discussions are presented almost exclusively through a binary and essentialist lens. *Men* and *women* are discussed with the assumption that these categories encompass the range of sex and gender experience. In addition to excluding the experiences of trans and nonbinary individuals, the statistics are rarely contextualized with discussions of transphobia and/or sexism. For example, *white race* and *male gender* are often listed as risk factors for death from suicide, but rarely do residents receive a rigorous sociopolitically informed exploration of these risk assessments. As an LGBTQ+ resident, you may see the implications of this in risk assessments documented throughout electronic medical records. More nuanced methods of assessing risk that do not rely on identity-based algorithms have not permeated the mainstream discourse. When LGBTQ+ concerns are discussed, structural oppression is often not named, which leads to the suggestion that the risk is conferred by these identities themselves.

Didactics replicate the cisheteronormativity of society and rarely interrogate it. Furthermore, overtly homophobic, biphobic, and/or transphobic material is still common. Stereotypes regarding various subgroups persist—of bisexual people as being "hypersexual," lesbians as "serial monogamists," gay men as "promiscuous," and trans people as psychotic and/or expressing their gender as a defense. You may experience a variety of challenging feelings in these moments, particularly if you identify as an LGBTQ+ resident, because you are put in the uncomfortable position of experiencing discrimination and simultaneously shouldering the burden of having to interrupt it.

There remains a dearth of LGBTQ+-specific curricula nationally. The creators of one anonymous cross-sectional survey sought to learn about LGBT-specific training from psychiatry program directors. Of the 233 program directors emailed, 72 responded and completed all items of the survey (30.8%). Fifty-six percent of these programs had 5 or fewer hours of LGBT-specific training (Hirschtritt et al. 2019). Another survey was distributed to psychiatry residents across the country in 2019 (Nowaskie 2020). The survey found a low number of annual LGBT curricular hours (mean=1.22, SD=1.59) and a moderate number of LGBT extracurricular hours (mean=10.79, SD=20.54). Although the residents reported very high affirming attitudinal awareness (mean=6.58, SD=0.72), they also reported moderate knowledge (mean=5.42, SD=1.28) and low clinical preparedness (mean=4.69, SD=1.23).

> As far as didactics, we don't have a lot of didactics on LGBTQ health or mental health. I'm struggling to think of any. This past year, the department has been trying to do more work around race and being more race conscious. It doesn't feel like they've been doing that work for sexuality or gender identity. The race work is brand new and not intersectional.
>
> —*Black, bisexual, cisgender woman, PGY-2 resident, East Coast*

Common strategies to cope with these challenges include the following:

- Find a community for emotional support. You may find community through LGBTQ+ affinity groups at your institution. If none are present, look to citywide, statewide, or national groups. The websites listed at the end of this chapter provide access to listservs that inform the wider community about social events, conferences, and social media pages.
- Organize with community members and augment didactic training. Most of the LGBTQ+-specific curricula are a direct result of solidarity between LGBTQ+ and supportive non-LGBTQ+ residents and faculty. These resources also can be found at the websites at the end of this chapter.

Elective Opportunities

Some residency programs offer elective opportunities for interested trainees. Such opportunities may be available in the form of programming that occurs during didactics, evenings (either program- or resident-driven), and/or clinical sites that see a higher proportion of LGBTQ+ patients. Outside residency programs, some national professional groups (see "Resources" at the end of the chapter) host talks, book groups, and panels. National conferences present another avenue for such content. Some psychoanalytic institutes also hold lecture series and study groups that are open to residents.

Clinical Training

The implications of the exclusion of LGBTQ+ concerns in the didactic curricula become apparent in clinical settings. You will likely experience and/or witness implicit and explicit forms of discrimination.

> I've seen abhorrent care for trans patients, including delayed admission to hospitals, frequent misgendering, and a certain shared delegitimizing that occurs behind the scenes. This has all been deeply concerning and has led me to question my decision to pursue allopathic medicine when the environment we are in feels so completely uninterested.
>
> —*White, cisgender, lesbian PGY-3 resident, West Coast*

You also might find it difficult to meet your training needs with respect to patient assignments.

> With respect to working with LGBTQ+ patients more generally, there is a risk of one of two extremes. On the one hand, some LGBTQ+ residents may find that LGBTQ+ patients tend to get diverted toward them, even if they have not requested this. On the other hand, LGBTQ+ residents may not get preference for working with these patients, even if they express a desire to do so.
>
> —*White, queer, genderqueer, larger-bodied inpatient and emergency psychiatrist, West Coast*

Furthermore, supervisors often are not equipped to supervise regarding concerns that may affect LGBTQ+ patients. Statistics regarding the proportion of psychiatrists (or even physicians) who identify as LGBTQ+ are not available, which itself reflects how challenging it can be to find them. Non-LGBTQ+ supervisors vary with respect to comfort and expertise.

> I was assigned a cisgender, gay community supervisor for my psychodynamic therapy cases. One of the patients I wanted to discuss was trans and the other was nonbinary, and this supervisor made some extremely transphobic remarks during our first session of super-

vision. I tried to discuss these issues with him, and he
became very defensive and angry.

*—White, queer, genderqueer, larger-bodied inpatient
and emergency psychiatrist, West Coast*

Some strategies to manage deficits you experience during clinical training might include the following:

- Supplement your training with supervision from faculty and peers who either have or are interested in developing this expertise. Some schools have "out lists" or mentorship databases that may assist in this process. Program directors are also a good source of information because they are typically asked these questions during recruitment. You may have to look to national organizations or other programs if such resources are not available at your institution.
- Engage in self-directed learning. Some resources are listed at the end of this chapter.

Resident as Educator

Given the lack of integrated curricula or available supervisors, LGBTQ+ residents may find themselves in the position of having to educate staff and their supervisors.

There was scant LGBTQ+ education in our formal residency curriculum. Our education was supplemented by myself and other residents committed to LGBTQ+ medical education who would provide lectures, journal clubs, and/or grand rounds on LGBTQ+ topics.

—Queer, transmasculine psychiatrist, East Coast

When I have had to train faculty members on the very basics of sexual orientation, gender identity, and gender expression, it was frustrating. It is not my responsibility to do this, and yet it always falls on queer people, particularly BIPOC [Black, Indigenous, and people of color] folks. Having to reprimand faculty members who use slurs against trans people. Correcting parents and providing education to use the right pronouns for their children.

—Black, queer, cisgender gay man, resident, East Coast

The role of resident as educator puts LGBTQ+ residents in the uncomfortable position of having to engage in uncompensated labor in an environment that is not supportive of them. It also puts them in situations where they encounter resistance from peers and people in positions in power. Such dynamics can be challenging for their training experience as well as their mental health.

Some strategies to manage the demands of educating might include the following:

- Leverage support from non-LGBTQ+ peers who can share some of the burden.
- Recognize that you also cannot educate everyone at all times. You deserve to make decisions about what you have the capacity for and take care of yourself accordingly.
- Refer residents and faculty to resources, some of which are listed at the end of this chapter.

MENTORSHIP

LGBTQ+ residents often struggle to find representation of their identities among the attending psychiatrists and other supervisors they work with. Even when there is representation of some part of their identities, many residents do not have the opportunity to work with anyone who shares their intersecting identities. The lack of connection and learning support that many LGBTQ+ residents feel can lead them to become disillusioned with their work despite having real feelings of excitement about the mental health field.

> [There is a] lack of mentorship for Black queer men, no spaces that are officially sponsored that feel safe to talk about Black queer issues.
>
> —*Black, queer, cisgender gay man, resident, East Coast*

> There was a lack of mentorship and career guidance throughout my time in residency. There were no trans or nonbinary attendings, and very few "out" LGB attendings.
>
> —*Queer, transmasculine psychiatrist, East Coast*

> I had a great mentor for LGB-related training, but there wasn't the same for trans-related issues…I had a lot of great mentors but not a single trans one.
>
> —*White, Hispanic, queer, trans psychiatrist*

Furthermore, residents are often acutely aware of politics within departments and witness discrimination against faculty members that affects their own sense of whether they are valued members of the hospital and residency community.

> There's this attending that I really looked up to…. They just left and it's commonly known that they were pushed out…. They always stood up for what was right and backed up what they were saying with well-studied facts. Their style was still seen as "abrasive."

—*Black, bisexual, cisgender woman, PGY-2 resident, East Coast*

Because many institutions have insufficient representation of LGBTQ+ psychiatrists, LGBTQ+ residents are burdened with seeking out mentorship on their own. It is common for residents to seek mentors by setting up rotations in clinics that cater to LGBTQ+ populations or by looking for research opportunities within the larger health care systems or universities where they are affiliated. If mentors are not available at your institution, you may need to turn to larger national organizations to fulfill your needs. See "Resources" for a list of some organizations that offer resources for LGBTQ+ trainees that include supplemental curricular material and events, mentorship opportunities, and social programming.

TRAINEE SAFETY

Despite broadening cultural acceptance and legal protection of LGBTQ+ individuals, harassment, discrimination, and assaults (verbal, physical, sexual), from patients and colleagues alike, remain extremely pertinent concerns for LGBTQ+ psychiatry residents.

> When [reporting verbal and physical harassment from an attending while doing a general medical rotation], I was…invalidated, gaslighted, and told there was nothing to be done. [After filing a] complaint [I] was contacted…and was strongly encouraged to drop my complaint so as not to "ruin" the perpetrator's career. I felt alone, invalidated, and unsafe but felt I had no choice but to oblige, which I have regretted ever since, as that attending harassed other residents after me before his relationship with the hospital system was terminated.

—*Queer, transmasculine psychiatrist, East Coast*

> [I've] been harassed by patients for my queer appear-
> ance and clothes and have not received support or
> guidance from faculty who witnessed these events.
> Pronouns are never discussed, and when I bring them
> up I'm often seen as the "woke police" or as an
> agitator.... There is truly no support by our faculty to
> guide us through these sorts of traumas.
>
> *—White, cisgender lesbian, PGY-3 resident, West Coast*

> Unfortunately, it is still common for some of our angry
> patients to use slurs about my sexuality (whether or not
> they actually know my sexuality), as well as my ethnic-
> ity, when expressing their displeasure with a treatment
> decision.... There wasn't [formal training] about how to
> handle harassment by patients...discriminatory or big-
> oted language directed toward me, or just frank threats
> to kill or gay bash me. I think the attitude is that psychi-
> atrists are just expected to take this harassment as part of
> the job of treating sometimes difficult patients.
>
> *—Asian American, gay, cisgender male psychiatrist, East Coast*

> Safety for me...is related to the invisibility.... I'm with
> a cisgender man and I also date outside of my relation-
> ship, including women. So my biggest fear has been
> "What if my program director or someone sees me
> with my nonprimary partner?" And the PD has said
> disparaging comments about nonmonogamy. So it's
> been worrisome to openly live my life.
>
> *—Black, bisexual, cisgender woman, PGY-2 resident, East Coast*

Nationally, LGBTQ+ people are more likely than non-LGBTQ+ people
to experience sexual violence (Chen et al. 2020; James et al. 2016; Katz-
Wise and Hyde 2012). One of our respondents who identified as a white,
cisgender lesbian with a chronic illness wrote about being sexually assaulted by a male veteran. She did not feel comfortable reporting this assault after witnessing the treatment of other patients and staff when
they reported such events. Reporting sexual violence (assault, harassment, abuse) is a personal decision. If you choose to report, protocols
vary by program. It may be helpful to find out if such protocols exist in
your program and to become familiar with them if they do. If you are
comfortable, it also may be helpful to involve trusted mentors and peers
for support. Some programs that are affiliated with larger university
systems may also offer confidential support services specific to such experiences. If you do not feel comfortable going through your program,

resources outside your program are also an option (e.g., the National Sexual Assault Hotline: 1-800-656-4673, pressing charges, emergency medical evaluations).

Some strategies to manage safety issues include the following:

- Become aware of programmatic reporting systems for such events.
- Identify emotional support resources relevant for such maltreatment.
- Identify the locations of gender-neutral restrooms and all-gender locker rooms, if available.
- Normalize use of pronouns in introductions (e.g., in general, on Zoom, in email signatures).
- Request gender-affirming ID badge name updates prior to legal name change proceedings.

HEALTH CARE FOR LGBTQ+ TRAINEES

Ideally, queer- and trans-affirming care should be accessible in all areas of medicine. Whether you are considering which program to apply to or to rank or you are already a trainee, consider exploring available health care options and associated training issues.

You might investigate medical care accessibility through questions such as 1) Are gender-affirming hormones covered? To what extent? 2) Which gender-affirming surgical procedures are covered? To what extent? 3) Which fertility services are covered? Does this coverage differ between cisgender and transgender or gender-expansive individuals?

> Our insurance program refused to cover basic health care needs of mine because I was trans.... It was decided that since it was a self-funded insurance program, the state rules of nondiscrimination did not apply. I had to wait until a couple years later in my residency for nondiscrimination to be added to the policy.
>
> —*White, Hispanic, queer, trans psychiatrist*

Medical leave policies are also essential to explore: How much paid and/or unpaid time is a resident allowed off for medical leave? How are missed rotations made up? How are missed call shifts made up or redistributed? What supports are in place for residents with medical leave needs? Often, if programs have not yet considered medical needs in the context of LGBTQ+ care (particularly gender-affirming care), policies already exist for other medical concerns and for parental leave.

> I was pleasantly surprised that I had no problems tak-
> ing leave from residency for top surgery, and my short-
> term disability through the residency program covered
> my leave.
>
> —*Queer, transmasculine psychiatrist, East Coast*

Mental health care services and crisis response services are also essential to health and wellness. Although mental health disparities for LGBTQ+ psychiatry residents have not been studied, LGBTQ+ medical students are more likely to report burnout, depression, anxiety, and harassment (Lapinski et al. 2016; Przedworski et al. 2015). This is reflected in the survey responses we received, highlighting the need for affirming mental health care services. For LGBTQ+ individuals in residency or fellowship training, this must include not only insurance coverage of therapy and psychiatry services but also access to queer and trans therapists and psychiatrists and those who specialize in caring for queer and trans patients.

RESIDENCY PROGRAM CLIMATE

Finally, institutional culture varies across the country by geography, time, and leadership. People occupying positions of power (e.g., department chair, program director, dean of medical education), faculty members, chief residents, and residents themselves all have an impact on program culture. Often, only a few faculty (if any) are tasked with leading LGBTQ+-specific teaching in a particular program, and the departure of such a faculty member can have a dramatic impact on the culture of the program. In addition, residents commonly lead cultural change in the absence of it coming from leadership. Because of the frequent rotation of residents, culture can change from year to year. A resident or potential resident looking to assess the climate of a given program likely would benefit from speaking to a wide array of people who are present at that particular institution at that specific point in time.

SPECIFIC CHALLENGES AND STRATEGIES

⌘ **I am overwhelmed by oppressive content in the curricula and/
or deficits in training on affirmative care for LGBTQ+ patients.**
Ask program leadership, faculty, and residents if they know of people
within the institution who share identities and/or interest in the material.
A wealth of material (see "Resources") is available that can be presented

to leadership and/or faculty if they have an interest in curriculum reform but do not know where to start. If there is scant support at your institution, this material is often accessible to all training levels for self-teaching. Prioritize community within and/or outside the profession for emotional support.

⌘ **I don't have access to career guidance and mentorship.** Start with your institution by speaking with anyone you view as an ally or observe doing LGBTQ+ work. Ask them about their careers and how they came to their current positions. Find out if they know anyone who could serve as a mentor to you. Be open to looking outside your institution if you are not successful within it. There may be potential mentors in your city or state. Connect with national organizations focused on LGBTQ+ health, such as the Association of LGBTQ+ Psychiatrists.

⌘ **I'm not sure how to access LGBTQ+-specific health care.** Reach out to your Graduate Medical Education office to discuss how residents in the past have navigated these issues and what support they might offer you. Also check with your insurance company to determine if out-of-network providers can be included in in-network rates because of a lack of available in-network providers.

SELF-REFLECTIVE QUESTIONS

1. What knowledge and skills do I need to be able to provide affirming care to LGBTQ+ patients? In what ways is my program meeting or not meeting these needs? How can I be in community with people who share my values, offer support, and/or keep me accountable?
2. What are my priorities for choosing a residency program? How do these priorities intersect with my LGBTQ+ identity? If I am already in residency, what are my priorities for future jobs?
3. What are the needs specific to LGBTQ+ psychiatry residents' daily well-being? How would I like to see psychiatry residency programs support those needs in the future?

RESOURCES

These resources include supplemental curricular material and events, mentorship opportunities, and social programming:

American Psychiatric Association Minority and Underrepresented (M/UR) Caucuses—LGBTQ: www.psychiatry.org/psychiatrists/cultural-competency/mur-caucuses

American Psychological Association: APA LGBT resources and publications: www.apa.org/pi/lgbt/resources

APA Task Force on Psychological Practice With Sexual Minority Persons: APA guidelines for clinical practice for lesbian, gay, and bisexual clients. Washington, DC, American Psychological Association, 2021. Available at: www.apa.org/pi/lgbt/resources/guidelines. Accessed September 20, 2022.

Association of LGBTQ+ Psychiatrists: www.aglp.org

Erickson-Schroth L, Ramos N, Hurley P, et al (eds): AGLP/GAP lesbian, gay, bisexual, transgender, and queer mental health: a curriculum for psychiatry residents. Dallas, TX, Group for the Advancement of Psychiatry, 2021. Available at: www.gap-lgbtq.org. Accessed September 20, 2022.

GLMA: Health Professionals Advancing LGBTQ Equality: www.glma.org

GLMA Provider Directory: https://glmaimpak.networkats.com/members_online_new/members/dir_provider.asp

Grossman G: Selected bibliography of gender and sexuality. New York, American Psychoanalytic Association, 2016. Available at: https://apsa.org/sites/default/files/BibliographyHomosexualityand Gender.pdf. Accessed September 20, 2022.

REFERENCES

Chen J, Walters ML, Gilbert LK, et al: Sexual violence, stalking, and intimate partner violence by sexual orientation, United States. Psychol Violence 10(1):110–119, 2020 32064141

Hirschtritt ME, Noy G, Haller E, et al: LGBT-specific education in general psychiatry residency programs: a survey of program directors. Acad Psychiatry 43(1):41–45, 2019 30430392

James S, Herman J, Rankin S, et al: The Report of the 2015 US Transgender Survey. Washington, DC, National Center for Transgender Equality, 2016

Katz-Wise SL, Hyde JS: Victimization experiences of lesbian, gay, and bisexual individuals: a meta-analysis. J Sex Res 49(2–3):142–167, 2012 22380586

Lapinski J, Yost M, Sexton P, et al: Factors modifying burnout in osteopathic medical students. Acad Psychiatry 40(1):55–62, 2016 26108394

Nowaskie D: A national survey of US psychiatry residents' LGBT cultural competency: the importance of LGBT patient exposure and formal education. J Gay Lesbian Ment Health 24(4):375–391, 2020

Przedworski JM, Dovidio JF, Hardeman RR, et al: A comparison of the mental health and well-being of sexual minority and heterosexual first-year medical students: a report from Medical Student CHANGE Study. Acad Med 90(5):652–659, 2015 25674912

CHAPTER 6

Professional and Personal Life

The International Medical Graduate Experience

Sanya Virani, M.D., M.P.H.

Oluwole Jegede, M.D., M.P.H.

Manal Khan, M.D.

Vishal Madaan, M.D.

International medical graduates (IMGs) are defined as physicians who received their initial medical degree from a medical school located outside the United States. It is the location of the medical school, not the physician's nationality or citizenship, that determines whether the graduate is an IMG. As a result, U.S. citizens who graduated from medical schools outside the United States are considered IMGs, whereas non-U.S. citizens who graduated from medical schools within the United States are not. The 2021 National Resident Matching Program report indicated that overall, 59.5% of U.S. citizen IMGs (U.S. IMGs) and 54.8% of non-U.S. IMGs matched successfully into postgraduate year 1 (PGY-1) positions (National Resident Matching Program 2020). According to the American Psychiatric Association's 2019 Resident/Fellow Census, the top three countries that contributed to the medical training of the non-U.S. IMG group from 2014 to 2018 were India (9.7%), Pakistan (3.95%), and Canada (2.79%) (American Psychiatric Association 2020).

IMGs constitute a formidable proportion and an essential component of the psychiatric workforce. Despite a steady decrease in IMG applications due to a multitude of factors, IMGs continue to be overrepresented in subspecialty fellowships and medically underserved areas as well as in the public sector. With a growing diversity of the U.S. population, the need for well-trained IMG physicians has never been more palpable. Each IMG journey has a unique trajectory yet follows a basic template full of trials and tribulations. For example, non-U.S. IMGs must not only learn psychiatry during training but also navigate immigration pathways while working through acculturation.

In this chapter we focus largely on non-U.S. IMGs because of the additional challenges faced by this group and provide a succinct overview of the interview and matching process, residency training experience, and postresidency fellowship and job environments. We explore various challenges to consider along the way, resources to review and support systems to tap into, and ways to make the journey meaningful and enjoyable.

KEY POINTS

- IMGs account for approximately one-third of the psychiatry workforce and are overrepresented in public psychiatry positions and subspecialty fellowships.

- With psychiatry lately evolving as a more desirable specialty for U.S. medical graduates, a steady decline in IMG application and match numbers has been noticed.

- IMGs undergo a triple learning process during training, with education not limited to psychiatry but also including navigation of immigration pathways and working through acculturation.

- Newer changes to United States Medical Licensing Examination (USMLE) scoring have the potential to have adverse impacts on IMGs and make the match more challenging.

- IMGs need mentorship for the specific challenges of acculturation and immigration.

INTERNATIONAL MEDICAL GRADUATES IN PSYCHIATRY: RECENT TRENDS

Historically, psychiatry residency has been particularly attractive to IMGs. This steady appeal may be related to the anecdotal evidence that psychiatry programs may be more likely to overlook the number of post–medical school graduation years for IMG applicants during selection. However, when compared with other sizable specialties, psychiatry saw the largest decrease in both U.S. IMGs and non-U.S. IMGs matching into PGY-1 positions in 2020, reflecting a 46.3% decrease from 2014 (30%) to 2020 (16.1%). Smaller decreases were reported in family medicine (22.3%), internal medicine (7.3%), surgery (4.6%), and neurology (4.6%), whereas pathology, pediatrics, and emergency medicine showed opposite trends, the reasons for which are unclear (Virani et al. 2021).

Comparing U.S. IMGs with non-U.S. IMGs in psychiatry, a recent study noted that on average, 10.8% of U.S. IMGs and a similar 9.7% of non-U.S. IMGs matched into PGY-1 categorical psychiatry programs (Virani et al. 2021). From 2014 to 2020, U.S. IMG numbers decreased by 41.5%, whereas non-U.S. IMG numbers decreased by 51.2%.

IMPACT ON IMGS: RECENT CHANGES IN THE U.S. RESIDENCY SYSTEM

With the USMLE Step 1 scoring changed to pass/fail and the number of attempts for each examination reduced, the match could potentially have more challenging downstream effects on IMGs, which will become clear over time. Doing away with the three-digit score in favor of the pass/fail grading system may align with the holistic method of reviewing applications, creating room for programs to pay more attention to and factor into their rankings reflections of subjective information about training, personalities, and life experiences of applicants. However, the Step 1 score has consistently been one of the most important factors considered when selecting applicants for interviews, with high scores potentially giving applicants an opportunity to distinguish themselves. The lack of such a clear and numerical data point may adversely affect IMGs' applications, especially because IMGs have traditionally scored higher on USMLE Step 1 compared with their U.S. M.D. and D.O. senior counterparts. In addition, although this change may alleviate the stress of securing a high Step 1 score, such concern may now shift to the Step 2 Clinical Knowledge score, which would remain the only available numerical data point.

Boulet and Pinsky (2020) reported that although there is limited evidence to suggest that Step 1 scores predict residency performance, the large numbers of applications forced many programs to use Step 1 scores as an initial screening mechanism in years past. With the change to the Step 1 examination in effect, IMGs will have to find other ways to distinguish themselves. A specific strategy to consider is planning elective rotations in the United States ahead of time, even during the second and third years in medical school, if the student has decided on psychiatry as a specialty choice by then. It might be very useful to start research projects during those rotations with potential long-term mentors and to maintain and nurture those relationships. This could also make it easier for mentors to assimilate information with specific data points and examples to include in letters of recommendation and the ability to point to an applicant's familiarity with the U.S. health care system.

On the other hand, it remains quite likely that in reviewing applications for markers of life events, experiences, extracurricular activities, and other interests, program directors might not find the details provided on a non-U.S. IMG's application as relatable as those from U.S. applicants. In addition, some IMGs may be identified for residency interviews on the basis of the reputation of their medical school and faculty. Unfortunately, this reputation says little about individual applicants' abilities. Although the Educational Commission for Foreign Medical Graduates (ECFMG) has been working toward creating a list of international medical schools accredited by the World Federation for Medical Education to allow training directors to feel more at ease with medical schools, the process has been delayed. Furthermore, it remains to be seen whether international medical schools or their regulatory agencies will participate in such an accreditation process, short of which their graduates may not be qualified to pursue U.S. residency training.

Past the stage of submission of applications, candidates then move on to the next set of challenges and opportunities encountered as a part of the interview process.

RESIDENCY INTERVIEWS: WHAT TO EXPECT AS AN APPLICANT

The interview day is usually preceded by a preinterview dinner and allows applicants to interact with residents in an informal setting. Because the interview is limited to a day, prepare to be available for a full day. An itinerary for the interview day is sent out to the applicants in advance. A typical interview day includes opening remarks by the program director, individual and panel interviews by faculty and residents, and a tour of various clinical sites.

Although interviews serve as an opportunity for the program and the applicant to get to know each other, they can also be stressful experiences. Non-U.S. IMG applicants can have additional challenges. For some applicants, this can mark their first international trip, a process that entails securing a visa and incurring travel and lodging costs without much social support in the United States. To limit financial strain, applicants should consider clustering interviews according to region.

Furthermore, non-U.S. IMG applicants have to familiarize themselves not only with the landscape of the United States but also with cultural nuances and linguistic colloquialisms. Some non-U.S. IMG applicants come from collectivistic cultures, and their indirect use of language, humility, and deference to hierarchy can, at times, be misinterpreted as lack of assertiveness. It may be helpful for applicants and programs alike to be aware of these cultural differences.

Regarding the interviewing experience, applicants can take steps to mitigate stress. After receiving an invitation to interview, applicants may professionally reach out to current residents of the program for informational interviews. The applicants also should familiarize themselves with the program and have questions prepared ahead of time. Although these connections are outside the structured interview day, applicants should be aware that residents may still give feedback to the program directors about the interaction. If the interview day itinerary specifies which faculty personnel will be interviewing the applicant, it is useful to look up their areas of expertise in advance to tailor the conversation and questions. Applicants also should go through their application thoroughly and be prepared to answer any questions pertaining to it. It can be useful to collect some common questions asked by residency programs and prepare well-thought-out talking points. Interviewers use adaptability and ability to converse well in English to assess a mutual fit, so applicants may find it useful to participate in mock interviews with mentors and colleagues. Applicants should consider recording their practice interviews to study their body language and verbal delivery.

The recommended dress code for the interview day is business formal. For preinterview dinners, applicants can wear business casual. It is important to arrive for the interview on time, so applicants should familiarize themselves with the directions to the interview site in advance. Applicants should know that the interview process begins with the preinterview dinner and continues until they leave the interview site. As a result, it is important to stay professional all along and to treat everyone in a respectful manner. Applicants are expected to ask a lot of questions regarding their potential workplace for the next 4 years because programs will regard this as a measure of the candidate's interest. After the completion of interview day, applicants can send brief thank you emails or cards to their interviewers highlighting salient features of their conversation.

Finally, in light of COVID-19's impact on recent match cycles, some programs might consider using a hybrid model consisting of both in-person and virtual interviewing. In the case of virtual interviewing, both the residency programs and applicants should be aware of unique challenges specific to non-U.S. IMG applicants. These can include an increase in the overall number of applications received by each program, which can be a disadvantage to IMG applicants. Other challenges include time zone differences, instability of internet connection in low- to middle-resource countries, and communication difficulties. It is important for programs to be aware of these challenges, and applicants also should be mindful of these issues and should strategize ways to circumvent them (e.g., by offering the program additional phone numbers for access ahead of time in case the internet connection is unstable).

VISAS

Non-U.S. IMGs must obtain an appropriate visa to participate in residency programs. The two most used visas for residency training are the H-1B (temporary worker) and the J-1 (exchange visitor)—both are nonimmigrant visas (Table 6–1). After completion of training, an individual may pursue permanent resident status for a longer stay within the United States.

ENTERING RESIDENCY

One of the major challenges for IMGs, particularly as they begin residency, is understanding and navigating the U.S. health care system culture and practices, which may be radically different from those of their home countries. The workplace culture of hospitals in the United States is highly reflective of the overall health care system, which is often more sophisticated, technologically and administratively, compared with most health care systems around the world. In addition, in terms of language and communication with patients and colleagues, the IMG's challenge is to understand the specific flavor and cultural context of conversations, including colloquial terms. Indeed, the literature suggests that IMG residents face major challenges and communication bar-

TABLE 6–1. J-1 and H-1B visa basics

	J-1 visa	**H-1B visa**
USMLE requirement	Not required	Passing essential
Where to obtain	ECFMG	Program or hospital system
Maximum length of stay	7-year limit	6-year limit
Who pays	No cost to training program	Employer pays filing fee of $3,000–$4,000 per GME trainee
Waiver requirements	The visa is sponsored contingent on the stipulation that the trainee will return to their home country for 2 years before applying for another visa; however, this requirement can be waived if appropriate waiver criteria are met	None
Permanent residency filing	Must complete waiver or home country requirement before filing for permanent residency	Can immediately file for permanent residency after completion of training

Note. ECFMG = Educational Commission for Foreign Medical Graduates; GME = graduate medical education; USMLE = United States Medical Licensing Examination.

riers based on the regional dialects of the community where the program is located, including cross-cultural differences in norms, values, and beliefs of such communities (Dorgan et al. 2009).

ACCULTURATION STRESS

Acculturation is a dynamic process that affects both the physical and mental health of people at individual and group levels. The dynamism of acculturation to a new host system depends on several contextual factors, the management of which may determine how successful an IMG is in thriving within the host system. Acculturation has been described as the psychological and behavioral changes that an individual may experience because of sustained contact with members of other cultural groups. Although initially described as a unidimensional construct, acculturation is probably more accurately depicted as a multidimensional process in which an individual maintains aspects or traditions of their

TABLE 6–2. Ecological framework of challenges facing the IMG physician

Individual	Interpersonal relationship	Community	Societal
Presence of chronic medical or psychiatric conditions	Network with family and friends	"IMG friendly" status of residency program	Region of residency (i.e., state)
Social isolation and discrimination	Marital status	Workload, burnout	Regional dialect
First language and accent	Work-life balance	Residency setting: community versus teaching/research hospital	Physician immigration status
Country of medical education		Medical specialty and residency track (e.g., clinical, research)	Ease of community integration
Economic and financial issues (e.g., housing, transportation)		Specific patient population	

Note. IMG=international medical graduate.

culture of origin while simultaneously adopting elements of the new cultural group (Schwartz et al. 2010). In this multidimensional, ecological framework (Table 6–2), individual experiences, interpersonal relationships, community, and societal factors all exert significant and observable influence on IMGs as they settle within the culture of the residency and the larger community where they now live, play, work, and raise their families (Chen et al. 2011).

Difficulties with acculturation and poor social support are predictors of mental health difficulties for IMGs during the process of adaptation into residency programs (Kirmayer et al. 2018). IMGs enter residency at different stages of cultural assimilation, which is a process of consistent integration whereby members of an ethnocultural group (e.g., immigrants, minority groups) are "absorbed" into an established, generally larger community. Assimilation can be the process through which people lose originally differentiating traits, such as traditional cultural outfits and speech particularities or mannerisms, when they encounter another society or culture. For most IMGs whose initial entry into the United States involves joining residency, this can feel like a cultural shock within a system to which they must quickly adapt to survive. Although losing one's cultural characteristics might be seen as a negative outcome of assimilation by some IMGs, it could also serve as an important survival trait for those who are well adjusted and assimilated.

TABLE 6–3. Examples of strategies to mitigate challenges faced by IMGs

1. Take advantage of support services provided by graduate medical education, including mindfulness, psychotherapy, counseling, and regular primary care.
2. Use vacation days for time off with friends and family, visiting new places, and relaxation.
3. Take an English as a foreign language class for physicians if necessary and ensure continuous practice outside work in the community.
4. Seek advice about payment of physician loans in your community, including opting for military reserve service.
5. Consider networking with current and past residents of your program to determine the program's IMG-friendly status.
6. Using various social media, continue networking with family and friends back home for support.
7. Consider other networking opportunities with your home country physician associations in the United States.

Note. IMG=international medical graduate.

Navigating such challenges can determine the IMG's success in residency and after residency. Table 6–3 identifies some examples of strategies to mitigate challenges faced by IMGs

FELLOWSHIPS

After completing psychiatry residency training in the United States, some IMGs may go on to pursue subspecialty training via fellowships. Data published in 2020 suggest that IMGs made up 16% of general psychiatry residents but 35% of child fellows, 40% of addiction fellows, and 47% of geriatric fellows (American Psychiatric Association 2020). Declining numbers of IMGs matching into psychiatry will have tremendous negative impacts on the fill rate of these fellowship programs. IMGs may prefer Accreditation Council for Graduate Medical Education (ACGME)-accredited fellowships in order to bolster their applications for a green card or to acquire "super specialty training" that may not be available in their countries of origin.

Psychiatry fellowships can be broadly classified as ACGME-accredited and non-ACGME-accredited (Table 6–4). Non-ACGME-accredited fellowships are available in the following areas (not an exhaustive list): global mental health, palliative care and psychosocial oncology, emergency psychiatry, behavioral sleep medicine, college mental health, psychotherapy, and research (clinical and translational research, health

TABLE 6–4. ACGME-accredited fellowships

Type of fellowship	Certification examination board	Fellowship length	Participation in ERAS match process
Addiction medicine	American Board of Preventive Medicine	1 year	No
Addiction psychiatry	ABPN	1 year	No
Brain injury medicine	ABPN	1 year	No
Child and adolescent psychiatry	ABPN	2 years	Yes
Consultation-liaison psychiatry	ABPN	1 year	Yes
Forensic psychiatry	ABPN	1 year	Plans under way for participation
Geriatric psychiatry	ABPN	1 year	No
Hospice and palliative medicine	ABPN	1 year	No
Sleep medicine	ABPN	1 year	Yes

Note. ABPN=American Board of Psychiatry and Neurology; ACGME=Accreditation Council for Graduate Medical Education; ERAS=Electronic Residency Application Service.

services research, basic sciences research, addictions research, and neuropsychopharmacology research).

EMPLOYMENT BEYOND RESIDENCY AND FELLOWSHIP

After completing residency and fellowship, IMGs pursue their careers in a variety of settings, which include joining public sector settings or academia and initiating private practice. Academic opportunities often involve serving on a clinician-only or clinician-educator track within an academic center and following requirements for promotion and tenure. Because IMGs must have permanent residency status to start independent private practice, recent non-U.S. IMG residency graduates often take on salaried positions. Similarly, non-U.S. IMGs on visas are ineligible for obtaining any federal grants, such as those from the National Institute of Mental Health and, as a result, may be underrepresented in research tracks.

TABLE 6–5. Permanent residency options

Family-based petition

Spouse of a U.S. citizen/legal permanent resident

Parent

Siblings

Employment-based petition

Labor certification/PERM

HPSA

EB-1: extraordinary ability with international recognition

EB-2: exceptional ability or national interest

Note. HPSA=health professional shortage area; PERM=Program Electronic Review Management.

IMG psychiatrists are overrepresented in public sector settings and among physicians serving the Medicaid and Medicare populations because these jobs may be a source for obtaining a J-1 waiver. The J-1 waiver eliminates the 2-year return to home country requirement that is associated with the J-1 visa if the physician agrees to work in a medically underserved area for 3 years after finishing training. Once waivers are completed, non-U.S. IMGs previously on a J-1 visa can apply for permanent residency. J-1 waivers may be requested on the basis of hardship or persecution and include but are not limited to interested government agency waivers (Conrad 30, Department of Veterans Affairs, or Department of Health and Human Services clinical waiver). Individuals on H-1B visas do not need to go through the waiver process. Regardless, employment positions for individuals on such visas or those requiring waivers are fairly limited in number, and as a result, a judicious, timely, and planned approach is required to meet regulatory timelines while simultaneously considering a good mutual fit for such an employment opportunity.

An immigrant visa (green card or permanent resident status) permits a foreign citizen to remain permanently in the United States. A lawful permanent resident may apply to become a naturalized U.S. citizen after living in the United States typically after 5 years (or 3 years if they are married to a U.S. citizen). Petitions to file for permanent resident status are often family based or employment based (Table 6–5). Some of the employment-based petitions are independent of a sponsor and are reliant on the physician's credentials (e.g., EB-1, extraordinary ability with international recognition; EB-2, exceptional ability or national interest).

SPECIFIC CHALLENGES AND STRATEGIES

⌘ **I am on a J-1 visa. How do I proactively manage it?** J-1 and H1-B visas are the most common visas used by IMGs for residency training in the United States. The J-1 visa is sponsored by ECFMG. The J-1 visa is accompanied by a DS-2019, which is a certificate of eligibility of J-1 status. The DS-2019 allows a person to request a J-1 visa to enter the United States. It also determines the length of a J-1 visa holder's legal stay in the United States. Residents on a J-1 visa should work closely with their training program liaison (TPL) to maintain their status. The TPL is usually a staff person in the residency office (such as the program coordinator). The TPL initiates an online appointment profile on a yearly basis via EVnet for the maintenance of the J-1 status for the resident. As per ECFMG, EVNet is described as "a secure, on-line platform through which TPLs can submit appointment details, upload supporting documentation, and manage various aspects of the J-1 sponsorship process" (Educational Commission for Foreign Medical Graduates 2022). The standard documents that are needed include a contract or letter of offer, form I-644, form I-94, and the training program description (if entering subspecialty training). This appointment profile is accepted by the resident via the On-line Applicant Status and Information System (OASIS), and additional documentation (if applicable) is provided. The resident should stay in touch with the TPL and determine a conservative timeline for annual renewal of the visa maintenance.

⌘ **My fellow residents really have no idea what my experience has been like in residency.** Residents have varied experiences, and the IMG cohort tends to have a unique perception of specific events and interactions during residency, especially when viewed through their own cultural lens. The first step would be to acknowledge that the experience of residency for an IMG is almost always inherently different from that of their counterparts, and that is not necessarily a disadvantage. Expecting U.S. medical graduate colleagues to fully comprehend the perception of that experience without open communication is somewhat unreasonable. However, educating colleagues about your experiences will expand their understanding of the challenges you face. Cultivate a broad and open mindset as you go along your residency path, always endeavoring to treat non-IMG counterparts as allies and not adversaries. With that foundation, you will be more likely to learn and adapt quickly and understand what the U.S. system really expects of you and become even more creative with paying attention to your unique strengths and using them to give back to your residency program. It is also wise to understand that some aspects of this lived experience might never be relatable, and discussing this in individual therapy sessions might be the best approach for an IMG to deal with a challenge in this area and to develop the appropriate coping skills necessary to accept differences.

Many psychiatry residency training programs in the United States recognize the toll of working as a trainee in mental health care and, hence, provide weekly process groups, which often are organized by postgraduate training level or class. In addition to process groups, some programs offer opportunities that are free of cost or include subsidized personal psychotherapy. A specific example of an organized group that aims to provide support to trainees is the Committee for Interns and Residents, which is a part of the Service Employees International Union.

At a programmatic level, engaging in supervision and seeking mentorship from both IMG and non-IMG mentors is beneficial (see Chapter 33, "Mentorship and Sponsorship"). It is also important to look at opportunities related to your culture, such as festival celebrations or movie screenings, within your city. In addition, country-specific psychiatry organizations, such as the Indo-American Psychiatric Association, may be additional sources of support and information.

⌘ **I feel like I'm losing part of myself as I train in the United States.** It is not uncommon for immigrants to ask this question as they integrate into a new culture and encounter new experiences such as living and practicing medicine in a new country, meeting new people, and essentially starting a new life, which can be experienced as foreign to ways in which they have been raised. Some reasons for this feeling may be the guilt of leaving behind family and friends and starting a new life in a new country or that one is not contributing enough to the health care of one's birth country. You must understand that 1) this process of acculturation is necessary and must be navigated in an adaptive way; 2) you can successfully integrate into the host culture while keeping your sense of cultural identity (i.e., you do not have to lose your sense of self as you embrace your new experience); and 3) your residency training is a way for you to improve yourself as a physician so you can be of more benefit to yourself, your family, and your community.

SELF-REFLECTIVE QUESTIONS

1. As an IMG, what unique perspective do I bring to my U.S. training, and how do I integrate that perspective into the practice of psychiatry here?
2. How do I hold on to the unique values and traditions of my culture while incorporating nuances of and contributing to U.S. culture?
3. How should I plan to navigate some of the immigration challenges I will face during the course of my career?

RESOURCES

American Association of Directors of Psychiatric Residency Training IMG Fellowship: www.aadprt.org/annual-meeting/awards-fellowships/award-detail?awardsid=70

American Psychiatric Association: Navigating psychiatric residency in the United States: a guide for international medical graduate physicians. Washington, DC, American Psychiatric Association, 2022. Available at: www.psychiatry.org/psychiatrists/international/international-trainees/international-medical-graduates-guide-to-u-s-residency. Accessed October 20, 2022.

American Psychiatric Association: A roadmap to psychiatry residency. Washington, DC, American Psychiatric Association, 2021. Available at: www.psychiatry.org/residents-medical-students/medical-students/apply-for-psychiatric-residency. Accessed October 20, 2022.

Association of Medical Colleges: Virtual interviews: tips for medical school applicants. Washington, DC, Association of Medical Colleges, 2020. Available at: www.aamc.org/system/files/2020-05/Virtual_Interview_Tips_for_Medical_School_Applicants_05142020.pdf. Accessed October 20, 2022.

Coalition for Physician Accountability's Work Group on Medical Students in the Class of 2022 Moving Across Institutions for Interviews for Postgraduate Training: Recommendations on 2021–22 residency season interviewing for medical education institutions considering applicants from LCME-accredited, U.S. osteopathic, and non-U.S. medical schools. Coalition for Physician Accountability, 2022. Available at: https://physicianaccountability.org/wp-content/uploads/2021/08/Virtual-Rec_COVID-Only_Final.pdf. Accessed October 20, 2022.

Conrad 30 waiver program, U.S. Citizenship and Immigration Services: www.uscis.gov/working-in-the-united-states/students-and-exchange-visitors/conrad-30-waiver-program

Educational Commission for Foreign Medical Graduates: ECFMG information booklet: www.ecfmg.org/2022ib/index.html

Educational Commission for Foreign Medical Graduates: Exchange visitor sponsorship program: www.ecfmg.org/evsp/about.html

Fitzpatrick E: An overview of ECFMG-FAIMER and international medical graduates in family medicine training. Philadelphia, PA, Educational Commission for Foreign Medical Graduates, 2018. Available at: www.aafp.org/dam/AAFP/documents/events/rps_pdw/handouts/res18-96-an-overview-of-ecfmg.pdf. Accessed October 20, 2022.

REFERENCES

American Psychiatric Association: 2019 resident/fellow census. Washington, DC, American Psychiatric Association, November 2020. Available at: www.psychiatry.org/File%20Library/Residents-MedicalStudents/Residents/APA-Resident-Census-2019.pdf. Accessed July 23, 2021.

Boulet JR, Pinsky WW: Reporting a pass/fail outcome for USMLE step 1: consequences and challenges for international medical graduates. Acad Med 95(9):1322–1324, 2020 32496289

Chen PG, Curry LA, Bernheim SM, et al: Professional challenges of non-U.S.-born international medical graduates and recommendations for support during residency training. Acad Med 86(11):1383–1388, 2011 21952056

Dorgan KA, Lang F, Floyd M, et al: International medical graduate-patient communication: a qualitative analysis of perceived barriers. Acad Med 84(11):1567–1575, 2009 19858820

Educational Commission for Foreign Medical Graduates: For J-1 host institutions. Philadelphia, PA, Educational Commission for Foreign Medical Graduates, July 19, 2022. Available at: www.ecfmg.org/evsp/resources-host-institutions.html. Accessed October 20, 2022.

Kirmayer LJ, Sockalingam S, Fung KP, et al: International medical graduates in psychiatry: cultural issues in training and continuing professional development. Can J Psychiatry 63(4):258–280, 2018 29630854

National Resident Matching Program: Charting outcomes in the match: international medical graduates. Washington, DC, National Resident Matching Program, July 2020. Available at: https://www.nrmp.org/wp-content/uploads/2021/08/Charting-Outcomes-in-the-Match-2020_IMG_final.pdf. Accessed August 29, 2021.

Schwartz SJ, Unger JB, Zamboanga BL, et al: Rethinking the concept of acculturation: implications for theory and research. Am Psychol 65(4):237–251, 2010 20455618

Virani S, Mitra S, Grullón MA, et al: International medical graduate resident physicians in psychiatry: decreasing numbers, geographic variation, community correlations, and implications. Acad Psychiatry 45(1):7–12, 2021 33469891

PART 3

Approaching Clinical Work

CHAPTER 7

Learning to Develop a Case Formulation

Phelan E. Maruca-Sullivan, M.D.

Rajesh R. Tampi, M.D., M.S., DFAPA, DFAAGP

Raziya S. Wang, M.D.

Case formulation serves as the foundation on which good psychiatric care is built; it identifies and organizes the core elements of a patient's illness into a coherent hypothesis. This important narrative then becomes the means through which psychiatrists understand, empathize with, and ultimately attempt to heal their patients (McWilliams 2011). It is an ever-evolving piece of work, consistently and carefully updated, as understanding of the patient grows. It is an essential part of comprehensive treatment planning. Ideally, the case formulation not only will illuminate the core issues contributing to your patient's distress but also will help you experience greater empathy and anticipate future challenges (Eells 2011). Good case formulation may also enhance your understanding of your own role in the therapeutic relationship, any implicit biases at play, and your capacity for self-reflection and self-awareness in the care of psychiatric patients.

KEY POINTS

- Formulation can enhance your understanding of your patient, help you articulate the complexities of your patient's illness, and ensure that you craft an effective and comprehensive treatment plan.

- Formulation is a skill that requires practice and can be made easier by relying on a trusted framework.

- The biopsychosocial model is a useful framework that incorporates the four Ps (predisposing, precipitating, perpetuating, preventative factors) of formulation.

- A thorough formulation also considers the cultural and structural factors contributing to your patient's illness as well as cultural differences and the potential for bias within the therapeutic relationship.

FUNDAMENTALS OF FORMULATION

Organization of the formulation may vary—style, length, and sequence are, in large part, at your discretion—but the task itself can contain inherent conflicts between efficiency and comprehensiveness and between simplicity of language and complexity of content (Eells 2011). Individuals in training may feel these conflicts most acutely. Regardless of style, a comprehensive formulation must include the following critical elements:

1. A diagnostic hypothesis and supporting evidence for that diagnosis
2. Discussion of the contributing biological, psychological, and social factors that predispose, precipitate, perpetuate, and protect against the illness
3. An appreciation of the cultural influences and structural factors at play
4. A comprehensive treatment plan, including a risk assessment, and the reasons for those choices

Although simple in its aim, in practice a formulation can be quite challenging and requires several prerequisite skills. Obviously, mastery of patient interviewing is essential; without it, a sophisticated formulation of the patient is just not possible. It will also require that you have a nuanced understanding of categorical diagnostics in psychiatry; are able to identify and comment on the psychological vulnerabilities, defenses, and personality traits at play; have a working knowledge of psychodynamic, cognitive-behavioral, and other psychological theories; and are able to appreciate the role of the patient within their social and cultural context.

Although usually a focus of training from early in postgraduate year 1 (PGY-1), formulation can take substantial time and effort to master and can feel intimidating at first. Learning the art of formulation is challenging, and you should seek guidance from faculty and prioritize self-reflection and patience as this task is mastered. That said, formulation may be made easier by regularly returning to a trusted framework.

TYPES OF FORMULATION

As described in the previous section, there are many different styles and approaches to the task of formulation. Table 7–1 summarizes some of these options and the pros and cons of each. You may draw from any of these styles or combine them to create the formulation. Keep in mind that formulation is a hypothetical understanding of the patient and should be confirmed or revised over time as more information about the patient becomes available, so some approaches may feel more relevant than others as your formulation evolves.

BIOPSYCHOSOCIAL MODEL INTEGRATED WITH CULTURAL AND STRUCTURAL FORMULATION

This section includes suggestions for designing and organizing each subsection of the biopsychosocial model and integrating the cultural and structural formulations. Not all features discussed will be relevant to every patient's case formulation, and emphasis should be given to the elements that are most salient to the patient's overall psychological functioning. To be sure that your formulation is complete, we suggest outlining the predisposing, precipitating, perpetuating, and protective factors (the four Ps) within each subsection. Table 7–2 provides a visual representation of this task and gives examples.

Biological Section

The biological formulation first determines the active symptoms for which the patient is seeking care and any associated symptoms (or lack thereof) that will inform your differential diagnosis. Following this, your biological formulation should discuss the relevant predisposing,

TABLE 7–1. Types of formulation

	Biopsychosocial formulation	Structural formulation	Cultural formulation	Psychodynamic formulation	Cognitive-behavioral formulation
Goal of formulation	To develop a comprehensive treatment plan	To supplement BPS formulation by enhancing understanding of the social, economic, and political roots of illness	To enhance understanding of the cultural context of illness	To guide the direction of psychodynamic therapy	To guide the direction of CBT
Pros	• Familiar, often taught in medical school • Easily communicated across multidisciplinary teams	• Allows levels of intervention at the patient level, the clinic level, and the community or policy level • Use of Structural Vulnerability Assessment Tool explicitly reduces provider bias with provider self-reflection	• Explicitly collaborative with the patient to reduce provider bias • Supplements the BPS formulation • Easily accessible in DSM-5-TR (American Psychiatric Association 2022) • Can be used in conjunction with structural formulation	• Extends beyond diagnostic categories to understand insight, agency, self-concept, capacity for relationships, and management of emotions	• Collaborative with the patient, so may be less influenced by provider bias • Incorporates understanding about the patient's emotions, thoughts, and behaviors with hypotheses about mechanisms • Facilitates development of a problem list and treatment agenda

TABLE 7–1. Types of formulation *(continued)*

	Biopsychosocial formulation	Structural formulation	Cultural formulation	Psychodynamic formulation	Cognitive-behavioral formulation
Cons	• May be influenced by psychiatrist's implicit bias • Must be considered hypothetical and be revised over time • Likely will not fully capture structural or cultural aspects of patient's experience	• Not as widely used as other formulations, so supervisors may be less familiar with it • Is best used in conjunction with cultural formulation because patients may experience cultural as well as structural issues	• May change over time depending on the patient's identity and experience and must be revised in collaboration with the patient • Is best used in conjunction with structural formulation because it does not explicitly incorporate questions about structural racism	• Subjective, inferential, more of an "art" • May be influenced by implicit bias • Must be considered hypothetical and be revised over time • Often exclusive of biological aspects or pharmacology	• Must be revised over time in collaboration with the patient • Often exclusive of biological aspects of case or pharmacology

Note. BPS=biopsychosocial; CBT=cognitive-behavioral therapy.
Source. Bourgois et al. 2017; Jacqueline and Lisa 2015; McWilliams 1999.

TABLE 7–2. Examples of the four Ps of psychiatric formulation

	Biological formulation	Psychological formulation	Social/cultural formulation	Structural formulation
Predisposing factors (intrinsic to a person)	• In utero exposures • Birth history • Developmental disorders • Family history • Temperament • Brain injury	• Attachment style • Family structure • Affect modulation • Cognitive style • Self-image/self-esteem	• Socioeconomic status • Childhood exposures/ trauma (e.g., maternal depression, domestic violence, late adoption) • Prior similar experience (e.g., loss, separation) • Social support network	• Exposure to discrimination • Racism • Access to care • Education • Literacy, language fluency • Food/housing insecurity • Insurance status • Immigration status • Being a member of an historically oppressed population
Precipitating factors (acute events that bring on or worsen symptoms)	• Medical illness • Physical injury • Substance abuse • Medication nonadherence	Stressors that trigger the following: • cognitive distortions • emotion dysregulation • grief • unconscious conflicts	• Loss of or separation from loved ones • Role transitions • Job loss or unemployment • Interpersonal trauma • Work, school, or financial stress • Loss of usual supports	• Loss of insurance or access • Loss of support services • Recent immigration • Homelessness

TABLE 7–2. Examples of the four Ps of psychiatric formulation *(continued)*

	Biological formulation	Psychological formulation	Social/cultural formulation	Structural formulation
Perpetuating factors (chronic issues that prevent recovery or make symptoms worse)	• Chronic illness • Chronic pain • Functional impairment • Learning disorders • Lack of appropriate treatment for medical comorbidity	• Internalized negative beliefs about self or the world and environments that reinforce them • Chronic maladaptive coping or defense mechanisms • Lack of insight • Personality traits • Traumatic reenactments	• Ongoing trauma or neglect • Poverty • Homelessness • Lack of culturally appropriate care • Chronic marital or other interpersonal discord • Isolation • Intergenerational trauma	• Systemic racism • Health care inequities or inaccessibility • Exposure to violence
Protective factors (intrinsic or external factors that may mitigate symptoms)	• Absence of comorbid medical or psychiatric illness • Absence of family history or in utero exposures • Adherence to medication	• Healthy emotional regulation • Impulse control • Coping skills • Self-image • Attachment style • Insight into illness	• Strong support system • Community connection • Religion • Financial security • Access to insurance, housing, and health care	• Policies to ensure health equity • Policies and legislation against discrimination

Source. Adapted from Barker 1995.; Selzer and Ellen 2914; Weerasekera 1993.

precipitating, perpetuating, or protective factors that may have a clear physiological basis or are attributable in part or in whole to concurrent medical illness.

The most basic biological factors that you should consider include the patient's age, in utero exposures, birth and developmental history, family history, and any potential genetic predispositions. Most important, the biological section considers the relationship between psychiatric and physical health. For example, you should be sure to comment on any concurrent medical illnesses that may

- Mimic psychiatric symptoms (e.g., hypothyroidism, anemia, arrhythmias)
- Have a bidirectional relationship with psychiatric symptoms (e.g., depression in dementia, multiple sclerosis, chronic pain, behavioral or cognitive symptoms in traumatic brain injury)
- Exacerbate or be exacerbated by psychiatric illness (e.g., depression after myocardial infarction, anxiety in chronic obstructive pulmonary disease)
- Be relevant to decision-making regarding somatic treatments (e.g., pregnancy, kidney or liver disease, diabetes, hyperlipidemia)

Consider potential medication side effects, many of which can contribute to symptoms otherwise easily attributed to psychiatric illness, such as fatigue, insomnia, cognitive symptoms, and restlessness. It also would be appropriate to comment on past drug trials for the current psychiatric illness, the effectiveness of these medications, and any side effects experienced. And, finally, think about the possible medical sequelae of psychiatric prescribing, such as the need for metabolic monitoring with antipsychotics or the risk of hyponatremia with some antidepressants.

Psychological Section

The psychological formulation should highlight the inherent, internal psychological contributors to the patient's presentation. You should gather data to inform the psychological formulation from your thorough psychiatric and social history but also from the experience of the interview itself and your own interactions with the patient. You should then consider how these data reflect some or all of the following:

- *Predisposing psychological vulnerabilities:* These vulnerabilities are usually the sequelae of disruptions in normal psychological development secondary to trauma, abuse, neglect, or significant loss (e.g., the impact of trauma on internal processing). Some examples might include difficulty trusting others, sensitivity toward rejection, low self-esteem, or difficulty tolerating the loss of control. These vulnerabilities may also be evident within the patient's history via recurrent difficulties in relationships with others or through the patient's own statements or reactions (or lack thereof) within the therapeutic relationship (Campbell and Rohrbaugh 2013).

- *Precipitating psychosocial stressors:* Events in the patient's life may lead to the activation or reactivation of maladaptive psychological functions that cause suffering and contribute to the patient's desire to seek care at the current time. For instance, stress or conflict at work or school can reactivate thoughts or feelings informed by experiences from childhood.

- *Perpetuating and/or protective psychological traits:* When a stressor hits on your patient's predisposing psychological vulnerabilities, extreme or uncomfortable emotional states may result, and these should clue you in to look more deeply for important themes within the psychological formulation. Often, patients in these states will display changes in their thinking or cognitive distortions that elucidate core beliefs about the self and others. In addition, patients will deploy defense mechanisms and coping strategies to keep these overwhelming emotional experiences at bay and their self-esteem intact. Defense mechanisms can vary widely in terms of their relative helpfulness, maturity, or adaptiveness and are usually employed persistently and in multiple contexts in the patient's life (McWilliams 2011). Patients also may employ helpful or harmful coping strategies that range from engaging in exercise or mindfulness to substance abuse or even self-harm. The patient's personal strengths, such as their resilience, insight, flexibility of thought, affect regulation, or positive sense of self, are all important protective factors, whereas absence of these strengths may perpetuate illness instead.

Social and Cultural Sections

Social factors might be most easily conceptualized as the external influences—those within the patient's social networks, communities, and relationships—that predispose, precipitate, perpetuate, or protect against mental illness. For instance, these factors might include your patient's family supports, friendships, religious communities, occupational or educational structures and supports, and legal involvement. Indeed, psychiatric illness is in many ways inextricable from the social context in which your patient lives.

A social formulation alone, however, is insufficient without consideration of the patient's culture. In this context, culture includes all the various communities or groups with which a patient identifies, such as gender, age, race/ethnicity, language, national origin, religion, sexual orientation, socioeconomic status, occupation, social and familial roles, disability, education, leisure activities, political involvements, and geographical region (Lewis-Fernandez et al. 2015). Your clinical interview should be designed to help you understand how various parts of your patient's identity impact their thoughts, behaviors, values, and experience. The Cultural Formulation Interview described in DSM-5-TR can help guide you in this regard and provide appropriate language for asking about these topics in a nuanced and culturally sensitive way (American Psychiatric Association 2022, pp. 862–871). In your cultural formulation, you should never make generalizations or assumptions about a patient based on their identification with any group; rather, you should seek greater understanding of the individual and the ways in which their group affiliations shape their experience (Lewis-Fernandez et al. 2015). For instance, your patient's culture may affect how they and their social support network talk about mental illness, how they explain its cause, how they perceive the nature and severity of symptoms within their own cultural norms, and what treatment they seek or will accept. In addition, a wealth of data shows the dangers of misinterpreting cultural phenomenon as other, often psychotic, disorders, and only a thorough cultural formulation will capture the complexity of some culture-bound syndromes (e.g., *ataque de nervios*, *taijin kyofusho*, ghost sickness).

In addition to understanding the patient within their own culture, you should also be cognizant of the ways in which your culture and the power dynamics inherent in the doctor-patient relationship may be influencing the therapeutic alliance and your formulation (Campbell and Rohrbaugh 2013; Lewis-Fernandez et al. 2015). Differences in race, ethnicity, gender, or religion may increase the chances of miscommunication or misinterpretation and should be considered carefully (Qureshi and Collazos 2011). Indeed, implicit bias within the therapeutic relationship is pervasive and well documented (Chapman et al. 2013). You should always strive to be aware of and combat your own biases, assume these biases to be present and affecting your perception of your patient, and approach your formulation from a race-conscious and antiracist perspective (see Chapter 8, "Working With Historically Oppressed Patient Populations").

Structural Section

The cultural formulation highlights the patient's own beliefs, behaviors, and community, and the structural formulation takes an even larger perspective and demands that you consider the social conditions, forces, policies, and institutions contributing to their presentation. Structural factors may be most easily understood as the forces within our communities that form barriers to care and often have impacts on certain groups over others. Examples include racism, sexism, income inequality, lack of opportunity, geographical inequities, and disparities within the health care system. These are critical predisposing, precipitating, perpetuating, and protective factors within your formulation and must be considered alongside the biopsychosocial model and the cultural formulation.

Structural barriers to care are often multiple and have a disproportionate impact on communities and patients of color. As displayed in Table 7–2, predisposing structural factors might include being a member of an historically oppressed group, exposure to discrimination, racism, and immigration policies. The loss of support services, insurance, or housing might all serve as precipitating structural factors. And perhaps most significantly, social factors such as systemic racism, sexism, systematized health care disparities, public policy, and intergenerational trauma (made more likely by these same structural forces) are frequent perpetuating factors in mental illness and should be recognized as such in your formulation. A good structural formulation takes into account the social, economic, and political underpinnings of illness in our society and encourages you to take both a patient-level and systems-level approach to treating mental illness (Metzl and Hansen 2018).

IMPACT OF THE FORMULATION

A comprehensive formulation affords several benefits for you and your patient. When appropriate, sharing aspects of your formulation with your patient and inviting their participation can foster patient engagement in care, decrease the impact of provider bias, and support the development of a comprehensive treatment plan. For example, sharing the diagnosis and formulation with a patient who has borderline personality disorder can be healing and destigmatizing when done with sensitivity and compassion. On the other hand, some patients may not be ready to hear or incorporate the full formulation because of the severity of their symptoms.

Importantly, a comprehensive formulation informs an assessment of risk and recommendations for an appropriate level of care. This step is vitally important given the responsibility you shoulder with respect to patient and community safety. The formulation should culminate in a synopsis of the recommended interventions, usually also organized by biological, psychological, social, cultural, and structural headings.

Biological interventions include any necessary workup for concurrent or contributing medical comorbidities, relevant studies required to assess the safety of psychiatric medications, and referrals to appropriate nonpsychiatric services. You should include all somatic treatment recommendations, including any pharmacotherapy recommendations, both stopping potentially offending medications and adding others. You also might make recommendations for changes in diet or other habits that lessen risk or improve overall well-being (e.g., modifications to lower risk of diabetes or hyperlipidemia, smoking or alcohol cessation, regular exercise). Recommendations in the biological treatment plan should include review of potential drug interactions and needed monitoring for the treatment proposed. It is also appropriate to include nonpharmacological somatic treatments such as electroconvulsive therapy, repetitive transcranial magnetic stimulation, and bright light therapy as well as psychological interventions for biological issues such as cognitive-behavioral therapy for insomnia or chronic pain.

Psychological treatment planning should also make specific recommendations with a particular goal in mind based on the hypotheses generated in the case formulation. Choosing from the multiple available psychotherapeutic modalities can be a challenge, but it is important to keep in mind that the overall goal usually remains the same: to assist the patient in gaining better understanding and acceptance of their vulnerabilities, the stressors that exacerbate these vulnerabilities, the resulting emotional states or cognitions, and the adaptive and maladaptive reactions the patient commonly employs in response and to improve the patient's overall resiliency, agency, self-esteem, and capacity for healthy relationships with others (Campbell and Rohrbaugh 2013; McWilliams 2011). This can be achieved through a variety of means, and many therapists use an eclectic approach to meet their patients' needs. To start, however, you should try to recommend a particular intervention (cognitive-behavioral therapy vs. psychodynamic therapy vs. dialectical behavior therapy), time frame (open-ended vs. time-limited), and format (individual vs. group) and to have a clear hypothesis about the achievable goals. Your patient's own therapeutic goals and preferences will further guide your recommendation.

A comprehensive social and cultural treatment plan often spans a wide range of potential interventions. These might include family meetings, social skills training, various types of group therapy (perhaps through the National Alliance on Mental Illness) or 12-step programs, referrals to social services agencies, educational or vocational counseling and advocacy, assistance with housing resources, assignment of fiduciary services or applications for financial assistance, evaluation and petitioning for conservatorship, liaising with other health care services to ensure adequate and meaningful access to care, child or adult protective services referrals if there are concerns of abuse or neglect, and referral for assistance with legal services. To be effective, the treatment plan must be developed within and be fully appreciative of the patient's culture and spiritual beliefs. The structural formulation provides an opportunity for you to consider issues of health equity and to contemplate opportunities for advocacy on individual, organizational, and community levels (see Chapter 32, "Advocacy").

Beyond treatment planning, completing a comprehensive formulation also has a positive impact on the evolution of your understanding of your patient. It is particularly important that you reconsider and rework the formulation regularly and avoid overconfidence in your formulation, which can prevent the incorporation of new information or information that contradicts the original formulation. In particularly difficult cases, especially for those patients whose presentations are complex or unusual or those whose progress in treatment has plateaued, discussion of the overall formulation with colleagues and/or supervisors may be most helpful.

Furthermore, it is imperative that you approach formulation with humility because it relates to the power differential and any cultural differences within the therapeutic relationship (Tervalon and Murray-García 1998). Failure to monitor and address your own implicit biases can contribute to the perpetuation of disparities in health care; present additional structural barriers for your patient; and prevent an appropriate, culturally sensitive formulation. Some steps you might take in this regard could include taking an implicit association test, consuming media that might help you better understand the perspective of patients who do not share your background, educating yourself about evidence-based strategies for embracing multiculturalism, and engaging in self-reflection and self-evaluation to promote cultural humility (Tervalon and Murray-García 1998; see also Chapter 8, "Working With Historically Oppressed Patient Populations").

DOCUMENTING THE FORMULATION

With the recent implementation of the Cures Act Final Rule from the Office of the National Coordinator for Health Information Technology, patients can now freely access all their electronic health information at any time (Office of the National Coordinator for Health Information Technology 2021). When considering documentation of a formulation in the patient's record, a general rule of thumb is to document concisely and include only the aspects that are confirmed or supported clearly by clinical data. However, as a resident, you might still find it useful to write down a full formulation outside the medical record for review with your supervisor. Keeping in mind that the formulation is always a work in progress, the practice of writing down your hypotheses allows you to think through your case more deeply and allows your supervisor to review and give feedback.

SPECIFIC CHALLENGES AND STRATEGIES

⌘ **It takes too much time to develop a formulation for my patient.** Expediency often comes only with experience, and you have several demands on your time that can make the type of comprehensive formulation described in this chapter feel burdensome. You may knowingly or unknowingly abbreviate a formulation—perhaps because of time constraints or lack of confidence or knowledge—or you might include too much unnecessary detail. Most residents would do well to formulate comprehensively and to discuss their formulation with supervisors. Practice leads to more efficiency over time.

⌘ **I'm not sure if this formulation is accurate; maybe I'm just making assumptions.** As you start out, formulation may feel as though you are guessing or trying to make the patient's illness fit things you have seen or heard before. You may feel a tension between generalization and individualization as you learn to formulate (Eells 2011). Both generalization and individualization can inadvertently lead you to mischaracterize the patient or mismanage their needs. It may help to remember that the formulation is always being updated. You are looking not for the "right" answer but rather for a working hypothesis that helps you understand your patient better. If that is the goal, then it is always acceptable to start more simply; write only what you are sure of and expand on it as your understanding of the patient improves over time.

⌘ **The psychological section is too difficult.** The psychological section can certainly feel intimidating and is often the most difficult part. However, it is a misconception to think that you must know multiple psychological theories in great detail or that the psychological section needs to be lengthy and complicated. The purpose of the formulation is to help you make sense of your patient, and starting with the basics of these theories and a few accessible texts on psychodynamics may be all you need.

SELF-REFLECTIVE QUESTIONS

1. Have I thoroughly considered the many biological, psychological, social, cultural, and structural factors that are contributing to my patient's presentation today?
2. Have I incorporated my patient's own perspective and experience into my formulation and sought my supervisor's feedback?
3. When considering my formulation, have I taken the time to reflect on my own biases?

RESOURCES

American Psychiatric Association: Cultural formulation, in Diagnostic and Statistical Manual of Mental Disorders, 5th Edition, Text Revision. Washington, DC, American Psychiatric Association, 2022, pp 860–871

Bourgois P, Holmes SM, Sue K, et al: Structural vulnerability: operationalizing the concept to address health disparities in clinical care. Acad Med 92(3):299–307, 2017 27415443

Campbell WH, Rohrbaugh RM: Outlined overview of the biopsychosocial formulation model (Figure 1.1), in The Biopsychosocial Formulation Manual: A Guide for Mental Health Professionals. New York, Routledge, 2013, pp 4–8

Gabbard GO: Long-Term Psychodynamic Psychotherapy: A Basic Text. Arlington, VA, American Psychiatric Association Publishing, 2017

Koffmann A, Walters MG: Introduction to Psychological Theories and Psychotherapy. New York, Oxford University Press, 2014

McWilliams N: Psychoanalytic Case Formulation. New York, Guilford, 1999

Selzer R, Ellen S: Formulation for beginners. Australas Psychiatry 22(4):397–401, 2014 24875370

REFERENCES

American Psychiatric Association: Diagnostic and Statistical Manual of Mental Disorders, 5th Edition, Text Revision. Washington, DC, American Psychiatric Association, 2022

Barker P: The Child and Adolescent Psychiatry Evaluation: Basic Child Psychiatry. Oxford, UK, Blackwell Scientific, 1995

Bourgois P, Holmes SM, Sue K, et al: Structural vulnerability: operationalizing the concept to address health disparities in clinical care. Acad Med 92(3):299–307, 2017 27415443

Campbell WH, Rohrbaugh RM: The Biopsychosocial Formulation Manual: A Guide for Mental Health Professionals. New York, Routledge, 2013

Chapman EN, Kaatz A, Carnes M: Physicians and implicit bias: how doctors may unwittingly perpetuate health care disparities. J Gen Intern Med 28(11):1504–1510, 2013 23576243

Eells TD (ed): Handbook of Psychotherapy Case Formulation. New York, Guilford, 2011

Jacqueline BP, Lisa ST: Developing and using a case formulation to guide cognitive-behavior therapy. J Psychol Psychother 5(3):179, 2015

Lewis-Fernandez R, Aggarwal NK, Hinton L, et al (eds): DSM-5 Handbook on the Cultural Formulation Interview. Arlington, VA, American Psychiatric Association Publishing, 2015

McWilliams N: Psychoanalytic Case Formulation. New York, Guilford, 1999

McWilliams N: Psychoanalytic Diagnosis: Understanding Personality Structure in the Clinical Process. New York, Guilford, 2011

Metzl JM, Hansen H: Structural competency and psychiatry. JAMA Psychiatry 75(2):115–116, 2018 29261822

Office of the National Coordinator for Health Information Technology: ONC's Cures Act final rule: 2021. Available at: www.healthit.gov/curesrule. Accessed August 18, 2021.

Qureshi A, Collazos F: The intercultural and interracial therapeutic relationship: challenges and recommendations. Int Rev Psychiatry 23(1):10–19, 2011 21338293

Selzer R, Ellen S: Formulation for beginners. Australas Psychiatry 22(4):397–401, 2014 24875370

Tervalon M, Murray-García J: Cultural humility versus cultural competence: a critical distinction in defining physician training outcomes in multicultural education. J Health Care Poor Underserved 9(2):117–125, 1998 10073197

Weerasekera P: Formulation: a multiperspective model. Can J Psychiatry 38(5):351–358, 1993 8348476

Working With Historically Oppressed Patient Populations

Nientara Anderson, M.D., M.H.S.

Michael O. Mensah, M.D., M.P.H.

J. Corey Williams, M.D., M.A.

Historical scholarship and contemporary research have shown that individuals from historically oppressed groups receive substandard care across the U.S. health care system, which is not designed to recognize or redress these disparities (Agency for Healthcare Research and Quality 2020). Consequently, it often falls on residents and fellows to advocate for equitable care for minoritized patients. In the United States, historically oppressed groups hold identities that are marginalized in a white supremacist, capitalist, heteronormative, and patriarchal society. These include people who are Black, Indigenous, or people of color (BIPOC); non-English speaking; undocumented; immigrants; women; or LGBTQ+ and those who have disabilities.

Crucially for psychiatry residents, people with mental illness or neurodivergence are also considered a historically oppressed group in the United States and are therefore marginalized within the health care system: Their complaints are often dismissed, and they have less access to care. They are also more likely to be misdiagnosed, to receive inferior care, and to be mistreated in the hospital (Nelson 2002).

KEY POINTS

- Structural vulnerability, historic oppression, and cultural context should always be considered part of patient care.

- Counteracting bias requires proactive, continual cultivation of individual introspection and systemic accountability.

- Historically oppressed patients may require extra advocacy, and as a resident, you must actively develop your skills in advocacy and activism.

CULTURAL HUMILITY AND STRUCTURAL COMPETENCY IN CLINICAL CARE

Working with diverse patients broadens and enriches your training, but traditional medical training often does not include the knowledge necessary to serve marginalized patients. Such understanding requires a lifelong commitment to learning and the active practice of cultural humility. Never assume that you are finished learning about the cultural and structural needs of marginalized groups. Do not be afraid to respectfully ask patients about their language and culture—not out of voyeurism but in order to understand their unique perspectives and needs. Cultural humility begins with recognition of the complexities of patients' multiple intersecting identities, including gender, sexual orientation, race and ethnicity, socioeconomic factors, immigration status, religious affiliation, geography, and politics.

Cultural context impacts every patient interaction. Roughly defined, culture comprises the history, beliefs, values, and customs of a particular social or ethnic group. For example, DSM-5-TR (American Psychiatric Association 2022) itself is a cultural construct. By recognizing that DSM-5-TR represents a Eurocentric worldview of human development and mental life that cannot be uncritically applied across global cultures, you will be able to leave space to validate and legitimize other forms of healing that patients may practice.

Cultural Formulation Interview

Interview techniques that elicit cultural valences foster more nuanced understanding of clinical presentations and more culturally responsive treatment. Recent changes to DSM-5-TR, especially the Cultural Formulation Interview (CFI), reflect a growing appreciation of cultural influence in psychiatry (American Psychiatric Association 2022). The CFI provides a process for eliciting pertinent cultural information by operationalizing Arthur Kleinman's (1980) explanatory model of illness to incorporate such domains as 1) cultural definition of the problem; 2) cultural perceptions of cause, context, and support; 3) cultural factors affecting self-coping and past help seeking; and 4) cultural factors affecting current help seeking. These domains evoke the patient's understanding of their condition and help you avoid making harmful assumptions. Below are examples of questions from each domain adapted from DSM-5 for a patient who presents with feeling "sadness":

1. *Cultural definition of the problem:* People often understand their problems in their own way, which may be similar to or different from how doctors describe a problem. How would you describe your sadness?
2. *Cultural perceptions of cause, context, and support:* What do others in your family, your friends, or others in your community think is causing your sadness?
3. *Cultural factors affecting self-coping and past help seeking:* Sometimes people have various ways of dealing with problems like sadness. What have you done on your own to cope with the sadness?
4. *Cultural factors affecting current help seeking:* What kinds of help do you think would be most useful to you at this time for your sadness?

Structural Vulnerability Assessment

Structural competency is another critical aspect of working with historically oppressed patients. Every patient represents a complex tapestry of structural vulnerabilities and protections. For example, consider a 27-year-old college-educated, cisgender, Black male patient who works as an engineer. His identity as a Black man in the United States makes him vulnerable to racial discrimination. However, being highly educated and having a high income is structurally protective because it increases his likelihood of having stable housing and health care. All these factors operate to influence his experience of the world, his risk of various health conditions, and the presentation of his illness.

Just as the CFI draws out cultural information, other tools provide questions to evaluate structural vulnerability. One popular tool is the Structural Vulnerability Assessment (SVA; Bourgois et al. 2017), which provides sample questions across eight domains of structural vulnerability: 1) financial insecurity, 2) residence, 3) risk environments, 4) food access, 5) social network, 6) legal status, 7) education, and 8) discrimination. In daily clinical practice, you would not be expected to complete fully structured interviews using the CFI or SVA. Rather, you should be familiar with these tools and incorporate them into your routine assessments as appropriate. For example, questions such as "Do you have a safe place to live?" or "Have you experienced discrimination based on your skin color?" can be included in a routine social history.

STRATEGIES FOR COUNTERACTING BIAS

Studies show that health care professionals have the same level of implicit bias as the general population (Hall et al. 2015). The culture of white supremacy in the United States has taught us to associate historically oppressed groups with negative stereotypes and to prefer whites over minority groups (Halberstadt et al. 2020). As a result, health care professionals may provide inequitable health care to marginalized groups. For example, in psychiatry, Black patients are diagnosed with schizophrenia more often than white patients are (Gara et al. 2012) and are more likely to be prescribed long-acting antipsychotics than white patients are (Aggarwal et al. 2012). A race conscious or antiracist approach can mitigate the influence of bias in your clinical practice. This approach rejects the notion of "colorblindness" (DiAngelo 2018). Instead, it acknowledges patients' oppressed identities, recognizes that bias is present in both the system and the provider, and helps you take proactive steps to address this bias.

Strategies to combat bias fall into two broad categories: cognitive strategies (changing thought patterns to influence behavior) and system-based strategies (changing institutional policies, practices, and norms). Neither strategy should be privileged above the other. Both cognitive and systems-based strategies are critical to fostering equity and justice in medicine.

Cognitive Strategies

Cognitive strategies to combat bias start with assuming that you have biases against historically oppressed groups. Volunteer experiences and diversity training do not shield anyone from the constant social conditioning that instills bias against marginalized groups. Cognitive strategies to counter bias could include attending workshops or diversity trainings, although these trainings have proven inadequate at producing systematic change (Noon 2018). More importantly, educate yourself about health disparities, then cultivate a routine practice of introspection at each phase of clinical care: rapport building, diagnosis, formulation, treatment, follow-up planning, and reflection. When diagnosing and designing treatment plans for historically oppressed groups, ask yourself: Am I being biased? What biases might I have against this patient?

Systems-Based Strategies

Resist the temptation to focus only on cognitive strategies against bias because systems-based strategies can be extremely impactful. Examples include reforming hiring and admissions practices or system-wide audits to assess disparities in care. For example, many electronic health record systems allow you to extract reports on disparities in diagnostic or prescribing patterns in marginalized groups. You could advocate for your medical institution to provide these types of audits (e.g., rates of restraints in patients from different racial or ethnic groups).

Edgoose and colleagues (2019) summarized cognitive-related and systems-based strategies for combating bias with the acronym IMPLICIT. In this approach, IMPLICIT stands for **i**ntrospection, **m**indfulness, **pe**rspective taking (considering the experience of the individual being stereotyped), **l**earning to slow down (pausing to reflect on your potential biases), **i**ndividuation (evaluating individuals on the basis of their individual characteristics rather than generalizations), **c**hecking your messaging (embracing evidence-based statements that reduce bias), **i**nstitutionalizing fairness (promoting change at the organizational level), and **t**ake two (practicing cultural humility and critical self-reflection).

ADVOCACY FOR HISTORICALLY OPPRESSED PATIENTS IN CLINICAL PRACTICE

Advocacy for patients from historically oppressed groups is a core professional responsibility (American Medical Association 2001; Vance et al. 2020). It is incumbent on the physician to advocate for patients as part of providing evidence-based, patient-centered care. You can advocate for patients on a variety of levels, including individual, clinical, organizational, community, and governmental/legislative (see Chapter 32, "Advocacy"). On an *individual level*, you might engage in cultural humility and examine your own biases. On a *clinical level*, you might engage in several actions as follows:

Draw attention to disparities in how patients are treated. Speak up about how supervisors, colleagues, and medical students discuss and treat minoritized patients. You might use concrete examples, such as "I noticed we did not call security when a white female patient hit a staff member, but we called security immediately when a Black patient verbally threatened a staff member." Raising such concerns during rounds and group settings rather than in one-on-one conversations minimizes the chances that the topic will be dismissed. However, you have to use your judgment about when to raise these issues. It can help to stay informed and come armed with citations. Read about historically marginalized groups and health care inequities and know which identities increase risk for discrimination in health care, such as race, gender, or socioeconomic status. If you are short on time (as many of us are), try podcasts, audiobooks, webinars, and other resources (see https://hslguides.med.nyu.edu/raceandracism). If a medical student has a presentation coming up, suggest the topic of health disparities or racism in medicine.

Promptly but courteously correct language that is discriminatory or stigmatizing. For example, if someone misgenders a patient, correct them in real time. Rectifying something immediately is more effective than trying to bring it up later. Trying to address racist or stigmatizing behavior after the fact leaves more room for misinterpretation and misunderstanding. Accordingly, if someone corrects your language, resist the impulse to defend yourself or rationalize your words. Do not excessively self-denigrate or overexpress remorse in a way that centers your guilt (DiAngelo 2018). Thank the person who corrected you and state that you will be more mindful in the future. Consider such corrections as gifts that help you provide more equitable care for your patients.

Support others when they are advocating for patients. Be a vocal ally to others when they advocate on behalf of patients from historically oppressed populations. Advocating for patients is often a lonely and intimidating task, so support from colleagues can be invaluable. Ask permission to join a conversation before offering your support.

Figure out reporting mechanisms for discriminatory incidents. Store this information on your phone or somewhere convenient so that it is easy to report incidents when they happen. During a busy day in the hospital, looking up reporting procedures can feel too burdensome, so it is best to have them on hand before you need them. Share this information with fellow residents and, if possible, post it where others can see it (see Chapter 39, "Handling Mistreatment and Discrimination").

Think about patients structurally as well as medically. Nonmedical structural interventions are an important form of patient advocacy (Kirmayer et al. 2018; Vance et al. 2020). This includes arranging transportation or connecting patients to legal advocacy.

You can also engage in *organizational and community levels* of advocacy. Advocacy for patients goes beyond the clinical encounter. Whenever possible, participate in hospital-wide, city, state, or national efforts to achieve equitable health care. You could organize grand rounds speakers, join diversity and equity committees, testify at community activist events, or attend racial justice protests. Consider subscribing to newsletters from local activist groups to find such opportunities (see Chapter 32).

SPECIFIC CHALLENGES AND STRATEGIES

The following vignette about Mr. X illustrates the application of cultural humility, counteracting internal bias, and practical advocacy strategies you can use as a resident.

Case Vignette

While in the psychiatric emergency room, you are assigned a patient named Mr. X who has been medically cleared by the emergency department (ED) and is being transferred to you for evaluation of "hallucinations." Mr. X's ED note describes him as "a 45-year-old Black male" who "only speaks Brazilian Portuguese." The note states that Mr. X "has a well-known history of schizophrenia and is having hallucinations for which he was sent to the ED on an involuntary hold by his primary care doctor."

⌘ **Strategy: Reject colorblindness.** Recognize Mr. X's historically oppressed identities (identifying or presenting as a Black person, being a non-English speaker, and having a psychiatric diagnosis) and how these identities increase his risk of receiving disparate care. Be mindful and counteract your own biases in your care for Mr. X.

⌘ **Strategy: Use a language interpreter and insist others do as well.** Always ask patients their preferred spoken or sign language. When using language interpreters, employ teach-back strategies to ensure patient understanding. If your institution's interpretation services are insufficient, advocate for better translation services. Even if you or another clinician feel competent to translate for a patient, do not do so unless you are a certified medical interpreter (Ramirez et al. 2008). If you observe others interacting with non-English-speaking patients without an interpreter, talk to them about it directly. Always indicate if your patient needs an interpreter in your notes or sign-out. Some electronic medical records (EMRs) include orders such as "nursing communication" where you can note that a patient needs translation services. Empower your patients by reiterating their right to a language interpreter or give them a written note that says, "I would like an interpreter."

Case Vignette *(continued)*

The ED note records Mr. X's systolic blood pressure at 200 and his blood glucose at 329 and describes him as "clearly medication noncompliant and a poor historian."

⌘ **Strategy: Draw attention to disparities in how patients are treated.** Mr. X's ED note contains disparaging phrases such as "poor historian" and "noncompliant" that are more often deployed toward minoritized patients (Park et al. 2021). These phrases may indicate physician biases against marginalized patients that can cloud clinical judgment and negatively impact patient care. It is important to discuss concerns about compliance directly with the patient instead of making assumptions. Look out for other red flag phrases such as "aggressive," "malingering," or "drug seeking" (Goddu et al. 2019; Park et al. 2021) in other providers' notes as well as your own; these may proliferate in the EMR and transmit negative bias against a patient to other providers.

Case Vignette *(continued)*

Speaking via the language interpreter, Mr. X reports that he lives alone and is functionally independent. He says, "I feel bad in my body; I am not normally like this." When asked about medication, Mr. X says his visiting nurse comes twice daily and he takes all the medications she gives him. Regarding his hallucinations, Mr. X says demons are present, but they are not bothersome and have not changed recently. He has no suicidal or homicidal ideation. Because Mr. X's psychiatric symptoms are not acutely exacerbated, you question whether he was only sent to the ED for hallucinations and wonder whether Mr. X needs additional medical workup.

⌘ **Strategy: If you do not agree with the way a patient is being managed, ask questions.** Perhaps there is sound reasoning behind a treatment decision, but if you have doubts, just ask. For example, "This patient seems to be at his psychiatric baseline. Is there another psychiatric question we can help with?"

Case Vignette *(continued)*

You approach the emergency medicine resident with your concerns, but he replies that no additional testing is warranted for a patient who is "poorly managed and definitely noncompliant with his meds." He adds, "We see this all the time; he's cleared for psychiatry," before walking away to see his next patient in the busy ED.

⌘ **Strategy: Get other team members involved.** Attending physicians can be allies. If your advocacy efforts for a patient are stymied, attendings can use their seniority to get things done. Especially when delayed care or unaddressed issues could seriously harm a patient, it is often more efficient to get a receptive attending involved than to struggle on your own. Medical students can also help with advocating for minoritized patients by speaking with family members to obtain past history or reviewing the medical chart for additional details. Collaborating with medical students on patient advocacy is also a valuable opportunity for teaching and learning in clinical practice.

⌘ **Strategy: Speak politely but directly when you think bias is affecting patient care.** Some bystander intervention and advocacy guides suggest challenging bias by asking questions as though you do not know that bias or prejudice is at play. However, trying to address biases by alluding to them indirectly or asking falsely naive questions can lead you in circles. It is better to address the topic head-on with tact and professionalism. By doing this, you will help normalize the examination and self-correction of discrimination in medicine.

Case Vignette *(continued)*

You tell your attending that you believe Mr. X needs additional medical workup. In clear, measured language, you say that you are worried he is not receiving adequate treatment because of bias against him as a non-English-speaking Black man with chronic psychiatric illness. You reference the stigmatizing language and false assumptions in his ED note to support your concern. Your attending then sees the patient herself, validates your concerns, and arranges for Mr. X to stay in the medical ED for further workup. He is later admitted to the neurology stroke service.

SELF-REFLECTIVE QUESTIONS

1. Do I engage in lifelong self-reflection and learning about my own biases?
2. Have I educated myself about systemic historical oppression in the United States of certain groups, including BIPOC, non-English speaking, undocumented, immigrants, women, LGBTQ+, and people with disabilities?
3. Have I educated myself about inequities in health care that are experienced by historically oppressed populations?
4. Do I practice individual and systems-level advocacy for equitable patient care?

RESOURCES

Bourgois P, Holmes SM, Sue K, et al: Structural vulnerability: operationalizing the concept to address health disparities in clinical care. Acad Med 92(3):299–308, 2017 27415443

Edgoose JYC, Quiogue M, Sidhar K: How to identify, understand, and unlearn implicit bias in patient care. Fam Pract Manag 26(4):29–33, 2019 31287266

Kennedy KG, Vance MC: Advocacy Teaching in Psychiatry Residency Training Programs. Washington, DC, American Psychiatric Association Publishing, 2018

Lewis-Fernández RE, Aggarwal NK, Hinton LE, et al: DSM-5 Handbook on the Cultural Formulation Interview. Washington, DC, American Psychiatric Publishing, 2016

New York University Health Sciences Library Subject Guides. Race and racism in medicine: books, videos, podcasts and websites. Available at: https://hslguides.med.nyu.edu/raceandracism. Accessed August 1, 2021.

Roberts DE: Fatal Invention: How Science, Politics, and Big Business Recreate Race in the Twenty-First Century. New York, New Press, 2011

Washington HA: Medical Apartheid: The Dark History of experimentation on Black Americans From Colonial Times to the Present. New York, Anchor, 2008

REFERENCES

Agency for Healthcare Research and Quality: 2019 national healthcare quality and disparities report. Rockville, MD, Agency for Healthcare Research and Quality, December 2020. Available at: www.ahrq.gov/research/findings/nhqrdr/nhqdr19/index.html. Accessed August 5, 2021.

Aggarwal NK, Rosenheck RA, Woods SW, et al: Race and long-acting antipsychotic prescription at a community mental health center: a retrospective chart review. J Clin Psychiatry 73(4):513–517, 2012 22579151

American Medical Association: AMA declaration of professional responsibility. Chicago, IL, American Medical Association, 2001. Available at: www.ama-assn.org/delivering-care/public-health/ama-declaration-professional-responsibility. Accessed February 17, 2007.

American Psychiatric Association: Diagnostic and Statistical Manual of Mental Disorders, 5th Edition, Text Revision. Washington, DC, American Psychiatric Association, 2022

Bourgois P, Holmes SM, Sue K, et al: Structural vulnerability: operationalizing the concept to address health disparities in clinical care. Acad Med 92(3):299–307, 2017 27415443

DiAngelo R: White Fragility: Why It's So Hard for White People to Talk About Racism. Boston, MA, Beacon Press, 2018

Edgoose JYC, Quiogue M, Sidhar K: How to identify, understand, and unlearn implicit bias in patient care. Fam Pract Manag 26(4):29–33, 2019 31287266

Gara MA, Vega WA, Arndt S, et al: Influence of patient race and ethnicity on clinical assessment in patients with affective disorders. Arch Gen Psychiatry 69(6):593–600, 2012 22309972

Goddu AP, O'Conor KJ, Lanzkron S, et al: Do words matter? Stigmatizing language and the transmission of bias in the medical record. Intern Med 34(1):164, 2019 30338470

Halberstadt AG, Cooke AN, Garner PW, et al: Racialized emotion recognition accuracy and anger bias of children's faces. Emotion 22(3):403–417, 2020 32614194

Hall WJ, Chapman MV, Lee KM, et al: Implicit racial/ethnic bias among health care professionals and its influence on health care outcomes: a systematic review. Am J Public Health 105(12):e60–e76, 2015 26469668

Kirmayer LJ, Kronick R, Rousseau C: Advocacy as key to structural competency in psychiatry. JAMA Psychiatry 75(2):119–120, 2018 29261839

Kleinman A: Patients and Healers in the Context of Culture: An Exploration of the Borderland Between Anthropology, Medicine, and Psychiatry. Berkeley, University of California Press, 1980

Nelson A: Unequal treatment: confronting racial and ethnic disparities in health care. J Natl Med Assoc 94(8):666–668, 2002 12152921

Noon M: Pointless diversity training: unconscious bias, new racism and agency. Work Employ Soc 32(1):198–209, 2018

Park J, Saha S, Chee B, et al: Physician use of stigmatizing language in patient medical records. JAMA Netw Open 4(7):e2117052, 2021 34259849

Ramirez D, Engel KG, Tang TS: Language interpreter utilization in the emergency department setting: a clinical review. J Health Care Poor Underserved 19(2):352–362, 2008 18469408

Vance MC, Kennedy KG, Wiechers IR, et al: A Psychiatrist's Guide to Advocacy. Washington, DC, American Psychiatric Association Publishing, 2020

CHAPTER 9

The Psychiatric Emergency

Clayton A. Barnes, M.D., M.P.H.

Juan David Lopez, M.D.

Case Vignette

As you arrive for your shift in psychiatric emergency services, you notice that the unit is uncharacteristically quiet. Everyone seems to have retreated to their own rooms or workstations, and neither staff nor patients are in sight. You and your attending physician learn during sign-out that just 5 minutes prior to your arrival, a patient assaulted a staff member, who is now receiving treatment in the medical emergency department (ED). Once the immediate needs of patient care have been addressed, you and your attending will facilitate a debrief and inquire as to what support team members need now and how the department could have prevented this assault.

In a psychiatry emergency unit, sometimes called psychiatry emergency service (PES) or comprehensive psychiatric emergency program, you will be working in a fast-paced, collaborative setting, caring for acutely ill patients. First and foremost, maintaining a safe environment for patients and staff will build the foundation for providing effective patient care. You will encounter patients who require management of their agitation and violence, at times necessitating involuntary medications and restraints; doing this in a respectful, compassionate, and trauma-informed way will require mindfulness and objectivity. Understanding what each team member needs will be vital to ensuring an effective and functioning unit during your shift. Finally, as you juggle the above clinical and emotional tasks, you will discover remedies to address your own burnout and compassion fatigue.

In this chapter, we detail the most important aspects for successful navigation of your rotation and how to create a safe and collaborative context in which to provide evidence-based care in a PES.

KEY POINTS

- Maintaining safety starts with an awareness of your behaviors, surroundings, and workflow.

- Care in the PES requires clinical decisions based on limited information while also taking into account the complexity of a patient's unique cultural context and developmental history.

- Clear, empathic, and inclusive communication with colleagues is essential in fostering a successful PES work environment.

- Sustainable, effective work in the PES requires you to learn how to care for yourself.

SAFETY

Forty to fifty percent of psychiatry residents will be assaulted during their residency training (Rueve and Welton 2008). To some extent, this statistic is a reflection of the patients we care for: patients seeking our help experience problems with impulsivity, anger, emotional lability, and paranoia. However, risks can be mitigated by how you approach your clinical duties in the PES. Your role includes not only treating patients but also setting boundaries, assessing risk, delivering difficult news, and initiating involuntary treatments.

In every care setting, it is important to be aware of your surroundings and positioning, but this is crucial in the PES. You will need to know the whereabouts of your colleagues and security staff and have a firm grasp of the layout of the unit (including exits) in order to act quickly in the case of a crisis. When interacting with patients, bear in mind that standing between a patient and a potential exit may make the patient feel trapped. In such cases, the patient may feel the need to regain a sense of control by escaping or fighting. It is important to know your role on the team: If a patient attempts to leave against medical advice from a locked unit, do not attempt to stop them yourself. Instead, use appropriate staff and alert systems.

It is also important to consider other aspects of your body language, such as your posture, facial expressions, and tone of speech. Patients present to the PES for a variety of reasons, and impairments of insight, judgment, and impulse control are common. As a general rule, patients experiencing paranoia are made uncomfortable by continuous and intense eye contact—it would be best to keep eye contact brief and indirect (always keeping the patient in view). Patients may interpret your hands behind your back or in your pockets as an effort to hide something. Instead, keep your hands in front of you in a nonhostile, open position. Speak with normal volume and cadence, or perhaps softer than usual, modeling for the patient a calm demeanor and expectations for an appropriate interpersonal interaction; this is most important for those patients who have lost control of their behaviors. Standing over a patient, whether they are sitting or lying down, may be experienced as dominating or infantilizing. However, if a sitting patient stands and begins to escalate (pacing or yelling), you should consider standing to ensure you can excuse yourself if you feel your safety is threatened.

A final aspect of safety is your workflow. Residents are often academically minded and eager to comb through charts and conduct literature reviews. This is entirely appropriate, although often not possible in the midst of clinical care. Histories, medication lists, and diagnoses may not be available and cannot always be incorporated into your clinical decision-making. The prioritization of your clinical care—evaluating patients, submitting orders, reviewing results—facilitates timely treatment and disposition. When you provide efficient, patient-centered clinical care, patients receive appropriate treatment on a reasonable time scale, thereby limiting the progression of any psychiatric decompensation and reducing the risk of violence.

PATIENTS

In a busy PES, you might be tempted to prioritize evaluation without taking the time to build a therapeutic alliance or consider the impact of bias on care. However, when you take the time to connect with the person in front of you with compassion and respect, you can often restore a patient's sense of humanity and dignity. In addition, building trust and connection will only enhance your capacity to make a therapeutic assessment and treatment plan.

Our patients face a variety of traumas: domestic violence, demeaning hallucinations, sexual assault, fear of deportation, homelessness, structural racism, and unemployment. There are multiple paths to the end points of despondency, paranoia, rage, substance use, and other presenting concerns. As a PES psychiatrist, you can approach patients holistically by simply paying attention to the culture, history, and dilemma of the person presenting to you for care and the impacts you can have on their situation.

We must bear in mind these trajectories and the impact they have on our patients' lives because otherwise, our implicit biases may unknowingly promote discriminatory and suboptimal patient care. For example, patients dysregulated by substance use who have also suffered recent sexual assault are likely to be further traumatized by the use of restraints. Additionally, many studies document the disproportionate psychiatric diagnosis of African Americans and Latinx Americans compared with Euro-Americans (Schwartz and Blankenship 2014).

Differences between the patient and psychiatrist must be acknowledged as well. If left unconsidered, language, race, age, sex, gender identity, culture, and socioeconomic status can all work to divide the patient and provider. An example of this is that physicians often spend less time with patients who speak a different language, presumably resulting in less informed, lower-quality care. There is also an inherent power dynamic between the patient and a psychiatrist who can potentially invoke involuntary hospitalization. Self-reflection on your personal biases as well as careful attention to the structural discrimination in clinical medicine are essential to making sure your treatment decisions are therapeutic, compassionate, and equitable. How we treat patients in these moments has the potential to either confirm their expectations of the world or provide a new, more therapeutic framework from which to grow.

COLLEAGUES

Regardless of whether you work within a dedicated PES or as a consultant to colleagues in the medical ED, caring for patients in psychiatric crises is 100% team based. When dealing with psychiatric emergencies, we rely on the wisdom, skill set, and comradery of our medical, nursing, social work, and security team members. Nurses are de-escalating patients nearly all day, every day. Social workers have extensive understanding of community resources and how to engage with overwhelmed families. Medical assistants anticipate and respond to the physical needs of patients in a timely manner. As a less experienced psychiatry resident, you will find that there is a lot to learn from more experienced team members, especially in violence assessment and de-escalation. As you become more proficient, this setting is a gold mine for your interdisciplinary leadership development.

In general, medicine is hierarchical, but in psychiatric emergencies, the hierarchy can fluctuate depending on the situation. Part of being an excellent leader is knowing when to take a step back. We do not get involved in helping to place restraints or administer intramuscular medications, but our colleagues look to us for guidance about *what to do*, *when to do it*, and *how to do it*. Rest assured, you are not expected to know it all. Even seasoned emergency psychiatrists seek consultation from colleagues. You can, however, always lead by example by demonstrating a calm and collaborative approach to care.

Additionally, an invaluable part of training is in the specialized skills of observation and therapeutic intervention. It is important to recognize that patients may feel more or less comfortable with different providers depending on demographic factors, life experience, or rapport from previous visits. Some team members may be more influential in engaging certain patients than others. Becoming a skilled leader of a multidisciplinary care team requires attention to the knowledge base, skill set, and personality qualities of each team member interacting with patients so that every patient encounter can be maximally therapeutic.

In addition to collaborating to treat patients, you will help multidisciplinary colleagues process difficult situations. With experience, you will get more comfortable tolerating the strong emotional experiences of colleagues as they look to you to help resolve the psychiatric crisis. A huge part of this work entails being able to hold these emotions and make sense of them for others. When you discuss a conceptualization of what has happened and how you can help, you actually help manage *everyone's* anxiety, anger, frustration, and sense of hopelessness by bringing a sense of clarity to the clinical situation and potential next steps in the treatment plan.

SELF

The PES will expose you to the trauma, pain, and injustice faced by humans. Feelings of sadness, rage, apathy, and overwhelm can arise, which are expected responses to these experiences. In one study, 13% of 212 residents met diagnostic criteria for posttraumatic stress disorder (Klamen et al. 1995), likely a byproduct of cumulative traumatic occupational exposures. As a psychiatry resident, you will learn that who you are—your history, preferences, traumas, and biases—can have a profound impact on the treatment of a patient in the form of countertransference.

It is human nature to have an intense countertransference reaction toward an individual who has made a disparaging remark or even threatened your life. Whenever you find yourself overwhelmed or activated emotionally, it is imperative to take a step back to help create some emotional space from what has transpired. That way, your clinical decisions will be based on the needs of the patient and will not be retaliatory in nature. Notably, even in the absence of a provocation from the patient, your personal bias may still have an impact on decision-making. Left unabated, these reactions can manifest as leaving a patient in restraints longer than necessary, providing intramuscular injections when a (previously agitated) patient has calmed and is willing to accept medications orally, or chemically sedating a patient who annoys you or makes you uncomfortable. The effects of acting on your countertransference or your personal biases can be damaging in the outpatient setting, but in the PES, allowing your judgment to be distorted is potentially life-threatening.

Educating yourself about the impact of structural racism and taking the time to consider your own biases are important for work in the PES. In addition, you may find that your strong emotional responses can be managed better if you make it a habit to engage in activities that provoke mindfulness and introspection such as personal psychotherapy, meditation, yoga, and journaling.

Maintaining a sense of groundedness and self care will be vital to your sustainability as a physician and psychiatrist; start these healthy practices now. While you are in the PES, if you need to take a moment to collect your thoughts, take it. Even just 30 seconds of helping to "close" a case before starting a new one can help to relieve the feeling of overwhelm. You also might try a ritual to ground yourself, such as repeating your name a few times after a challenging situation or taking several deep breaths. For additional support, it may be helpful to have a regular, intentional space with colleagues to process bad outcomes, compassion fatigue, and burnout; some programs offer vicarious trauma support groups, but if not, working with a therapist individually is an excellent option as well. Thankfully, psychiatric emergency work is time limited; the shift work nature of it can be liberating, so when you leave for the day you should feel welcome to leave the work behind.

SPECIFIC CHALLENGES AND STRATEGIES

⌘ **I find it hard to learn in a fast-paced environment.** The PES is a rich source of exposure to interesting presentations, psychopharmacology riddles, and psychodynamic conundrums. Unfortunately, the pace of the work is such that you are unlikely to be able to research and review questions not immediately relevant to clinical care during your shift. Identify a strategy for learning during off hours that also respects your time off. One strategy is to carry a note card during each shift, and when a particularly salient question arises, write it down for review later. Limit the number of questions to two or three to ensure adequate time for rest. Alternatively, bring these interesting presentations into didactics to solicit feedback from peers and lecturers.

⌘ **I find it challenging to pay attention to early learners.** As is expected elsewhere in residency, you will need to balance learning, clinical care, and teaching in the PES. This is always a difficult task, but the acuity of this environment makes having a teaching plan imperative. Working with medical students in the PES can be mutually rewarding because there are ample opportunities to see patients together and discuss diagnostic impressions and treatment plans. Allowing medical students and PGY-1 or PGY-2 residents to interview complex patients lets you assess their skills while also generating hypotheses about the patient and a potential course of treatment. More skilled trainees can be tasked with interviewing independently. Additional enrichment for learners could include drafting notes, obtaining collateral information, and presenting case formulations to the interdisciplinary team.

⌘ **The information I have seems too limited to make decisions about my patient's treatment plan.** Occasionally, patients in the PES are not capable of providing or willing to provide history. Collateral information can be vital and should be obtained whenever possible. You must use all of your resources—the electronic medical record, the patient, the patient's belongings, the outpatient team—in order to expand the data included in your formulation. If collateral is unobtainable, supplement your assessments by using epidemiological facts, longitudinal observation, and laboratory data. With limited data, we are more likely to rely on our mental shortcuts to generate hypotheses, referred to as type 1 thinking; availability bias (judging a certain diagnosis as more likely because you have seen it recently) and anchoring (the tendency to use only information obtained earlier in presentation and not incorporate new information) can be more common in emergency settings. In the PES, you must make decisions based on limited information. However, the goal is to ensure that your decision-making is fact based, deliberate, and continuously revised.

⌘ **The ED attending and I disagree on the treatment plan.** You have experience in evaluating psychiatric disorders—trust it. If a disagreement arises, share sound clinical reasoning and specific concerns with both your supervisor and the ED attending. For example:

I've visited the patient three times, and his level of consciousness has differed each time. I spoke with the patient's wife, and his behavior change is acute over the previous day or two. He has no history of psychosis. New-onset psychotic disorder is unlikely given his age, history, and clinical presentation. I think this patient would benefit from further medical workup, and psychiatry is happy to follow along for consultation.

Whenever there is a disagreement between services, it is wise to check in with your psychiatry attending early in the process for guidance and assistance. Recognize that your goals are both to provide the best patient care and to maintain a professional relationship with the ED provider. Be collegial while emphasizing concern for the patient.

SELF-REFLECTIVE QUESTIONS

1. How do I feel about the power differential between the psychiatrist and a patient experiencing a mental health crisis?
2. How could I improve my collaboration skills?
3. How have I incorporated learning and teaching into previous rotations? How can these be applied to the emergency setting?
4. What habits (physical, vocal) do I have that might make a patient uncomfortable, afraid, uncertain, or angry?
5. What patients do I work really well with? What patients do I struggle with?
6. How do I care for myself?

RESOURCES

Burke C, van Dernoot Lipsky L: Trauma Stewardship: An Everyday Guide to Caring for Self While Caring for Others. San Francisco, CA, Berrett-Koehler, 2009

Knox D, Holloman G: Use and avoidance of seclusion and restraint: consensus statement of the American Association for Emergency Psychiatry Project BETA Seclusion and Restraint Workgroup. West J Emerg Med 13(1):35–40, 2012 22461919

Maloy K: A Case-Based Approach to Emergency Psychiatry. New York, Oxford University Press, 2016

Ravindranath D, Riba MB: Clinical Manual of Emergency Psychiatry. Arlington, VA, American Psychiatric Association Publishing, 2016

Richmond J, Berlin J, Fishkind A, et al: Verbal de-escalation of the agitated patient: consensus statement of the American Association for Emergency Psychiatry Project BETA De-Escalation Workgroup. West J Emerg Med 13(1):17–25, 2012 22461917

Shea SC: Psychiatric Interviewing: The Art of Understanding, 3rd Edition. New York, Elsevier, 2017

Wilson M, Pepper D, Currier G, et al: The psychopharmacology of agitation: consensus statement of the American Association for Emergency Psychiatry Project BETA Psychopharmacology Workgroup. West J Emerg Med 13(1):26–34, 2012 22461918

Wilson MP, Nordstrom K, Anderson EL, et al: American Association for
Emergency Psychiatry Task Force on Medical Clearance of Adult
Psychiatric Patients part II: controversies over medical assessment,
and consensus recommendations. West J Emerg Med 18(4):640–646,
2017 28611885

REFERENCES

Klamen DL, Grossman LS, Kopacz D: Posttraumatic stress disorder symptoms
in resident physicians related to their internship. Acad Psychiatry
19(3):142–149, 1995 24442586

Rueve ME, Welton RS: Violence and mental illness. Psychiatry (Edgmont)
5(5):34–48, 2008 19727251

Schwartz RC, Blankenship DM: Racial disparities in psychotic disorder diagnosis: a review of empirical literature. World J Psychiatry 4(4):133–140, 2014
25540728

CHAPTER 10

On Call and Night Float

Melissa M. Ley-Thomson, M.D.

Cybèle Arsan, M.D.

Christine T. Finn, M.D.

Gillian L. Sowden, M.D.

Covering clinical services after hours or on weekends is typically referred to as being *on call*. Psychiatric residents may have many different responsibilities on call, and there are various ways to schedule on-call coverage, including night float, which typically will be a single person covering overnight for multiple nights in a row. Regardless of how it is scheduled, most residents might say that they do not really want to *take* call, but looking back, most psychiatrists are glad that they *took* call. As a resident, you want to have a sense of mastery and confidence at the conclusion of residency, and managing the clinical and interpersonal situations that arise on call can help you achieve that goal. The Accreditation Council for Graduate Medical Education has outlined different supervisory levels to be achieved during residency, paving the way to autonomous practice (Accreditation Council for Graduate Medical Education 2020). Early in residency, on-call experiences can sometimes feel overwhelming. Residents may be asked to manage high-acuity and high-volume clinical situations, with the highest levels of independent practice often occurring in the on-call setting. As a result, these experiences are valuable to the professional development of each resident.

Moreover, on-call duties often provide opportunities to supervise medical students and residents early in their training, helping you prepare for future supervisory roles. In this chapter we highlight important considerations for making the most of your on-call experiences.

KEY POINTS

- Prepare for call by reviewing common clinical scenarios and questions.

- Recognize the importance of the handoff process and listen for anticipatory guidance.

- Staff members are your allies—align goals and develop rapport early and often.

- When in doubt, ask for help—you are never alone.

- Take care of your body and mind before, during, and after call.

- However onerous call may seem, attending physicians retrospectively see it as a time of significant professional growth.

EFFECTIVELY MANAGING CLINICAL WORK ON CALL

Call is the epitome of experiential learning, and in the beginning, you will constantly be confronted with unfamiliar experiences. You simply cannot know everything, and no one expects you to. The following subsections provide tips for managing your work more effectively.

Identify Common Clinical Scenarios, Relevant Medications, and Protocols

Familiarizing yourself with some of the more common clinical scenarios and questions that you might encounter can help to alleviate some of your uneasiness. For instance, you can expect to be called with questions about how to manage agitation, suicidality, withdrawal, and insomnia, and familiarizing yourself with relevant medications and protocols can help to build your knowledge base and lessen your anxiety. Compiling a "cheat sheet" with dosing of emergency medications and instructions regarding the use of restraints can also help to temper your nerves when nursing calls to report a patient's increasing agitation and insists that you do something immediately.

Execute Handoffs Well

Executing handoffs well is vital to preventing medical errors and provides another opportunity to anticipate and begin to develop contingency plans for issues that may arise on your shift. When receiving a handoff on call, be sure to obtain relevant information, such as the patient's legal status (Is there a guardian involved? Under which condition can the patient leave against medical advice in the middle of the night? Is an involuntary hold due to expire?), recent medication changes and side effects, medical issues, or behavioral plans in place. Anticipatory guidance (i.e., *if this happens, then do this*) is of great value when you are covering patients who are unfamiliar to you. Develop a system to keep track of to-dos and active patients. Becoming familiar with the handoff tool used at your institution and how information is organized in the written and verbal handoff is recommended. Using check boxes for to-dos can save a lot of mental energy, and checking off boxes can be oddly satisfying.

Triage Effectively

Learning how to triage effectively is essential to providing good patient care on call. When you are being paged to multiple patients and services at once, it is important to have an organized and structured response. Prioritization is a must, with agitated patients, acute safety concerns, and patients at risk for medical decompensation being the top priority (Figure 10–1). Beyond clinical acuity, programmatic or institutional expectations will help guide workflow on a busy call shift (e.g., is it a higher priority to admit a patient or to see a new emergency department consult?). Notes often come last, and learning efficient charting is useful. For situations in which a note is required to help guide care (e.g., agitated patients, emergency department patients needing discharge), you can consider writing a brief note in the chart delineating any important information and recommendations and including the annotation "full note to follow," then updating the chart with additional information later in your shift.

Cross-Cover Colleagues' Patients

Depending on availability of other providers overnight and on weekends, the on-call resident also may be responsible for taking calls directly from patients who are cared for in the outpatient practices. Ideally, you will be able to access the electronic medical record and review a recent clinical note and medication list before or during your conversation with a patient. When available, crisis plans or other docu-

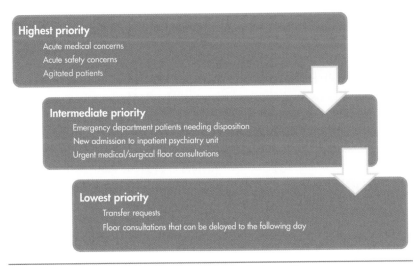

Highest priority
- Acute medical concerns
- Acute safety concerns
- Agitated patients

Intermediate priority
- Emergency department patients needing disposition
- New admission to inpatient psychiatry unit
- Urgent medical/surgical floor consultations

Lowest priority
- Transfer requests
- Floor consultations that can be delayed to the following day

FIGURE 10–1. Example of priority triage during call.

ments that outline behavioral management provide valuable information for after-hours decision-making. Quickly establishing whether a patient is experiencing a psychiatric crisis (e.g., suicidal ideation, psychosis) and managing acute safety concerns are important. Managing safety may include securing help for the patient from a family member or friend, calling a local mobile crisis service, or calling 911 to bring help directly to the patient. Beyond acute management, prolonged phone calls with patients are generally not advised, and nonacute issues should be deferred to the outpatient team. For patients who call repeatedly after hours (and sometimes as a means of avoiding scheduled outpatient appointments), it can be particularly helpful to follow an established behavior plan provided by the clinical team or if one does not exist, to bring the situation to the attention of your supervisor. Closing the loop with outpatient providers via messaging or forwarding documentation is essential, especially for situations requiring timely action on their part.

Manage the Quiet Pager

Instances in which your pager is unusually quiet can be anxiety inducing. Calling the operator or checking the online paging system to confirm that your pager is working and receiving forwarded pages appropriately can assuage any concerns that technology is to blame. Once you have confirmed that your pager is functioning properly, you can use this time to update documentation, place hold extensions, and complete some of the other less urgent tasks that were signed out to you. If you manage to check off all of your to-do boxes and your pager is still not alerting you to new business, listening to music, catching up on reading, going for a walk, or practicing sun salutations or other yoga poses can help to reduce your stress.

SUCCESSFULLY MANAGING AND LEVERAGING RELATIONSHIPS ON CALL

As a resident who may feel less than confident about your own knowledge or skills, you may find it hard to recognize that you know more about psychiatry than anyone from nonpsychiatry services with whom you will be interacting, including more senior residents and attendings. It can be difficult to disagree with someone whom you perceive to be "more experienced" than you, but remember that you are bringing a different viewpoint and expertise to the encounter. Reminding everyone that you are all working toward the same goal by using a prefacing statement such as "I think it is in the patient's best interest to..." makes it hard for someone to disagree with you and aligns everyone along the same goals.

Establish Good Rapport With Staff

Nurses on the floor can be under a lot of pressure. Although it is not included in the specific job description of a resident, establishing good rapport with all staff will save time and energy in the long run. Nurses can be your best allies. They may be more experienced in managing certain clinical situations and often are skilled in the art of de-escalation. Additionally, nurses may have institutional knowledge or logistical information that residents do not. Proactively spending a few minutes of face-to-face interaction with nursing staff reviewing plans and contingencies for active patients may improve patient care and have the additional benefit of saving you many pages in the middle of the night, which in turn may lead to more uninterrupted sleep. Failure to achieve a good working alliance with other team members, including nursing, nonpsychiatric residents, emergency department staff, security, and attendings may lead to problems. A summary of potentially challenging interactions between residents and other staff members and proposed solutions is shown in Table 10–1.

Work With Your Supervisor

Another important relationship for a resident on call is with your supervisor, who is typically a more senior resident or psychiatry attending

TABLE 10–1.   Strategies for navigating potentially challenging interactions between residents and other staff members

Characteristic of paging staff	Helpful on-call/night float resident responses
Anxious—pages frequently	• Check in at the beginning of your shift and before going to the call room and let nursing or other staff know where you will be. • Make clear your availability and how best to reach you. • Plan to be present on the unit on a regular basis, even if you have not been called. Just knowing you are around can help alleviate staff anxiety.
Difficulty taking initiative—pages frequently	• Empower other staff to intervene in patient care within the scope of their professional knowledge. • Design multistep plans for implementation by staff.
Does not page enough	• Outline situations in which you want to be notified, such as significant patient agitation, attempted elopement, or a change in medical status.
Does not know the patients	• Be very specific about what information you want provided. • When coming to see a patient, direct the staff member what to review and have ready for you when you arrive.
Unprofessional interactions	• Recurring issues with any staff members, unprofessional behaviors, or demeaning attitudes should be reported to your direct supervisor and specific hospital reporting systems. Make a note of the name and situation.

physician. Supervision overnight and on weekends provides a unique challenge because it is frequently indirect, performed by phone, text, or other digital formats (Raj and De Golia 2019). Unlike other supervisory relationships, supervision on call is highly variable, often with a supervisor with whom you do not have a long-standing relationship or may have never even met. Thus, the inherent basis of trust that usually accompanies other forms of supervision is often lacking with on-call supervision.

Strong communication is key to any successful supervisory relationship. Reaching out and contacting your supervisor at the beginning of the shift to introduce yourself, especially if you have not worked together before, can go a long way to improving the quality of the experience. Clarifying expectations, such as when to call and how to present cases, can also help avoid potential ruptures in the supervisory relationship and optimize patient safety.

Your supervisor may have helpful advice on the clinical situations you encounter during your call shift. However, some residents may feel uncomfortable contacting their supervisor while on call, feeling that their institution has a "do not call" culture or residents may think that these are things that they *should* know already. Interestingly, a study found that when given hypothetical call situations, supervisors reported wanting to be called more often than residents felt comfortable calling (Benson et al. 2019). Not calling your supervisor could have negative consequences if an adverse event were to happen, especially if it could have been avoided with input from a more experienced clinician. If a supervisor indicates a reluctance for you to call, this would be important to address with your chief resident or program director because having easy access to a supervisor when on call is essential and a requirement of residency.

On busy call nights, residents may feel they do not have time to call their supervisor. Knowing your institution's expectations regarding when to call your supervisor is important. Overnight and weekend call can be a particularly anxiety-provoking and sometimes lonely experience. The age-old adage "a problem shared is a problem halved" is never truer than while on call. Whenever in doubt, never worry alone. *Learning to ask for help not only is essential for patient safety and for minimizing burnout, it is an important skill to master during residency.*

In addition to clinical issues, dealing with interpersonal challenges can be part of the call experience. Some situations on call can be particularly challenging, such as being the recipient of microaggressions from patients or staff (see Chapter 39, "Handling Mistreatment and Discrimination"). A supervisor can be a useful support for processing these events both in real time and after the fact. Similarly, if you find yourself in conflict with an attending on another service, it can be helpful to involve your supervisor not only to process the situation but also to consider the need for an attending-to-attending discussion.

It is the rare resident who has never experienced a situation of not being able to reach their supervisor on call. If this happens during an emergent situation, it can be particularly disorienting and can put patient safety at risk. Given that these situations can occur with some frequency, it is always important to have a backup supervisor available. Whether this is a backup supervisory system, your program director, or other identified clinician responsible for the patient, knowing whom to call in an emergency when you cannot reach your primary supervisor is essential. Confirming the best ways to reach your supervisor at the start of your shift, as well as potential times when they may be difficult to reach, and what to do if an emergency were to arise during that time period, can help mitigate this issue altogether.

SELF-CARE WHEN TAKING CALL

Call interferes with the everyday aspects of your life, such as family dinners, workouts, and sleep. Further, it complicates the less routine aspects, such as caring for a sick child or celebrating the holidays. Rather than passively accepting (and then perhaps resenting) these interferences, actively request assignments that do not coincide with your daughter's dance recital or your family's visit. Recognizing that not everyone can have Thanksgiving off and everyone works some shifts they prefer not to, you can plan ahead and request to work specific weekends, nights, and holidays that provide the minimum disruption to your particular circumstances, or you can make approved call swaps as needed. Prioritize events that will help you to build and maintain the important relationships in your life and seek call assignments that accommodate them.

Lack of sleep and fatigue are an inevitable part of overnight call. Acute sleep loss starts approximately 17 hours after continuously being awake (Institute of Medicine 2009). Helpful strategies to combat these issues are outlined in Table 10–2.

SPECIFIC CHALLENGES AND STRATEGIES

⌘ **I am so anxious, I dread call.** Anticipatory anxiety about call is normal and can be quelled with expectation setting. Early in your residency career, much of this anxiety may stem from fear that you will not know how to manage a situation. It is important to remember that your primary job is to get patients through the night. You may be the sole physician caring for a large number of patients who are cared for by multiple distinct teams of physicians and social workers during the day. It can be helpful to remind yourself that you are one person and you do not have a magic wand. You simply cannot simultaneously be an expert diagnostician, therapist, and discharge planner at 2 A.M. When you find yourself on the receiving end of unrealistic expectations, actively listening for 3–5 minutes, rephrasing both the content of and the affect contained in the message, and calmly explaining your plan to pass this on to the day team can go a long way toward diffusing tense situations and resetting expectations. In cases in which your anxiety may be interfering with your per-

TABLE 10–2. Strategies for a successful call

	Before	During	After
Call	• Pack an overnight bag with food, toiletries, multicolored pen, phone charger, a change of clothes, eye drops, pajamas, earplugs, sleep mask, and your favorite podcast or meditation • Adapt your caffeine intake by changing timing or quantity • Prepare for sleep loss by trying to get good sleep on the days prior to call	• Strategic napping • Take a break for meals (high protein and high fat tend to sustain you) • Take a shower	• Sleep • Exercise • Spend time with loved ones
Night float (multiple nights in a row)	• See above • Arrange coverage for daytime clinical duties • Plan ahead for daytime sleep: identify a cool, dark location, purchase earplugs and sleep mask	• See above	• Sleep in cool, dark location • Use earplugs and sleep mask • Turn off cell phone and sign out pager

formance on call, talking with chief residents or your program director is recommended.

⌘ **My pager will not stop going off.** Even when you are armed with cheat sheets and realistic expectations for your role, anxiety will likely mount as you receive your fourth new consultation in an hour and floor pages are piling up faster than you can return them. Although the natural inclination may be to race off to begin seeing these consults, taking a few minutes to recalibrate can save time and increase productivity in the long run. Completing four cycles of box breathing (inhale for four seconds, hold for four seconds, exhale for four seconds, hold for four seconds to complete one cycle) can noticeably reduce heart rate and muscle tension and have a calming effect. Taking a short amount of time to organize and prioritize can also help you feel more in control. In the event that you are responding to a time-sensitive emergency that does not permit this, taking a 10-

to 20-second breather before entering the patient's room can help to ground yourself and refocus. Additionally, it is important that you familiarize yourself with your program's policies for calling in assistance. Do not hesitate to call your attending physician or senior resident to discuss prioritization of work and the potential need for on-site backup.

⌘ **My supervisor disagrees with me.** On-call clinical scenarios are often high acuity, which can create unease for many supervisors who have not met the patient themselves and are relying solely on your assessment to make difficult decisions. Discharging a suicidal patient whom you have never met can be anxiety provoking for even the most experienced of supervisors. Sometimes a supervisor's on-call responsibilities are not necessarily in their area of practice or expertise. If the supervisor's decision seems actively unsafe, you may need to voice your concern to the supervisor or reach out to another person in authority. For example, you might say to the on-call attending, "I may have misunderstood at the time, but this decision seems contrary to what I was taught on [inpatient rotation/consult rotation/didactics]. Would it be OK if I call Dr. Smith and run this by her for additional input?" If the disagreement does not endanger patient care, you may want to go along with the supervisor's plan at the time but give feedback to them at the end of the shift. Ultimately, the supervisor is responsible for the care that you provide, so complying with their preferred plan and making sure that you understand the rationale behind it is recommended.

⌘ **Other staff are directing their anger at me.** At times, you may be called to help manage emergent or other emotionally charged situations where patients and staff are feeling unsafe, angry, or otherwise overwhelmed. In these circumstances, you need to become an "affect sponge," absorbing affect and helping others regain their self-control and equilibrium. You cannot do this if you are also feeling unsafe, so first taking steps to ensure safety (e.g., security presence, asking families or staff to remove themselves) may be necessary. Looking for ways to validate concerns, never arguing (even if you disagree), and generally using clinical de-escalation techniques are recommended.

⌘ **I cannot unwind after my call shift is over.** Finding a way to effectively debrief and not take call home with you is as important as developing a helpful system to prioritize the pages you receive throughout the night. Time permitting, it may be helpful to carve out a formal debrief immediately following clinical sign-out in the mornings. Some programs employ *process rounds*, which are led by a senior psychiatrist and provide a safe space for the overnight resident to bring up challenging interactions and unclear clinical presentations and the emotions they elicited overnight (Beach et al. 2017). Alternatively, if you are all talked out by the end of a call shift and prefer to write down your reactions to various incidents overnight and then shred this paper, that can serve as an effective way to rid yourself of any negative emotions and cognitions prior to going home to sleep or interact with family.

SELF-REFLECTIVE QUESTIONS

1. Is there anything I can do to modify my sleep environment to promote sleep postcall?
2. What makes me uncomfortable about calling a supervisor at night?
3. What skills do I need to work on that the on-call experience is particularly helpful for?
4. What sense of mastery have I gained from being on call?
5. When supervising a resident early in their training or a medical student on call, what qualities do I most want to model?
6. What actions can I take to optimize my relationships with others on the clinical team?

RESOURCES

Cleveland Clinic: How you can sleep better if you work the night shift. Cleveland, OH, Cleveland Clinic, December 2014. Available at: https://health.clevelandclinic.org/how-you-can-sleep-better-if-you-work-the-night-shift. Accessed March 15, 2021.

Krischke M: 5 easy ways to prepare for night-shift nursing. Onward Healthcare, February 28, 2018. Available at: www.onward healthcare.com/resources/blog/travel-nursing-tips/5-ways-to-prepare-for-night-shift-nursing. Accessed March 15, 2021.

University of St. Augustine for Health Sciences: How to work the night shift and stay healthy: 12 tips. St. Augustine, FL, University of St. Augustine for Health Sciences, July 2020. Available at: www.usa.edu/blog/how-to-work-night-shift-and-stay-healthy. Accessed March 15, 2021.

REFERENCES

Accreditation Council for Graduate Medical Education: ACGME program requirements for graduate medical education in psychiatry. Chicago, IL, Accreditation Council for Graduate Medical Education, July 1, 2020. Available at: www.acgme.org/globalassets/pfassets/programrequirements/400_psychiatry_2020.pdf. Accessed June 8, 2022.

Beach SR, Taylor JB, Kontos N: Teaching psychiatric trainees to "think dirty": uncovering hidden motivations and deception. Psychosomatics 58(5):474–482, 2017 28602447

Benson NM, Taylor JB, Bird SA, et al: "Call me, maybe": supervisor and resident comfort with indirect supervision in psychiatry training. Psychosomatics 60(5):474–480, 2019 30685118

Institute of Medicine: Residency Duty Hours: Enhancing Sleep, Supervision and Safety. Washington, DC, National Academies Press, 2009

Raj KS, De Golia SG: Night float, working with supervisees remotely, in Supervision in Psychiatric Practice: Practical Approaches Across Venues and Providers. Edited by De Golia SG, Corcoran KM. Washington, DC, American Psychiatric Association Publishing, 2019, pp 139–146

CHAPTER 11

Nonpsychiatry Services

Grace Lee, M.D.
Diana Willard, M.D.

Now that you have selected your career specialty, you may dread returning to a nonpsychiatry rotation in your first year of psychiatry residency. This may especially be the case if your nonpsychiatry rotations are scheduled toward the end of your intern year or if the services are more demanding than what you experienced in medical school. You may have already begun a nonpsychiatry rotation and feel isolated from your residency program or your identity as a psychiatrist. If you are experiencing nerves before or during a nonpsychiatry rotation, remember that your goal (and others' expectations) is not for you to become a neurologist or an internist. Although individual goals will vary, an overarching one is to gain sufficient medicine and neurology knowledge and skills to provide excellent, comprehensive care to your patients as a psychiatrist. These rotations will serve you well in your career—more than you might realize now.

In this chapter we refer to the neurology and medicine rotations as nonpsychiatry services, although we recognize that some residents will rotate through other services, such as pediatrics, emergency medicine, and/or palliative medicine. We provide you with insights into why these services are relevant to your future in psychiatry, as well as strategies for doing well on them and for incorporating self-care along the way.

KEY POINTS

- Approach your nonpsychiatry rotations as an opportunity to broaden exposure to psychiatric differential diagnoses; potential consequences of psychiatric treatment; and a wide range of colleagues, patient populations, and treatment settings.

- Think through your learning goals prior to beginning a nonpsychiatry rotation.

- Consider reviewing key pathologies, diagnostic tests, physical examination skills, and treatment options in medicine in advance of your rotations.

- Learn which team members and residency supports can help you navigate difficult situations arising on nonpsychiatry rotations.

- Stay connected to your support system and psychiatry coresidents while on nonpsychiatry services.

ADVANTAGES OF NONPSYCHIATRY SERVICES

Nonpsychiatry rotations are opportunities to build foundational knowledge for your future psychiatric practice. Reflecting on the value added by the rotations will yield a more intentional and rewarding experience. Benefits from a robust medicine and neurology training include being better able to identify and manage adverse sequelae of medications and medical causes of psychiatric issues, preparation for consultation-liaison psychiatry, and enhanced ability to navigate medicine or neurology consultations, as well as preparation for in-training and board examinations.

Identification and Management of Adverse Medical Sequelae of Psychiatric Medication

Atypical antipsychotics are notorious for inducing adverse metabolic changes and are an example of psychotropics linked to medical side effects. In such cases, you may need to initiate treatment for hyperlipidemia and/or mild diabetes, particularly in rural geographies with a dearth of primary care providers or clinics serving patients with severe mental illness. Mental health clinics are frequently the only point of contact that patients with severe mental illness have with health care, despite their shortened life expectancies due to genetics, limited health-promoting behaviors, and psychotropic side effects (Haupt 2006). If you are not managing the medical conditions yourself, your medicine rotation will still prepare you to monitor laboratory results, encourage behavioral changes, and enlist resources to connect patients with a primary care physician as needed.

Identification of and Addressing Medical Causes for Psychiatric Issues

Anti-*N*-methyl-D-aspartate receptor encephalitis, seizures, anemia, brain masses, and hypothyroidism are examples of conditions that can manifest as psychiatric symptoms. Learning how to screen for a root medical cause enables you to create a robust formulation and initiate the appropriate interventions for your patients.

Preparing for Examinations

The inclusion of neurology content on psychiatry exams, including Step 3 of the United States Medical Licensing Examination, reflects how these fields intertwine. For example, patients with Parkinson's disease may present with psychosis; patients with a recent stroke may experience emerging depression; and new-onset psychosis in an emergency department patient could be a result of schizophrenia, encephalitis, or a seizure disorder. Neurology topics compose 13%–19% of the psychiatry board exam and 15%–20% of the Psychiatric Resident-In-Training Examination (PRITE) (American Board of Psychiatry and Neurology 2020; Shalev and Jacoby 2019). Experiential learning and multiple exposures through patient encounters on your nonpsychiatry rotations are powerful ways to consolidate and store new information that you want to retain for examinations (Carey 2014). You can deepen this learning by reading up on your patients. For example, for a patient with new-onset complex partial seizures, review seizure types, etiology, and examination and electroencephalogram findings.

Preparing for Consultation-Liaison Psychiatry, Where Medicine and Psychiatry Intersect

Building a strong grasp of medical and postoperative conditions, laboratory findings, and medication interactions will aid you in providing more comprehensive recommendations as a consultant to the nonpsychiatric primary team. On the nonpsychiatry rotations, you also will witness the psychological impact of medical and neurological illnesses as you care for patients. Knowing firsthand the toll taken by severe illness, hospitalization, and diagnostic and prognostic uncertainty can help you better understand the stressors patients and their loved ones experience when you are in the role of a psychiatric consultant or therapist. Further, while on nonpsychiatry rotations, you can also give team members insight into what the psychiatry service contributes, enabling them to place informed psychiatry consultations.

Learning When to Place Medicine or Neurology Consultations for Psychiatric Patients

On the nonpsychiatry services, you will encounter both bread-and-butter and fringe consultations that your nonpsychiatry team members accept and manage, which will help you manage medical issues yourself and better navigate whom to consult for which issues on behalf of your psychiatry patients. You also will learn when the input of more specialized providers is indicated. Building positive relationships with your co-interns and senior residents while on nonpsychiatry rotations will later help you feel more comfortable curbsiding them or clarifying whether a formal consultation is more appropriate for your patient's care. Across services, consultants may at times push back on a request they deem inappropriate, and establishing rapport with nonpsychiatry team members will ease interactions when you share mutual patients with them in the future.

DIFFERENCES BETWEEN NONPSYCHIATRY AND PSYCHIATRY SERVICES

Although you have had exposure to nonpsychiatry services in medical school, it can be helpful to review some of the differences, including culture, structure, and logistics. Of course, these aspects will vary across training programs.

Schedule and Pace

On nonpsychiatry inpatient rotations, anticipate earlier mornings, longer hours, formal rounds, and a fast pace. Approach your responsibilities systematically to maximize efficiency and prioritize rest and enjoyable activities during time off to bring a sense of balance to your rotation. It can also be helpful to minimize energy-expending commitments outside work and simplify tasks and chores during your inpatient months. Find easy ways to take care of meals and save nonurgent to-dos for a lighter month. Nonpsychiatry outpatient rotations tend to be more similar to psychiatric clinics in schedule and pace, with variations related to clinic setting and other individual factors.

Rounding Expectations

Expect to be managing a high volume of information for each of your nonpsychiatry patients, including vital signs, overnight events, diagnostic results, consultant recommendations, and examination findings. Ask your attending physician how they prefer this information be presented during rounds and develop a system to keep track of the information. We present examples of systems you can use in the section "Logistical Preparation." Your attending also may ask you questions about your patient's pathology, workup, and treatment options to test your understanding, so be prepared by consulting *UpToDate* or your preferred reference before rounds.

Team Structure

Although interns tend to work directly with the attending on psychiatry services, inpatient neurology and medicine teams often include more team members, with the addition of senior residents who assume a supervisory role. Although you will see your attending for rounds and other meetings, your senior resident is the person consistently on the ground fielding consultations, assigning new patients, and ensuring that all urgent and important tasks are under way. The senior resident is a good initial point of contact for issues that arise and will escalate matters to the attending as needed. Team structure can vary widely between services and institutions, so when in doubt, ask questions to clarify whom you need to report to for what.

Teaching Methods

Busy nonpsychiatry inpatient rotations typically have morning reports or scheduled didactics that use an interactive, question-and-answer format focusing on interesting cases. In contrast, teaching on psychiatric services is often structured differently, focusing more on high-level discussions about biopsychosocial context and both pharmacological and nonpharmacological interventions. As you experience different teaching methods, identify which ones resonate with and engage you best and find ways to creatively incorporate them into your residency training as you learn (and also teach medical students).

PREPARING FOR A NONPSYCHIATRY ROTATION

Getting ready for a rotation includes logistical and clinical preparation. Often, interns are apprehensive about their clinical preparation, but logistical preparation can be equally important for rotation success.

Logistical Preparation

Imagine yourself starting your new rotation. Where will you go? What will your schedule and duties be? Whom will you work with? What tools will you need? Keep these questions in mind when reviewing written guides or discussing the rotation with other residents to help you focus on the most salient information. Consider jotting down a cheat sheet with important information, such as locations, key codes, schedules, and team members' names and contact information.

Each day, you will need to manage large amounts of patient information and your own to-do list. Having a system to organize this information from the beginning of your rotation will be of tremendous help to you. Common options include the following:

- Printing and annotating the electronic medical record's patient list—depending on the system, you may be able to concisely print each patient's daily laboratory results, vitals, and medication list and keep track of daily to-dos in the margins
- Using an index card for each patient that you update daily
- Folding a regular-size piece of paper into a grid of rectangles, one for each patient, that you update daily
- Creating a one-half- or one-quarter-page template in Word that you can print out and fill out by hand, folding a part of the page over to list to-dos on the back page (Figure 11–1).

Clinical Preparation

Your need to prepare will depend on your level of comfort with the material, the amount of time since your last rotation in the field, and time constraints. If you do not have time prior to the rotation to review, don't panic. You will experience plenty of on-the-job learning, and simple bookmarking of resources for quick access later can be very helpful. See Table 11–1 for helpful topics to review before your rotation.

Take a few minutes to brainstorm your short- and long-term learning goals. Having a clear sense of your learning goals can guide your individual study and help you obtain the most relevant training during the rotation. You could mention these topics to your attending as areas of interest for tailored teaching or let your attending or senior resident know if there are any particular patient presentations you would like to be assigned.

Remember: the goal of any prerotation preparation is not for you to feel completely prepared. It is normal to feel nervous prior to a nonpsychiatry rotation (or any rotation). Your upcoming rotation is a chance for

Date:	Admission date:		Room #:
Pt ID:			
S: Interval events:		**Subjective:**	

O: Vitals: T   Tm   HR
        BP   R   PO2
I/O: IV   PO   UOP   BM
 	
PEx:
 	
Labs:
 	
    $\times$ $+\!+\!\!<$ Ca Mg Ph
 	
Results (micro/path, EKG, imaging, etc.):
		Medications/PRNs:
		
		A/P by problem:	

		Dispo plan:	

FIGURE 11–1. Sample prerounding template.

Source. Adapted from Medfools 2001.

TABLE 11–1. Topics to review for different services

Service	Topics to review
Internal medicine	• The complete physical examination • Interpretation of important studies and laboratory results (e.g., ECG, hematocrit/hemoglobin, acid/base status) • Commonly used lines, tubes, and drains
Neurology	• The physical examination, with focus on the neurological examination • The NIHSS (or other tool your institution uses) • Relevant neuroanatomy to localize lesions, such as dermatomes and common patterns of sensory or motor loss
Pediatrics	• The physical examination and newborn examination • Key developmental milestones • Normal vital signs by age
All services	• Common "bread-and-butter" pathologies seen on the service and their presentations, workup, and treatment • Acute emergencies (e.g., cardiac arrest, stroke) and their management algorithms

Note. ECG=electrocardiogram; NIHSS=National Institutes of Health (NIH) Stroke Scale.

you to learn: if you had already mastered all the content of the rotation, there would be no need for you to do the rotation.

FIND YOUR RESOURCES

When joining a new team, interns often have a wide range of questions. This is completely normal. Finding ways to efficiently get your questions answered without disrupting your or others' workflow can be very helpful (Table 11–2).

STAYING CONNECTED TO PSYCHIATRY

Being on a nonpsychiatry rotation can lead to feelings of being disconnected: from your co-interns, your residency program, the field of psychiatry, or your identity as a psychiatrist. Long hours, a field that you did not specifically choose, and separation from your usual supports in residency can produce feelings of discontent, frustration, or burnout. These experiences are very common. All interns have the experience of being separated from their residency and co-interns during nonpsychiatry rotations. Most, if not all, of your nonpsychiatry team will have done an off-service rotation during their own residency and may be able to relate.

Think creatively about ways to reconnect with your residency, coresidents, or the field of psychiatry. Carve out time to check in with co-interns, take an extra few minutes to just chat with a patient and provide supportive therapy, or set aside a few minutes to do some psychiatry-related reading—whatever fills your cup.

Another approach is to *become* a neurology or medicine intern for the duration of the service, joining the team both professionally and interpersonally. Get to know your team members, do something fun to support your team, or dive into the content area. Finding a sense of satisfaction within the nonpsychiatry rotation can help with feelings of disconnection or burnout.

SPECIFIC CHALLENGES AND STRATEGIES

⌘ **I feel nervous about my performance compared with my medicine co-intern.** Feeling unsure about your performance on nonpsychiatry rotations is very common. Interns often compare themselves with members of their nonpsychiatry team, who may come across as incred-

TABLE 11–2. Finding the appropriate resources

Type of question	Example question	Possible resources
Logistical	What will my general schedule and duties be?	• Rotation guide (if available) • Outgoing psychiatry intern
	How can I best incorporate myself into the team?	• Team (teams appreciate this)
	How do I present at rounds?	• Attending physician
	How do I sign out?	• Residents
	How do I place this order?	• Any team member for specific, straightforward tasks • Senior team member for more complicated or sensitive tasks (e.g., placing admission orders or other complicated order sets)
Clinical	What is the differential and workup for this symptom?	• UpToDate for general clinical questions (download app on your phone; take 10–15 minutes daily to review relevant topics)
	How do I interpret this finding?	• UpToDate for general guidance • Senior resident or attending physician for specific issues related to an individual patient
Personal	How are days off scheduled?	• Rotation guide or orientation for standard logistical questions about the rotation • Nonpsychiatry interns for common logistical issues (team members will often stagger days off to maintain a smoothly functioning team and minimize impacts on patient care)

TABLE 11–2. Finding the appropriate resources *(continued)*

Type of question	Example question	Possible resources
Personal *(continued)*	What if I need additional time off?	• Senior resident or attending physician for individual situations • Psychiatry chief resident or training director for delicate topics that may be difficult to approach (they may need to start thinking about coverage options in parallel)
	What are my options if I'm feeling overwhelmed or burned out?	• Psychiatry co-interns for support • Attending physician or senior resident for how to navigate intern year • Trusted team member, psychiatry chief resident, or training director to discuss your feelings and explore options

ibly knowledgeable and competent. Two things may help rein in these feelings: a quick reality check and shifting to a growth mindset.

The reality check: remember that nonpsychiatry co-interns, residents, and attendings have been developing their knowledge and skills for months or years, whereas you have just started. We often think of our first day of residency as the first day of a new job. However, residency usually involves short blocks or rotations that each could be considered a new job, with a new team, location, and set of knowledge and skills.

Despite this reality, interns often expect themselves to be fully up to speed within hours of starting a new rotation. This mindset can lead to real struggles when you inevitably do not know the answer to a question or how to perform a task. Instead, shift to a growth mindset: "The passion for stretching yourself and sticking to it, even (or especially) when it's not going well..." (Dweck 2006, p. 7). You are a beginner, and that is exactly what you are supposed to be. In this mindset, every question, challenge, or mistake is a chance for powerful new learning. When you find yourself in this situation, recognize it as a chance to grow and remember to reach out to your resources for help. This beginner mindset allows people to thrive during some of the most challenging times in their lives (Dweck 2006).

⌘ **I feel uncomfortable performing procedures.** While on nonpsychiatry rotations, you may encounter a situation in which your upper-level resident or attending physician asks if you would like to perform a supervised procedure such as a lumbar puncture or paracentesis. For some psychiatry interns, this is a highly welcome and exciting prospect. For others, the idea may provoke feelings of discomfort and concern. If you have concerns about the procedure, know that many before you have felt the same way, and feel free to alert the upper-level resident on your team, who can then play a more hands-on role in guiding you.

Although stepping outside your comfort zone is encouraged (so long as close supervision is in place), your ability to be a well-regarded intern or a future competent psychiatrist does not rest on these procedures. Be present and attentive throughout, ask questions, and assist with setup and breakdown. Rather than mastering procedural skills, the expectation on these rotations is that you are engaged, reliable, and invested in patient care and your responsibilities.

⌘ **I sense I am treated differently from my neurology co-interns while on nonpsychiatry rotations.** Differential treatment on nonpsychiatry rotations can manifest in numerous ways and for a variety of reasons. For example, some teams may assign only patients with comorbid psychiatric presentations to the psychiatry intern, whereas other teams assume psychiatric interns would rather avoid patients with psychiatric presentations.

Depending on the context, differential treatment may feel positive, neutral, or negative to you. If differential treatment feels negative, it may be informed by past experiences with other psychiatry interns having communicated this preference or by how the team member would want to be treated. Regardless of the underlying reason, if you encounter instances of differential treatment that you deem worthwhile to address, try expressing your thoughts and suggestions to your teammate in a respectful manner. If any treatment makes you uncomfortable, do not hesitate to reach out to a trusted advocate from your nonpsychiatry team or your psychiatry residency. When in doubt, consult your fellow psychiatry interns or chiefs to process the situation and hear their insights.

SELF-REFLECTIVE QUESTIONS

1. What thoughts and feelings arise as I think about the upcoming nonpsychiatry rotations in my intern year?
2. What type of psychiatry practice setting do I envision entering, considering geography, patient demographics, the health care system, and my role? How might a firm grasp of internal medicine and neurology aid me in this setting?

3. How comfortable am I with telling supervising residents or attendings that I don't know the answer to their questions or that I feel underprepared to perform a procedure?

4. How important is it to me to remain connected with my psychiatry intern cohort while I am on nonpsychiatry rotations? What are ways I can stay in touch with my cohort while on nonpsychiatry rotations?

RESOURCES

Preparation for Medicine Rotations

Geeky Medics: OSCE guides and OSCE stations [videos], https://geekymedics.com/category/osce

Goldman L, Schafer AI: Cecil Textbook of Medicine, 26th Edition. New York, Elsevier, 2019

Kasper D, Fauci A, Hauser S, et al (eds): Harrison's Principles of Internal Medicine, 19th Edition. New York, McGraw-Hill Education, 2015

OnlineMedEd: Crash course in medicine, https://onlinemeded.org/spa/crash-course-in-medicine

Sabatine MS: Pocket Medicine, 7th Edition. New York, Wolters Kluwer, 2020

Stern SDC, Cifu AS, Altkorn D: Symptom to Diagnosis: An Evidence Based Guide, 4th Edition. New York, McGraw-Hill Education/Medical, 2019

UpToDate: www.wolterskluwer.com/en/solutions/uptodate

Preparation for Neurology Rotations

Lowenstein DH: The neurologic screening exam [video], in Harrison's Principles of Internal Medicine. New York, McGraw Hill, 2014. Available at: www.youtube.com/watch?v=OKz8-OFaxpc. Accessed October 4, 2022.

OnlineMedEd: Neurology, https://onlinemeded.org/spa/neurology

UpToDate: www.wolterskluwer.com/en/solutions/uptodate

Resources to Stay Informed on Medicine and Neurology Topics After PGY-1

McCarron RM, Xiong GL, Keenan CR, et al: Preventive Medical Care in Psychiatry: A Practical Guide for Clinicians. Arlington, VA, American Psychiatric Association Publishing, 2015

Weiner WJ, Goetz CG, Shin RK, et al (eds): Neurology for the Non-Neurologist, 6th Edition. Philadelphia, PA, Lippincott Williams & Wilkins, 2010

REFERENCES

American Board of Psychiatry and Neurology: 2021 ABPN content specifications in psychiatry certification. Deerfield, IL, American Board of Psychiatry and Neurology, 2020. Available at: www.abpn.com/wp-content/uploads/2020/10/2021_Psychiatry_CERT_Content_Specifications.pdf. Accessed August 19, 2021.

Carey B: How We Learn: The Surprising Truth About When, Where, and Why It Happens. New York, Random House, 2014

Dweck CS: Mindset: The New Psychology of Success. New York, Random House, 2006

Haupt DW: Differential metabolic effects of antipsychotic treatments. Eur Neuropsychopharmacol 16(3)(suppl 3):S149–S155, 2006 16872808

Medfools: Medicine H&P card. Medfools, 2001. Available at: www.medfools.com/downloads/michals-medicine-ward.pdf. Accessed August 20, 2021.

Shalev D, Jacoby N: Neurology training for psychiatry residents: practices, challenges, and opportunities. Acad Psychiatry 43(1):89–95, 2019 29777396

CHAPTER 12

Inpatient Services

Amy Gallop, M.D.

William Newman, M.D.

On acute psychiatric units, you will treat patients struggling with complex issues such as psychosis, suicidality, and behavioral dyscontrol. You will work with interdisciplinary teams, including some combination of nursing staff, security guards, medical students, psychologists, and social workers. Your roles involve coordinating communication between team members, managing medications, coordinating care, and determining patients' legal status. This is in addition to interviewing patients, clarifying diagnoses, and performing suicide and homicide risk assessments to guide decision-making and treatments. The environment requires cognitive flexibility and awareness of your surroundings. Many situations you encounter are emotionally draining, so peer support is paramount.

The focus of this chapter is on acute inpatient units, which differ from state-operated psychiatric hospitals. Since the push for deinstitutionalization in the 1960s, inpatient units have been used for stabilization, with average length of stay gradually decreasing. In this chapter we provide general resources to help prepare you for your inpatient psychiatry rotation.

KEY POINTS

- Get to know your staff. Use their expertise and involve all team members in regular communication.

- Become familiar with the layout of the unit and available options for managing agitation.

- Consider how you will balance patient autonomy with safety. You will have to balance the complex dynamics of being in a position of authority while providing care for the patient.

- You will be caring for a sick and vulnerable patient population, and using compassion and empathy in their care will be crucial.

- Be aware of the legal aspects of civil commitment and substituted decision-making, which vary by jurisdiction.

COMMUNICATION WITH TEAM MEMBERS

You will be working on a team with nursing staff, social workers, therapists, security, and medical students, among others. Navigating communication with them will be important in providing consistent and comprehensive care. Depending on your hospital, you also may encounter clergy, unit clerks, and interpreters.

Nursing Staff

As a resident, you will be on a rotating schedule. In contrast, nursing staff commonly work on inpatient units full time. Their observations and suggestions can be of tremendous value. Seek their input frequently. Prior to sharing difficult or upsetting news with a patient, inform the patient's nurse so they can anticipate the response. You also can plan for staff to be available for support after the patient receives the news.

Social Workers

Regular communication with social workers allows for efficient disposition planning and helps you understand patients' needs. It is also important to familiarize yourself with the region's mental health and case management services. Frequent communication with patients' inpatient and outpatient social workers helps optimize outcomes.

Psychologists and Therapists

Depending on the facility, you may be working with other mental health providers who have evaluated the patient. Regular meetings with the therapist will help develop your understanding of the patient's behaviors on the unit and needs on discharge, such as specific types of therapy. Psychological testing may also be an available resource.

Security

Depending on unit acuity, security may be consistently or intermittently present. Introduce yourself to security staff and maintain communication. You should speak to security about potential behavioral issues before they arise because this will make de-escalation measures more efficient and effective.

Medical Students

Medical students often have fewer patients and therefore can spend more one-on-one time with their patients. Allow them to play an active role in their patients' care and to be involved in substantive patient conversations when possible. You also will be responsible for teaching medical students. It is helpful to create two to three handouts on high-yield topics that you can provide to the students. You should also incorporate informal teaching related to the medical student's patient care.

Residents

There likely will be resident cross-coverage. It will be important for you, the primary psychiatrist, to formulate a plan and convey it to covering residents. This plan should include medication adjustments, disposition plans, and medical issues. It is often helpful to make the covering resident aware of possible behavioral issues and provide recommendations for medication and behavioral management by using "If, then" statements. For example, "*If* Mr. N remains agitated and starts posturing around other patients, *then* please speak to his nurse about administering another 10 mg prn."

SAFETY ON THE INPATIENT UNIT

Especially in inpatient psychiatry, you will be working in a setting where patients may be acutely agitated. Mental health staff experience higher rates of workplace violence than do other areas of health care. According to the U.S. Department of Justice's National Crime Victimization Survey, mental health workers are victims of crimes at 5.5 times the rate of the average population and are more than 3 times as likely to be the victim of a crime compared with other health care professionals (Duhart 2021). Because of the high acuity of this patient population, it is important to remain aware of de-escalation techniques, consider causes of agitation, and discuss ways to improve outcomes.

Awareness of Your Emotions

You will be interacting with patients who may easily escalate. They may respond in unexpected ways to your presence. You need to remain mindful of your potential responses and actions. When talking to agitated or paranoid patients, you may feel uneasy or on edge. You should not ignore your own response and can terminate the interview if you feel uneasy. Supervision, either formally arranged through your residency program or informally arranged with senior residents or faculty, will be a helpful venue to process your emotional response to this heightened setting. Finding ways to decompress outside work and maintaining existing hobbies will also be important.

Entrance and Exit

When rotating on an inpatient unit, familiarize yourself with the entrances, exits, and procedures for requesting assistance in case of an emergency. Be aware of which patients hover by the doors or may be an elopement risk. Be mindful of trip hazards as well for a situation in which you may need to exit a space quickly.

Interview Location

Prior to interviewing patients, review the patient's chart and ask the staff about recent problematic behaviors. If the patient has been agitated or holds persecutory delusions involving staff, you may need to conduct an interview in a public area or with an escort. While interviewing a patient, ensure that you are not blocked into the room by the patient. It is helpful to leave equal space between you, the patient, and the exit.

Attire

Avoid articles that could be used as weapons, including neckties, purses, pagers, or dangling jewelry. Avoid dressing in a manner likely to attract unwanted attention from patients. When possible, adapt religious clothing to be safe for the inpatient unit (such as hijabs without safety pins). It may be helpful to speak to your hospital's de-escalation and restraint trainers in order to consider specific accommodations related to religious or cultural attire.

Medical Student Orientation

This rotation will be the only exposure to inpatient psychiatry for many students. Orient the students to safety considerations. You may initially have students shadow you as they grow familiar with the setting. Encourage them to terminate interviews immediately if they become concerned about safety or a patient is becoming agitated.

Responding to Agitated Patients

Your role as the unit resident will include discussions with staff, ordering medications, and assessing the outcome of interventions. Although you may receive self-defense training through your residency program, typically you are not asked to restrain patients or administer medications. Make sure you are familiar with unit policies about hands-on interventions.

1. *Verbal de-escalation* is the first line when dealing with agitation. When patients behave aggressively, they may benefit from time to reflect. A member of the team can encourage them to take a break in their room. When talking to a patient, it is important to use a quiet or calming voice and be mindful of your own body language. You can give the patient a choice between two options to calm down so they can have some control over the situation. If they continue making threats or behaving aggressively, other interventions may become necessary.
2. *Chemical restraints*, such as intramuscular antipsychotic medications, represent a potential alternative to seclusion or restraint. Studies have reported less trauma by patients with chemical restraints than with physical restraints (Barnett et al. 2012). If patients refuse oral medications or remain too aggressive for that option, the team needs to decide whether a parenteral medication is indicated for acute dangerousness. If a patient is hurting themselves, attempting to destroy property, or threatening others and is not redirectable with verbal de-escalation, chemical restraints may be needed. You should offer oral medication first, but if the patient refuses or is unable to comply because of their level of agitation, intramuscular injection can be used. A therapeutic hold, in which a patient must be physically restrained, often by a nurse or security guard, would likely be used in this situation. Be mindful of your bias and biases of the staff because bias may play a role in use of restraints (Payne-Gill et al. 2021).

3. *Seclusion and isolation rooms* may be preferred to medication by patients at times because they may be viewed as less coercive (Chieze et al. 2019). These rooms generally have padded walls and a window for staff to observe the patient for safety. Following as-needed medication administration, patients may benefit from a short period of isolation. Removing agitated patients from the milieu may be beneficial to maintain calm across the unit because one agitated patient can be disruptive and distressing to other patients.

4. *Physical restraints* are often a last resort and typically are used if a patient remains at acute risk of harm to self or others after other interventions. Because of the risk of physical harm (strangulation, rhabdomyolysis, lacerations) and mental harm from restraints (Kersting et al. 2019), you will be required to check on the patient periodically and have a plan for step down to less restrictive measures.

Debriefings

Following episodes involving agitated patients, a debriefing session can be helpful for discussing strengths and weaknesses of the de-escalation process and ways to improve the process. It can be valuable to gather as many staff as possible in a secure location to discuss their observations in a nonaccusatory manner. It is also important to check in with fellow residents and medical students regarding their emotional reactions to addressing agitated patients.

INVOLUNTARY CIVIL COMMITMENT

Involuntary civil commitment is a relatively new protection. In the 1800s, it was relatively accepted that patients in mental institutions lacked global capacity and were unable to refuse treatment (Gold and Frierson 2018). Prior to the 1960s, need for treatment was based largely on the principle of the *parens patriae* doctrine, by which the "state protects those unable to protect and care for themselves" (Gold and Frierson 2018).

In the 1960s, the standard shifted to a *dangerousness* standard. This required a level of danger, either to the patient (such as suicidal ideation with intent) or to others (such as targeted persecutory delusions) in order to involuntarily commit an individual (Testa and West 2010). In 19 states, the dangerousness standard includes *grave disability*, meaning the individual is unable to provide basic necessities for survival. In 45 states, dangerousness must be due to a mental illness; 5 states do not specifically require a mental illness (Hedman et al. 2016).

You will be determining legal status while balancing patient autonomy with safety considerations. For example, if a patient voices willingness to be admitted but is acutely psychotic with limited insight, they may lack the capacity to consent to voluntary admission and may need to be admitted involuntarily. States define an initial observation and treatment period that lasts from 23 hours (North Dakota) to 10 days (New Hampshire and Rhode Island), with an average of 72 hours (Hedman et al. 2016). In some jurisdictions, patients may refuse nonurgent medications without having a hearing. Furthermore, other extended involuntary holds beyond the initial observation period are available for suicidality, homicidality, and/or gravely disabled status, depending on the state. You need to familiarize yourself with local laws.

As a resident, feeling as though you are usurping patients' civil rights can be difficult and lead to moral injury. As you gain experience in the decision-making process, you will better understand the complexities of the decision. Ultimately, psychiatrists should believe that civil commitment is in the best interest of the patient to address ongoing risk.

Substitute Decision Makers

You may encounter substitute decision makers on your inpatient psychiatry rotations. It is important to familiarize yourself with the laws in your jurisdiction.

Advance Directives

Patients may have completed an advance directive to appoint a surrogate decision maker (referred to as a power of attorney in some states) for medical decisions if the patient is unable to make those decisions. If this person has not been appointed ahead of time, 35 states have established a surrogacy hierarchy, which includes spouse, child, and parent in the highest-priority category (DeMartino et al. 2017). The specific regulations, requirements, and documents vary across states (American Bar Association 2019). Some jurisdictions allow a person to specify psychiatric treatment preferences in an advance directive.

Psychiatric Advance Directives

Twenty-five states have specific psychiatric advance directives, legal documents that appoint a surrogate decision maker and include preferences for psychiatric care. This does not supersede involuntary commitments, but the psychiatric advance directive may be followed for medication decisions (Swanson et al. 2003).

Guardianship

You may encounter patients with or in need of a guardian. In contrast to power of attorney, which is used when a person is temporarily incapacitated, a guardian replaces a person's authority to make decisions because of an illness. The requirements that necessitate guardianship vary across states (Barton et al. 2014; Kelly et al. 2021).

Limited Guardianship

Full guardianship differs from limited guardianship, which is used in some states. In limited guardianship, the court decides the extent of the guardian's role in decisions for the ward (Barton et al. 2014). If there is a threat of immediate harm to the incapacitated person, temporary or emergency guardianship can be pursued.

Emergency or Temporary Guardianship

Emergency guardianship is often used in the medical setting following a catastrophic event, such as a stroke, after which the patient is unable to make decisions for themselves regarding further care or disposition. Emergency guardianship typically lasts less than 6 months.

The following example illustrates one potential use of temporary and full guardianship.

Case Vignette

Ms. P has been involuntarily hospitalized in psychiatric units in various states 12 times in the past year. She has a history of bipolar 1 disorder and has been using illicit substances, at times turning to the sex industry to support her substance use. She has been unable to hold a job and is homeless. A judge has granted her parents a 6-month temporary guardianship because of her inability to care for herself. If Ms. P continues to require hospitalization for uncontrolled bipolar 1 disorder, remains homeless, and continues engaging in high-risk behaviors, full guardianship may be considered.

Payees

If a person has difficulty managing their finances, they may benefit from assigning a payee to receive that person's benefits and use them on the beneficiary's behalf. A payee may be established through the social security office (Social Security Administration 2019). For example, a person may receive monthly disability benefits to cover their living expenses but be unable to maintain stable housing because of difficulty with managing finances. If a long-term pattern is established, a payee may be appropriate. In this case, the individual continues making their own medical and mental health decisions. It is important that you remain mindful of potential abuses of payee status and report abuses if necessary.

BOUNDARY SETTING

Communication With Patients

Consider what information you are willing to share when patients inquire about elements of your personal life. Before disclosing information, it is helpful to evaluate if this information is going to help the patient in some way, such as strengthening the alliance and reducing stigma. If not, it is best to avoid disclosing information that may blur professional boundaries or would not benefit the patient's care.

Treatment

It may be taxing to you as a new resident to prescribe patients medications they do not want, such as an antipsychotic. Weighing patient autonomy with safety will be paramount. With serious mental illness, such as schizophrenia, patients may experience anosognosia or limited insight into their mental illness (Lehrer and Lorenz 2014). Although they may disagree with the treatment, it is important to remember that you are acting in their best interest regarding safety and long-term stability.

Families

Each family will have varying preferences regarding the amount of communication they receive. Providing frequent updates is appropriate, but you should set clear expectations with family members regarding the frequency and content of communications. In highly involved families, it may be advisable to designate a primary contact for routine updates who can then communicate with other family members. Periodic family meetings can also foster positive communication with the team. Collateral information can always be collected in emergency situations, such as when conducting triage assessments in the emergency department. You will need to familiarize yourself with consent policies on the inpatient unit.

Staff

It is important to maintain professional relationships, but it is additionally important to establish boundaries between work and personal life. Avoid giving medical advice or prescribing medications to staff because this will compromise the professional relationship. You should immediately raise concerns if you receive unwanted or problematic communications from staff outside your professional capacity.

There may also be patients who split between psychiatrist and nurses. For example, a patient may make frequent demands and rude remarks to the psychiatrist while joking in a friendly manner with nursing staff. Communication with nursing staff about this splitting and enforcing boundaries during these patient interactions are important to remain a united front.

SPECIFIC CHALLENGES AND STRATEGIES

⌘ **My patient's psychosis improved, but we could not find adequate support for them on discharge, so they were still admitted.** With each patient, begin considering disposition challenges, including housing and outpatient support, at the beginning of their hospitalization. For example, if a patient with schizophrenia who is experiencing homelessness gets admitted for exacerbated psychosis, discussing disposition options early may prevent delays in discharge and also improve your patient's mental health. Become familiar with your region's resources and support systems and collaborate with case managers to support therapeutic discharges.

⌘ **I'm so stressed on the inpatient unit.** Emotions may run high on the inpatient unit because of patient vulnerability, distrust, and anxiety. You will likely experience countertransference and be affected by patients' frustrations. Finding colleagues and supervisors with whom to discuss difficult experiences will be crucial in preventing burnout. In addition, reflecting on your own emotional response and taking a deep breath can give you additional capacity to respond therapeutically to challenging situations.

⌘ **How can I improve the patient's hospital stay?** Taking time to discuss your patient's comprehension of their diagnoses and treatment will be helpful in strengthening the therapeutic alliance and will give you an opportunity for psychoeducation and inclusion of the patient's preferences in the treatment plan. You should seek to understand how your patient identifies their values, beliefs, and culture and how your patient finds meaning and enjoyment in life and ways these aspects can be incorporated into their care. Figuring out ways to help the patient communicate effectively with family or other supports also can improve outcomes.

SELF-REFLECTIVE QUESTIONS

1. Do I understand the application of civil commitment criteria to clinical situations in my institution?
2. How will I balance staff concerns with my own clinical judgment?
3. What is my natural response when I feel threatened? How do I respond in highly emotional situations?

RESOURCES

Barton R, Lau S, Lockett LL: The use of conservatorships and adult guardianships and other options in the care of the mentally ill in the United States. Arlington, VA, Family Members as Guardians for Mentally Ill Patients World Guardianship Congress, May 29, 2014. Available at: www.guardianship.org/IRL/Resources/Handouts/Family%20Members%20as%20Guardians_Handout.pdf. Accessed September 14, 2020.

Sattar SP, Pinals DA, Din AU, et al: To commit or not to commit: the psychiatry resident as a variable in involuntary commitment decisions. Academic Psychiatry 30(3):191–195, 2006 16728764

Substance Abuse and Mental Health Service Administration: Civil Commitment and the Mental Health Care Continuum: Historical Trends and Principles for Law and Practice. Rockville, MD, Office of the Chief Medical Officer, Substance Abuse and Mental Health Services Administration, 2019

REFERENCES

American Bar Association: State health care power of attorney statutes. Washington, DC, ABA Commission on Law and Aging, 2019. Available at: www.americanbar.org/content/dam/aba/administrative/law_aging/state-health-care-power-of-attorney-statutes.authcheckdam.pdf. Accessed January 5, 2021.

Barnett R, Stirling C, Pandyan AD: A review of the scientific literature related to the adverse impact of physical restraint: gaining a clearer understanding of the physiological factors involved in cases of restraint-related death. Med Sci Law 52(3):137–142, 2012 22833483

Barton R, Lau S, Lockett LL: The use of conservatorships and adult guardianships and other options in the care of the mentally ill in the United States. Arlington, VA, Family Members as Guardians for Mentally Ill Patients World Guardianship Congress, May 29, 2014. Available at: www.guardianship.org/IRL/Resources/Handouts/Family%20Members%20as%20Guardians_Handout.pdf. Accessed September 14, 2020.

Chieze M, Hurst S, Kaiser S, et al: Effects of seclusion and restraint in adult psychiatry: a systematic review. Front Psychiatry 10:491, 2019 31404294

DeMartino ES, Dudzinski DM, Doyle CK, et al: Who decides when a patient can't? Statutes on alternate decision makers. N Engl J Med 376(15):1478–1482, 2017 28402767

Duhart D: Bureau of Justice Statistics Special Report National Crime Victimization Survey December 2001, NCJ 190076 Violence in the Workplace, 1993–99. Washington, DC, Bureau of Justice Statistics, 2021

Gold LH, Frierson RL (eds): The American Psychiatric Association Publishing Textbook of Forensic Psychiatry, 3rd Edition. Arlington, VA, American Psychiatric Association Publishing, 2018

Hedman LC, Petrila J, Fisher WH, et al: State laws on emergency holds for mental health stabilization. Psychiatr Serv 67(5):529–535, 2016 26927575

Kelly A, Hershey L, Marsack-Topolewski C: A 50-state review of guardianship laws: specific concerns for special needs planning. Journal of Financial Service Professionals 75(1):59–79, 2021

Kersting XA, Hirsch S, Steinert T: Physical harm and death in the context of coercive measures in psychiatric patients: a systematic review. Front Psychiatry 10:400, 2019 31244695

Lehrer DS, Lorenz J: Anosognosia in schizophrenia: hidden in plain sight. Innov Clin Neurosci 11(5–6):10–17, 2014 25152841

Payne-Gill J, Whitfield C, Beck A: The relationship between ethnic background and the use of restrictive practices to manage incidents of violence or aggression in psychiatric inpatient settings. Int J Ment Health Nurs 30(5):1221–1233, 2021 34180128

Social Security Administration: A guide for representative payees. Publ No 05-10076. Woodlawn, MD, Social Security Administration, 2019. Available at: www.ssa.gov/pubs/EN-05-10076.pdf. Accessed January 5, 2021.

Swanson JW, Swartz MS, Hannon MJ, et al: Psychiatric advance directives: a survey of persons with schizophrenia, family members, and treatment providers. Int J Forensic Ment Health 2(1):73–86, 2003

Testa M, West SG: Civil commitment in the United States. Psychiatry (Edgmont) 7(10):30–40, 2010 22778709

CHAPTER 13

The Psychiatric Consultation

Carrie Ernst, M.D.

Metin Cayirolgu, M.D.

Antoine Beayno, M.D.

The consultation-liaison (CL) psychiatry rotation offers a unique opportunity for you to gain exposure to the subspecialty that focuses on the psychiatric care of medically ill patients. During the rotation, you will learn how to diagnose and treat psychiatric disorders in complex medically ill patients, how to detect the influence of chronic medical conditions on psychiatric symptoms, and how psychological factors can potentially affect physical conditions. The rotation will last at least 2 months and will take place in the inpatient and/or outpatient medical-surgical settings. Some of the unique features of the CL psychiatry rotation, strategies you can use to prepare for the rotation, and approaches that will be helpful in navigating the clinical responsibilities and educational goals of the rotation are included in this chapter.

KEY POINTS

- You can prepare for the CL psychiatry rotation by clarifying how the role of the consultant differs from that of the primary psychiatrist, reviewing learning objectives, and using resources to increase clinical knowledge.

- Direct verbal communication with the primary team can help you clarify the consult question, including the explicit versus implicit request, by direct verbal communication with the primary team.

- Conducting a thorough chart review ensures that you understand the presenting complaint, reason for admission, and main events from the current hospital course.

- Planning your approach in advance, establishing rapport, and performing a comprehensive history and physical examination will ensure a successful interview.

- You should keep your assessment and plan informative and practical, while at the same time maintaining the broadest possible understanding of the patient, which optimally should include pertinent biological, psychological, and social contributors.

- You should directly communicate recommendations to the consulting team, taking a curious and collaborative rather than judgmental or oppositional approach if there is disagreement and document your consult note clearly and concisely, weighing completeness versus confidentiality.

PREPARING FOR THE CONSULTATION-LIAISON PSYCHIATRY ROTATION

In contrast to most patients seen by residents in other rotations, the patients seen in the CL psychiatry setting are, for the most part, not hospitalized for primarily psychiatric reasons or etiologies, and the psychiatrist's goal is to determine whether there is also a psychiatric diagnosis or a role for a psychiatric treatment. Patients are generally acutely ill and medically complex, and they are seen in unfamiliar and physically suboptimal medical, surgical, or obstetrical spaces, which may require a flexibility in approach so as to conduct a psychiatric assessment practically, confidentially, sensitively, and safely. Interruptions may be frequent, distractions may be present, and privacy may be limited; patient physical discomfort may additionally shorten the encounter.

The role of the psychiatrist on the CL psychiatry rotation is not to serve as primary provider but rather to provide an expert opinion and a subsequent recommendation for the medical, pediatrics, surgical, or obstetrical team who is responsible for the patient's care. Practically, this means that the psychiatric consultant's intervention will be in the form of a verbal and/or written recommendation, and the decision to implement it will be that of the primary team. In most institutions, the psychiatry team does not write the orders in the patient's electronic medical record, although this may vary in some programs or institutions. This would be important to clarify at the beginning of the rotation.

In the consultant role, you will find that providers, not patients, request the psychiatric assessment in most cases, so clarification of the patient's awareness and acceptance of the consult will be helpful in fostering patient engagement and rapport. Generally, it is important that the patient consents to the psychiatric assessment, except in situations where there is an acute safety concern or where the patient might lack decision-making capacity.

In contrast to the shift work of the psychiatry emergency service, the prescheduled appointments of the outpatient clinic, and the patient cap of the inpatient psychiatric service, the workflow and workload on the CL rotation are highly unpredictable. In fact, consults are placed by primary teams at various times of the day, which might include "late" consults (i.e., consults that are placed later in the afternoon and need to be seen that same day because of clinical acuity). You may end up with large caseloads of patients with varying levels of acuity and will need to work with supervisors to determine how often each patient should be seen and for what duration. Maintaining a flexible schedule, limiting external commitments, and being prepared for either an unusually slow or a busy day will best help you navigate the rotation.

Prior to the start of the rotation, you should expect to receive learning objectives and orientation materials from the rotation director or program leadership. These materials may contain readings or web-based resources that you may want to review prior to or during the rotation. Additionally, a few important resources can be found in the "Resources" section at the end of the chapter that may be helpful in preparing for the CL psychiatry rotation or in supplementing clinical work throughout the course of the rotation.

SEEKING ATTENDING SUPERVISION

Not only is attending supervision necessary for optimal patient care and from a medicolegal and hospital administrative standpoint, it is also a cornerstone of your educational experience on the clinical rotation. Although the CL service can be busy and finding adequate time for teaching and supervision is challenging, you can take a number of steps to optimize your educational experience. Reviewing expectations at the start of the rotation is important for clarifying the service workflow and supervisory process, the learning goals and objectives, and attending availability. Clarify with the supervising attending physician in advance how and when the attending would like to supervise each case and how best to reach the attending for urgent clinical questions. Some attendings prefer to see the patient from start to finish with the trainee, whereas others request that the trainee see the patient alone first and present the case later for discussion, especially if the trainee has had more CL psychiatry experience. In the latter situation, you may gain more from the supervision if you have taken some time in advance of meeting the supervisor to prepare the case presentation, develop an initial formulation and treatment plan, and review pertinent literature. With increased preparation on your part, the attending may be able to hone in on teaching more advanced skills. In an on-call situation, the attending may be available only for phone supervision, and the focus of the supervision likely will be addressing acute safety concerns.

You may need to familiarize yourself with the format, opportunities, and challenges of *bedside* or nursing station supervision; the CL rotation may be the first psychiatry training experience where this type of supervision is used. Although less structured and in many ways more challenging, bedside supervision provides a learning opportunity that is patient centered and that provides for more role-modeling and autonomy development than do other more traditional forms of (closed-door) psychiatric supervision. During the rotation, you should avail yourself of the opportunity to observe supervisors both interviewing patients and speaking with consulting teams as well as have the supervisor observe you doing the same. Feedback should be requested after individual clinical encounters and during periodic intervals throughout the rotation.

CLARIFYING THE CONSULT QUESTION

When the psychiatric consultation is received, the most fundamental initial step is to clarify the *consult question*. This should be done through direct verbal communication with the primary team. Clarity on what type of help is being requested will determine how best to approach the consultation and how targeted of an assessment is required. Although it is important to determine what the team's explicit (stated) question is, it is also helpful to consider what the implicit (unstated) question or request might actually be. Sometimes, the consult question is very obvious and specific (e.g., "Should we continue this patient's home prescription of sertraline while they are in the hospital?"); other times, the question is broader (e.g., "Is the patient depressed?"). In some cases, consulting teams have a general sense that they need or want psychiatric assistance with a challenging patient, but they need help articulating the question. When the consult question is overly vague or is not a question that can be answered realistically given the particular circumstances of the case, the psychiatric consultant often can help identify a more appropriate or accurate question. See Table 13–1 for examples of explicit and implicit consult questions.

TABLE 13–1.	Examples of explicit and implicit consult questions or requests	
	Explicit (stated) consult questions or requests	**Implicit (unstated) consult questions or requests**
Diagnostic issues	• Evaluate new emotional or behavioral symptoms for a psychiatric disorder • Determine the etiology of an acute change in mental status	• Assist with obtaining collateral and psychiatric records and completing the medication reconciliation
General treatment	• Provide medication recommendations for an acute psychiatric symptom • Provide psychotherapy to assist the patient with coping with illness	• Provide a supportive space to assist the team with coping with a complex patient
Psychopharmacology in the medically ill	• Provide a safer alternative treatment for the patient's chronic psychiatric disorder given current acute medical problems	
Safety	• Assess patient for suicidal ideation or homicidal ideation	• Provide reassurance to team members who feel frightened of a patient
Legal issues	• Assess decision-making capacity	• Give permission to discharge or decline further workup for a patient

TABLE 13–1. Examples of explicit and implicit consult questions or requests *(continued)*

	Explicit (stated) consult questions or requests	Implicit (unstated) consult questions or requests
Substance use	• Assist with management of intoxication or withdrawal	
Behavior	• Manage agitation • Assess psychiatric reason for treatment nonadherence	• Share responsibility for the management of a difficult patient • Help referee a conflict between the primary team and the patient • Make an intervention to improve the patient's adherence
Treatment referrals	• Provide referral for outpatient psychiatric follow-up	• Help resolve a complicated psychosocial situation that is preventing discharge • Facilitate transfer of a difficult patient to psychiatry

Source. Adapted from Ernst 2020.

REVIEWING THE CHART

A thorough chart review is an important early step in the consultation process. The chart review will help you obtain data that are required for a comprehensive and accurate case formulation and also will help you avoid duplication of history taking that has already been done. Because patients often experience frustration with providers who have not reviewed the chart prior to an evaluation, some patients may be easier to engage if they are confident that the provider is familiar with their history. You should make sure that you understand the presenting complaint, reason for admission, and main events from the current hospital course. It is often helpful to begin to outline the note while reviewing the chart. In addition to reviewing daily progress notes from the current admission, essential and helpful elements of the chart for the consultation psychiatrist are summarized in Table 13–2.

TABLE 13–2.   Important elements of the chart review for the consultation psychiatrist

Chart element	Details
Notes	Previous psychiatry and/or neurology notes
	Nursing notes (behavior, sleep, activity level)
	Social work notes (functional status, social supports, living situation)
Data	Brain imaging
	Laboratory results, including, if applicable: TSH, B_{12}, and folate levels; RPR; HIV testing; blood or urine toxicology screens; CSF studies
	ECG: QTc interval
	EEG if done
	Vitals: signs of withdrawal, infection, hypoxia, adverse effects of medication
Medications	Psychotropics
	Medications with neuropsychiatric side effects (e.g., opioids, steroids, anticholinergics, antihistaminergics)
	Medications with potential drug-drug interactions
	Medications that can prolong the QTc interval
External information	State controlled substance database
	External hospital or outpatient records
	State database of mental health encounters

Note.   CSF=cerebrospinal fluid; ECG=electrocardiogram; EEG=electroencephalogram; RPR=rapid plasma reagin; TSH=thyroid-stimulating hormone.

FINDING THE PATIENT AND OPTIMIZING THE INTERVIEW SETTING

Sometimes the patient may not be in their hospital room because of testing or treatment in a specialty unit. Delays in finding a patient often lead to frustration and inefficiency for consultation psychiatrists. Check with nursing staff or the primary team to locate a patient and, if possible, bring the patient back to the room or conduct some of the psychiatric assessment in the other location. Locations to check when a patient is not in their room include the unit or floor lounge, the hemodialysis unit, radiology, and the pre-op or post-op holding area. Long waits for tests in the hospital and lengthy procedures such as dialysis provide an opportunity for you to perform the most important aspects of the assessment.

Because you may be unfamiliar to staff in some of these settings and unaware of unit procedures, you should first introduce yourself and inquire if it is appropriate to interview the patient. Be mindful of limited privacy when interviewing a patient outside the patient's hospital room. You may find it appropriate to return later or on a different day to complete some of the more sensitive components of the assessment. If the patient is physically unavailable for assessment for an extended period (e.g., in the operating room or undergoing a procedure), you should review next steps with the primary team. Depending on the urgency of the consultation, options might include postponing the consultation until the following day, signing out the consultation to the on-call or next-shift psychiatrist, or performing a curbside or electronic consultation (in which general recommendations are provided on the basis of chart review and information gathering from collateral).

Optimizing the physical space for a psychiatric assessment may be challenging even at the bedside within the patient's room. The patient will likely have roommates, staff may enter and leave the room throughout the encounter, and the noise level in units such as the ICU may be high. Interventions that may enhance comfort or privacy include closing the curtain, turning down the volume on televisions and monitors (if deemed appropriate by the nursing staff), speaking quietly, sitting close to the bedside, acknowledging the suboptimal privacy, and giving the patient permission to decline to respond to more sensitive questions. In some situations, you may be able to interview ambulatory patients in a unit lounge or conference room, if available.

INTERVIEWING AND EXAMINING THE PATIENT

Following a series of steps that start with planning your approach and establishing rapport will increase your likelihood of obtaining a comprehensive history and mental status examination.

Planning Your Approach

Planning your approach to the interview prior to meeting the patient is a crucial step to a successful interview. Consideration of the consult question, information obtained from the chart review, and discussion with the primary team will help to formulate the optimal interview approach to obtain the information required to complete the diagnostic assessment and answer the consult question. In most cases, a general approach will enable a full psychiatric assessment, but sometimes a more focused interview and brief observation will be appropriate. Additionally, if the patient is acutely agitated, you must be able to assure the safety of the patient, yourself, your team, and other health care staff and must always plan for a way to end the interview safely if necessary (e.g., never block your exit route, give the patient space).

Establishing Rapport

It is well known that therapeutic rapport is extremely helpful in evaluation and treatment, and much focus should be placed on building appropriate rapport with the patient. This task is critically important given how stressful an inpatient hospitalization may be for the patient, but it also is particularly challenging in the general hospital setting because of such factors as lack of privacy, external distractors, physical discomfort, concerns about confidentiality, lack of familiarity with a new psychiatrist, team-based care, and, for many patients, the unexpected nature of a consult that was not self-initiated.

Treat the patient with respect. Introduce yourself, describe your role, and explain the reason for the consult, as well as provide the names and roles of other members of the consult team. Confirm that you are meeting with the correct patient by asking their full name and date of birth. It is also helpful to inquire as to whether the patient was informed about the consult and whether the patient feels that a psychiatric consultation might be helpful. Acknowledging and addressing (to the extent possible) any privacy or confidentiality concerns can help to build trust and comfort.

Although a busy workload, high acuity, and the sterile environment of the hospital setting can result in a more impersonal approach, you should be sure to demonstrate sensitivity and empathy at all times, validating the feelings of the patient and reflecting on any potential barriers to care that may result from transference or countertransference. An approach that resembles more of a curious, active listening role rather than the usual abstractor of information will enable the patient to feel more comfortable sharing information and will improve your capacity to serve the patient well.

Prior to diving into the questions that must be asked for a complete psychiatric evaluation, address any concerns or barriers to the interview such as current physical discomfort or other symptoms that may not allow the patient to fully participate in the interview. The environment should be optimized for privacy, and steps should be taken to ensure that the patient has hearing or visual aids, water, and an interpreter if needed. If visitors are present in the room, the patient should be asked if they are comfortable with having them there, and if not, those individuals should be asked to leave for at least the initial portion of the interview.

History Taking

You are familiar with the basic psychiatric history and mental status examination, but there are some unique aspects of the history and exam that should not be missed in this type of consultation. It is best to start by asking the patient how they are currently feeling and what their most pressing concerns are at this time. More often than not, patients are happy to discuss their current status, and much information can be obtained from this open-ended approach. If the patient is unwilling or unable to do so (e.g., is unable to speak because of a recent stroke or is somnolent because of a delirium), then you can use a more close-ended interview approach. In taking the history, it is generally less frustrating to patients for the physician to first summarize known information and then ask the patient to correct misinformation, rather than asking the patient to retell the entire story. Unique components of the CL psychiatry history of present illness include the reason for the current hospitalization; the patient's understanding of their medical and psychiatric history and the current treatment plan; and the patient's assessment of the impact of their illness on their daily life, relationships, and roles.

Once the history of present illness has been established, you can conduct a formal review of symptoms to evaluate whether the patient is experiencing any psychiatric symptoms or whether any symptoms are being exacerbated by the patient's current presentation. In order to avoid missing a potential psychiatric symptom or diagnosis, the review of systems should be broad, even if the consult question is narrow. A risk assessment is vital to every psychiatric interview and should include an appropriate suicide and violence risk assessment, an assessment of self-care, and assessment of substance use and potential withdrawal.

For a comprehensive psychiatric formulation and treatment plan rather than one based on an overly biological or medical model, it is imperative to consider the temperament and personality style of the particular individual; presentation under normal circumstances without the stress of illness; and core aspects of identity, such as culture, religion, family role, gender, race, and ethnicity, all of which will help you to understand the personal meaning of the illness to the affected individual. Exploration of the person's resilience in dealing with adversity, historical coping mechanisms and defense styles, meaningful relationships, areas of accomplishment, and sources of pride can be important components of a supportive psychotherapeutic approach and may help to predict resilience in the face of the current illness. Additionally, assessing for structural vulnerabilities, such as discrimination faced and food, financial, and housing insecurity, will ensure that your formulation and plan address the social determinants that may be contributing to the current clinical presentation.

If appropriate to the situation, end-of-life concerns should be discussed openly and with empathy. You also should explore religious or spiritual beliefs and practices, discrimination and adversity experienced, and any additional aspects of the patient's identity that the patient would like to share. Although it is important to respect a patient's privacy regarding spiritual beliefs or aspects of personal identity and to avoid imposing your own beliefs on others, supporting spirituality or addressing specific sources of distress may greatly help the patient during the crisis of an illness. Referrals to hospital chaplains or community resources may be useful for the patient.

In addition to the standard psychiatric mental status examination, a formal cognitive examination should be included in the CL psychiatrist's assessment. A cognitive examination is especially important for patients who are at high risk for a neurocognitive disorder such as delirium. A standardized assessment tool such as the Montreal Cognitive Assessment (MoCA) or Folstein Mini–Mental State Examination (MMSE) can be particularly helpful and provides an important baseline for future presentations. Explain the purpose of the cognitive examination because some patients may feel insulted if not provided with some context.

Physical Examination

Selected aspects of the physical examination, including the neurological examination, will be helpful in identifying potential side effects and toxicity of medication, assessing for withdrawal symptoms, clarifying neurological or metabolic versus psychiatric etiology of a symptom, and diagnosing syndromes such as catatonia.

Wrap-up Visit

After gathering all of the pertinent information, you should begin to wrap up the interview, sharing preliminary thoughts and recommendations with the patient and providing space for the patient to ask any questions or voice concerns. Although you have not yet gathered all the information or come to a final recommendation, it is particularly helpful for you to leave the patient with something concrete, such as a case formulation, a follow-up time, or treatment resources (Yager 1989). This step increases trust and collaboration between you and the patient.

IDENTIFYING AND OBTAINING COLLATERAL INFORMATION

Obtaining collateral information is an essential step in any psychiatric evaluation, especially when evaluating medically complex patients who may not be able to provide a complete or accurate history. Information from family members, partners, friends, and other health care providers can be helpful in assessing accuracy of the patient's history, establishing risk level, and clarifying the course of symptoms. The patient's nurse likely will be able to provide especially helpful information regarding the patient's symptoms and behavior in the hospital. Collateral sources also can be helpful in providing a clear description of the patient's baseline cognitive, emotional, and functional status prior to the hospitalization.

Confidentiality must be respected when obtaining collateral information. Therefore, in most situations, the patient's consent must be obtained first. Exceptions include emergency situations, when concerns about safety are a factor, or when the patient is incapacitated.

DEVELOPING YOUR ASSESSMENT AND PLAN

After gathering all of your data and evaluating the patient, seek out attending supervision to develop your assessment and plan.

Assessment

You will already be familiar with the general process of developing a psychiatric formulation, and much of the assessment process will remain the same for the CL psychiatry rotation, with some variations and additions. Given the limited opportunity to evaluate the patient over an extended period of time, it is prudent to maintain the broadest possible understanding of the patient, which optimally should include pertinent biological, psychological, and social contributors, including cultural and structural formulations (see Chapter 7, "Learning to Develop a Case Formulation"). Rather than a long narrative, the assessment should answer the consult question; contain a balance between oversimplification and overly technical language; and be clear, direct, concise, scientific, professional, informative, and practical without excess use of jargon or abbreviations. It is acceptable to say that more data are needed in order to clarify the diagnosis or establish the treatment plan. Depending on the consult question, the consultant may need to assess whether the presenting symptoms are due to a psychiatric or nonpsychiatric condition, include a risk assessment if there are acute safety concerns, and make a recommendation about the disposition plan. Assessments should be devoid of any reference to diagnosing the consultee's behavior or undermining the current treatment.

The task of the CL psychiatrist is often to determine either 1) the extent to which psychiatric symptoms are being caused or exacerbated by a physical condition or medication or 2) whether the patient's behavior represents a psychiatric disorder or a normal response to the stress of illness. Reading more about potential neuropsychiatric effects of the patient's particular disease or treatments and speaking to the treating team will help make this determination.

Although outside the direct expertise of the consultation psychiatrist, the assessment also might address adequacy of pain or somatic symptom management if pertinent to the presentation. Severe undertreated somatic symptoms will make it difficult to engage the patient in the psychiatric evaluation and will contribute to mood, anxiety, and insomnia symptoms; asking the primary team to address these symptoms will often go a long way toward alleviating the related psychiatric symptoms.

Recommendations

The recommendations may be the only section read by the consultee, so they should be informative and practical, and the recommendations should be listed in clear, concise order. In some circumstances and in deference to the primary team (who is ultimately responsible for the patient's care) or to another consulting team, you may choose to provide suggestions rather than explicit recommendations or directives. If applicable, recommendations should address any acute safety concerns, and input from nursing staff and hospital security may be needed to help mitigate risk. Additional specific recommendations that may be included might consist of further workup to clarify diagnosis (e.g., laboratory results or tests, collateral, additional consultations), practical strategies for managing a patient with challenging behavior or maladaptive coping mechanisms, and pharmacological or behavioral strategies for addressing any acute or chronic psychiatric symptoms. Delineation of which aspects of the plan will be the responsibility of the consultant versus the primary team is also important. The recommendations should include a clear follow-up plan, specifying whether and how often you plan to return to see the patient, whether you are signing off after the initial consultation, and what type of psychiatric care the patient will require after medical clearance. The note should always include information about how to get in contact with you in case of questions, concerns, or new symptoms. A nice final gesture is to thank the consulting team for the consult and express appreciation for the referral (Garrick and Stotland 1982).

COMMUNICATING RECOMMENDATIONS

Because busy consulting team members often do not read chart notes in a timely or complete manner, one of the most important components of the psychiatric consultation is directly communicating recommendations to the primary team and to the patient or family.

To the Team

After formulation of a treatment plan, recommendations should be discussed and communicated directly with the consulting team. If possible, in-person discussion is preferable to avoid any miscommunication and to foster discussion of the thought process behind the recommended treatment plan. Additionally, much of the liaison work is done in the team setting, which typically includes education of the primary team about pertinent psychiatric information and facilitation of improved communication between the primary team and the patient. If an in-person discussion is not possible, a phone call should be used as an alternative. Using a Health Insurance Portability and Accountability Act of 1996 (HIPAA)–secure texting platform is suboptimal but may suffice for some nonemergent recommendations.

To the Patient and Family

A private setting should be used to relay medical information and treatment recommendations to the patient, family, or other supports. Medical jargon should be avoided as much as possible, and you should take time to ensure that the family is comfortable with the information provided and that their questions have been addressed. Ideally, this should be done in person, but it also can be done via a phone conversation. Prior to disclosing private health information, you should be sure that the patient gives permission for you to do so.

HANDLING DISAGREEMENTS WITH THE PRIMARY TEAM

Learning to embrace the role of the consultant and manage scenarios in which the primary team or another consultant disagrees with your recommendations is an important goal of the CL rotation. In this type of situation, take a curious and collaborative rather than judgmental or oppositional approach, exploring the reasoning behind the disagreement and determining if any outstanding concerns could be addressed that would increase acceptance of the recommendations. Although openness, flexibility, and collaboration are valuable attributes of a consultant, you should not change clinically appropriate recommendations because of pressure or guilt, nor should you be afraid to discontinue unnecessary psychotropics or refute a chart-documented psychiatric diagnosis if appropriate (Kontos et al. 2003). Using supervision may be helpful in setting firm boundaries with dissatisfied consulting services and accepting that the primary team retains final responsibility for the patient and can therefore make the choice to accept or reject the consultant's recommendations. You may choose to sign off on the case if the recommendations are not being followed but should remain available without malice for any follow-up questions or requests for follow-up evaluations.

DOCUMENTING YOUR CONSULTATION

The consult note must serve the function of answering the consult question. Keep in mind that in contrast to most psychiatric notes (which have an added privacy and confidentiality status in some health care settings), this note must be designed to be viewed and used by the entire treatment team, and it is more easily available to the patient to review. You must therefore decide which details are essential information for the entire team to know to successfully care for the patient. This entails carefully weighing completeness versus confidentiality versus immediate clinical relevance (Garrick and Stotland 1982). It is important to avoid too much psychiatric jargon and keep the note well organized and succinct.

FOLLOWING UP

To identify and resolve all problems pertaining to a consultation, a single visit sometimes may not be sufficient, and several encounters may be needed. Additionally, the patient's mental status and overall presentation or the consult question might change and evolve during the hospitalization. Patients requiring psychiatric one-to-one observation (e.g., suicidal, agitated, violent, or acutely psychotic patients) should be seen daily. In other situations, patients can be seen on an as-needed or less frequent basis depending on the psychiatric problem and consult question being addressed. If a new psychiatric medication is recommended, the patient should be seen for a follow-up visit to assess response and tolerability.

SPECIFIC CHALLENGES AND STRATEGIES

⌘ **My patient refused the consult.** Generally, it is important that the patient consents to the psychiatric assessment, except in situations where there is an acute safety concern or where the patient might lack decision-making capacity. If you are able to do so, explore the patient's concerns about the consult and rationale for refusing. Many patients initially refuse but will accept evaluation after you explain the reason for the consult, provide empathic listening, and acknowledge their frustrations. Ask a member from the consulting team to join you in explaining to the patient the reason for the consult and enlist the help of family members and friends if available. Suggest to the patient that you might return at a more convenient time to try again. If the patient continues to refuse but has a better relationship with the primary team, it may be appropriate to guide the primary team in performing their own assessment (e.g., of capacity). For some consult questions, you also may be able to provide recommendations based on chart review and discussion with collateral.

⌘ **The primary team wants me to fix a difficult patient.** In a situation like this, attempt to understand both the team's and patient's concerns and work to build a therapeutic alliance with the patient. Identify any contributing psychiatric symptoms or structural vulnerabilities. Provide support for both the patient and the primary team, while at the same time setting appropriate limits with the patient and reasonable expectations with the primary team as to how you can be helpful. Once you have fully assessed the patient, educate the primary team on the reason for the difficult behavior and provide several strategies for how they can best manage it, modeling a more therapeutic interaction or helping to write a behavior plan if appropriate.

⌘ **The primary team requests that a difficult patient be transferred to psychiatry.** Frustration, helplessness, and fear of difficult patients often lead to a consultation request to transfer the patient to an inpatient psychiatric unit. Using a collaborative and empathic approach, explore the reasoning behind the team's concern because the team may have additional information or observations that might change your assessment. Explain the clinical criteria for inpatient admission and the realistic therapeutic goals that can be accomplished on an inpatient psychiatric unit and review management strategies for acute versus chronic psychiatric symptoms. Do not change clinically appropriate recommendations because of pressure or guilt, and use supervision to help you set firm boundaries. Rather than signing off on the case, continue to work with the primary team and the patient to provide appropriate management strategies for the remainder of the inpatient medical-surgical admission and assist with a postdischarge psychiatric follow-up plan if appropriate.

SELF-REFLECTIVE QUESTIONS

1. When I think of the times that I have called medicine or other specialty consults on my patients, which strategies for communicating with the consultant worked well and which did not?
2. What type of work am I good at, and what type of work has been challenging for me?
3. How might I best prepare myself to handle the unpredictable CL psychiatry service workflow, complex patients, and demanding liaison role?

RESOURCES

Textbooks

Ackerman K, Dimartini A: Psychosomatic Medicine (Pittsburgh Pocket Psychiatry Series). New York, Oxford University Press, 2015

Fogel BS, Greenberg DB: Psychiatric Care of the Medical Patient, 3rd Edition. New York, Oxford University Press, 2016

Levenson JL: The American Psychiatric Association Publishing Textbook of Psychosomatic Medicine and Consultation-Liaison Psychiatry, 3rd Edition. Washington DC, American Psychiatric Association Publishing, 2019

Philbrick KL, Rundell JR, Netzel PJ, et al: Clinical Manual of Psychosomatic Medicine: A Guide to Consultation-Liaison Psychiatry, 2nd Edition. Washington, DC, American Psychiatric Publishing, 2011

Stern TA, Freudenreich O, Smith FA, et al (eds): Massachusetts General Hospital Handbook of General Hospital Psychiatry, 7th Edition. New York, Elsevier, 2017

Classic Papers

Garrick TR, Stotland NL: How to write a psychiatric consultation. Am J Psychiatry 139(7):849–55, 1982 6979943

Kontos N, Freudenreich O, Querques J, et al: The consultation psychiatrist as effective physician. Gen Hosp Psychiatry 25(1):20–3, 2003 12583923

Mermelstein HT, Wallack JJ: Confidentiality in the age of HIPAA: a challenge for psychosomatic medicine. Psychosomatics 49(2):97–103, 2008 18354061

Schiff SK, Pilot ML: An approach to psychiatric consultation in the general hospital. AMA Arch Gen Psychiatry 1:349–57, 2008 14442743

Yager J: Specific components of bedside manner in the general hospital psychiatric consultation: 12 concrete suggestions. Psychosomatics 30(2):209–12, 1989 2710920

Online Resource

Academy of Consultation-Liaison Psychiatry: C-L curriculum for psychiatry residents. Bethesda, MD, Academy of Consultation-Liaison Psychiatry, 2022. Available at: www.clpsychiatry.org/training-career/resident-curriculum. Accessed October 16, 2022.

Journals

Journal of the Academy of Consultation-Liaison Psychiatry
General Hospital Psychiatry

REFERENCES

Ernst CL: Academy of Consultation-Liaison Psychiatry how to guide: doing a consult. Bethesda, MD, Academy of Consultation-Liaison Psychiatry, October 9, 2020. Available at: www.clpsychiatry.org/wp-content/uploads/ACLP-How-To-Guide-Doing-a-Consult-2020.pdf. Accessed on February 11, 2022.

Garrick TR, Stotland NL: How to write a psychiatric consultation. Am J Psychiatry 139(7):849–855, 1982 6979943

Kontos N, Freudenreich O, Querques J, et al: The consultation psychiatrist as effective physician. Gen Hosp Psychiatry 25(1):20–23, 2003 12583923

Yager J: Specific components of bedside manner in the general hospital psychiatric consultation: 12 concrete suggestions. Psychosomatics 30(2):209–212, 1989 2710920

CHAPTER 14

Working in a Multidisciplinary Team

Sourav Sengupta, M.D., M.P.H.

As you walk up to the main desk, the unit clerk greets you, and you introduce yourself. What do you call yourself? You go with your first name and say you are one of the residents starting your new rotation. You make sure to note the clerk's name. She introduces you to the charge nurse, who is busy getting the report from the overnight shift and handing out nursing assignments for the day. After she finishes up, she shows you around the unit and introduces you to different members of the team and their roles. At one point, you note that she is mispronouncing your name. Do you correct her now or hold off? You decide to introduce yourself directly the next time you meet a new team member, offering a clear pronunciation and using a little humor to defuse the situation. You meet one of the other nurses passing medications, a milieu technician preparing to lead a group on problem-solving skills, and a therapist discussing strategies with the team on engaging a neurovegetative patient. As you get your bearings, your attending physician walks up and welcomes you to the team. You take time to acclimate yourself to your new patients and begin your rounds. You are now part of a new multidisciplinary team working together to improve the lives of your patients.

KEY POINTS

- Get to know the members of your multidisciplinary team—who are they and what are their roles?

- In situations in which you are not fully empowered (yet), be prepared to gather and wield influence in the best interests of your patients, team members, and yourself.

- Communicate in a kind and respectful manner that clearly conveys your thoughts while valuing and supporting those of others.

- Although we can and should acknowledge challenges with the medical hierarchy, finding ways to better understand your supervisors and how they work can improve team functioning.

- The Golden Rule helps in navigating challenges that inevitably arise in training and clinical work.

THE MULTIDISCIPLINARY TEAM

Why work in teams, anyway? As a psychiatrist, you will be working with patients who are often vulnerable, underserved, and functionally impaired. Most patients struggling with significant mental health challenges benefit from many modalities of support. They may need to work with a psychotherapist to address an impairing emotional pattern of avoidance or interpersonal communication difficulties. They may need the assistance of a social worker to help them connect to important community social services. They may need the guidance of an occupational therapist to learn a new adaptive skill or a physical therapist to improve their conditioning after a period of prolonged inactivity. They may need the support of a nutritionist to help them understand new dietary restrictions or healthy eating strategies. Providing excellent health care relies on experts with the skills and knowledge in these broad and disparate disciplines working together to benefit the patient (Nancarrow et al. 2013; White et al. 2018). Your role as the psychiatrist is often to ensure that the multidisciplinary team is working well together toward the improved functioning and well-being of the patient. At the same time, especially during residency training, working in a multidisciplinary team is an opportunity to learn a wide range of knowledge and skills from a broad diversity of perspectives. Although you may not ultimately function as the primary psychotherapist or case manager when in practice, you may need to assist or supervise team members, coordinate with them, and at times advocate for them to change course. Residency training is an excellent opportunity to learn and develop the skills to function well within and to lead multidisciplinary teams.

GET TO KNOW YOUR TEAM

Working well in a multidisciplinary team requires getting to know your teammates. Be sure to introduce yourself to and remember the names and roles of different team members. You might want to even jot down a few details when you first start on a team to help you remember who is who and who does what. In your first few team meetings, as participants go around the table introducing themselves, make a diagram of names and roles for yourself. Some team members will ask you more about yourself. If you are comfortable sharing a bit about yourself, reciprocate by learning a bit about them as well. Asking about their children in school or an ailing parent or a favorite pet can go a long way toward establishing that you want to know them as individuals and not just for what they can or must do for you. Take the time to learn what each member's role is in the clinical work of the team. If you are unsure, ask others or the team member directly to clarify for you. As you continue to work with the team, you will begin to understand individuals' strengths and challenges. Note and positively reinforce others' strengths and do your best to support others in their challenges. If your coresident or a unit social worker skillfully diffuses a tense family meeting but struggles to organize competing team priorities, highlight their impressive family engagement skills in morning conference and privately "run the list" with them twice a day to make sure you are both on the same page in terms of priorities and strategies.

POWER VERSUS INFLUENCE

As a trainee, you will not necessarily be or feel empowered to make as many decisions as you might like in your daily work. Your attending physician might set the time for rounding. The charge nurse might not support your plan to take a patient off the unit. A family might have other ideas about a complex patient's treatment or disposition plan. Although some aspects of this decision-making power will likely change as you progress in your career (someday soon, you will get to decide when the team rounds), you might be surprised at how often you will not hold all the cards. Sometimes, this is really as it should be. While on call covering multiple units, you might quickly assess a patient and wonder if they might benefit from being taken off one-to-one observation status, although that decision may be better suited to the team currently working with that patient. Other times, perhaps you could or even should be able to make a particular decision but will not be allowed to do so. Utilization review and prior authorization challenges come to mind. Often enough, during the early years of your residency, you will be variably included in decisions on which you would like to weigh in. In situations in which you do not have the power to make the decision, it can be just as, if not more, important to learn to wield *influence.* Develop a reputation for being helpful, accessible, skilled, knowledgeable, and willing to speak up for others, and team members will naturally include you in decision-making. Learn to concisely and compellingly share your perspective and flexibly support a decision or direction that is not your preference. Pitch in regularly to help with the work of the team. Frequently give credit to others for their positive work. Share your appreciation when others help or support you.

From time to time, you will encounter situations in which you are asked to be involved in a process with which you disagree. These may be clinical issues (e.g., medication or disposition decision), academic concerns (e.g., the final grade assigned to a rotating medical student), or ethical quandaries (e.g., the decision to disclose the full details of a negative outcome to a patient's family). Try to determine if this is an issue of low, medium, or high importance. For low- and medium-importance issues, practice wielding the influence and/or power that are available to you to shape the outcome. For issues of high importance, we sometimes have to find ways to influence the outcome that are unrelated to the power or influence you have in a system. Although this does not mean that you have to sacrifice your career trajectory for every major challenging decision, it does mean that sometimes living up to your ideals can carry a cost. Some battles are worth the costs, whereas others are not. For these challenging issues that are of high importance to you, consider the "mirror" test. At the end of the day, will you be able to look at yourself in the mirror and be satisfied that you did all that you could to ensure that the team adopted your perceived right course of action? If not, reassess the situation to see if you can do more now or in the future to shape the process or outcome. Be sure to value your efforts to do all that you could to positively influence the process, regardless of the outcome. Speaking up for a colleague who feels unheard, advocating to address a patient's psychosocial challenges, or shielding a less experienced trainee from harassment—the process of taking action in line with deeply held beliefs can be incredibly meaningful for you and your team.

This challenging dance between power and influence can also be the domain in which implicit bias and systemic discrimination can rear their heads. We all can work to examine our implicit biases (take a self-assessment at Harvard's Project Implicit: https://implicit.harvard.edu/implicit). If you are in a position of influence, power, or privilege, invest the time and energy to be an ally and encourage the input and agency of less empowered team members. Note and bring up challenging process dynamics when working with your supervisors. For example, if you note a female colleague's input being ignored by a team leader in favor of a male colleague's similar input, make an effort to credit her contribution.

SUCCESSFUL TEAM COMMUNICATION

You have probably heard of the saying "It's not what you say, it's how you say it." As you progress in your psychiatric training, you will spend a great deal of time and energy developing knowledge and skills in "how you say it" with patients and families. But equally important is how we communicate with our colleagues in a multidisciplinary team setting. Kindness with and respect for every single member of the team is critically important. Saying "please" and "thank you" goes a long way. Taking the opportunity to close the loop by reflecting back what you understand of others' perspectives helps others feel heard. Asking others' opinions while advocating for yours demonstrates your interest in other perspectives. Making a specific effort to credit others' contributions and achievements shows that you value the important contributions of all, from nurses to aides, from clerks to custodians.

Communicating successfully during team encounters and meetings is critical to collaborating in the successful care of your patients. You want to ensure that you are encouraging and receptive to the observations and opinions of other team members. If a team member has been overlooked or has not had the opportunity to contribute, be the one to invite them into the discussion. While taking care to be responsive to and not to interrupt others, be sure not to miss your opportunity to offer your perspective. In a busy team meeting, this may mean nonverbally signaling your interest in offering your impression with your face, hands, or body posture. Take a moment to consider whether your non-verbal signals are indicating interest and engagement in the discussion. Similarly, as you advance in your training and begin to lead multidisciplinary discussions, be sure to invite the participation of all relevant team members. Although some decisions ultimately need to be made by a team leader, most decisions tend to develop by consensus. If you are participating in a discussion that seems to be stagnating (e.g., multiple perspectives complaining about the same issue), see if you can move the discussion forward by summarizing the primary issues, asking if there are differing opinions, and progressing toward the next stage in the decision-making process.

Some communications work well in written or electronic formats, whereas others do not. A quick question to your patient's social worker about collateral history or disposition planning may be perfect for the brief, sequential style of communication of an email. A difference of opinion about the formulation for a complex personality issue may lend itself better to a live, in-person discussion with key team members. Giving feedback, especially negative or constructive, should always be done in person and in private, with sincere and authentic observations about areas of strengths as well as areas for improvement (with specific suggestions for how to improve) (Patterson et al. 2022). In general, for matters where there may be a difference of opinion, a complaint or concern, or other situation that may present an opportunity for some conflict or confrontation, you may be better off meeting to discuss in person. For example, you can soften constructive criticism with nonverbal communication signals that you understand that this is a challenging process (e.g., head tilt or leaning in), that you regret having to bring up the subject (e.g., shrug of the shoulders), and that you still care for and value the other team member (e.g., a smile, a thumbs up, a wave goodbye).

Managing Up

As you progress through your professional development journey, you will take on varying levels of autonomy and leadership. As you move into more senior roles, look for opportunities to progressively take on more leadership roles, although you will often be in a middle management role. You may be responsible for managing the clinical and educational needs of medical students or running the clinical logistics of your consultation-liaison team. Simultaneously, you will need to take direction from your attending around coordinating and completing clinical documentation, treatment planning, and complex disposition challenges. For better or for worse, our medical training system is an apprenticeship model. You will benefit from learning how to "manage up" (Zuber and James 2001).

It can be useful to discreetly learn more about your supervisors' and superiors' values and priorities, strengths and challenges, and preferred clinical and work patterns. Although your values and priorities do not have to align exactly with those of your supervisor, understanding where they are coming from and what drives them can help you find win-win strategies or understand where you are likely to view issues from a different perspective. Discreetly determining a supervisor's challenges can allow you to find ways to be supportive in a complimentary fashion, and understanding the supervisor's strengths can help you determine what set of knowledge, skills, and attitudes you can best learn from them. For example, help a chronically tardy attending who has a masterful grasp on cognitive-behavioral therapy (CBT) by organizing your rounds efficiently, allowing you more time to develop more advanced CBT skills with them. Finally, learning how your supervisor prefers to work clinically can offer opportunities to improve the functioning and efficiency of the team. At times, if and when you think you could manage certain workflows better or more efficiently, gauge whether your supervisor may be open to this feedback and, if so, make a pitch. But do not feel bad if a busy clinical attending seems set in their ways that do not seem ideal to you. After all, sometimes what you can take away is how you want to do things differently when you are in a more senior role.

SPECIFIC CHALLENGES AND STRATEGIES

⌘ **A surgery attending just consulted me frantically for a patient found crying in the bathroom after major surgery. How should I handle this consult?** Throughout your residency, you will intermittently have to navigate challenging situations, from clinical crises to serious team conflicts. There will be times when a nonpsychiatric team member's crisis will not appear as acute to you. In these situations, remember to be professional and kind while trusting your impulses to not be overly reactive. When navigating crises and conflicts, try to remember the Golden Rule: Treat others as you would want to be treated.

⌘ **Loud shouts ring out from a patient room down the hall from me while clinicians and staff from all over the unit rush there to help. What should I do?** In more acute situations, remember the general advice in any crisis: Take a moment to center and orient yourself before diving in. What is actually happening? What can you offer to assist? Try hard to communicate clearly and professionally, directing others as appropriate, taking care of the responsibilities that fall within your role. Afterward, check in with team members to see if they need to process what happened, if any amends need to be made, and if anything can be learned from the experience to improve future crisis responses.

⌘ **An emergency department physician is pushing back on my desire to discharge a patient who is well known to my outpatient clinic team and threatens to call my attending.** When things are feeling unsettled, remember the ultimate goal of keeping patient safety and well-being at the forefront of your priorities. Communicate your viewpoint calmly and confidently. Ask others to explain their concerns, even if you suspect you may disagree. Search for potential compromise. Remember that sometimes, doing the right thing bears some cost, but one that may be well worth it.

SELF-REFLECTIVE QUESTIONS

1. Do other members of the multidisciplinary team know me better than I know them? If so, can I invest some time to get to understand them and their role better?
2. Thinking of the last significant team conflict I was involved in, how could my communications or actions contribute to a more positive outcome in the future?
3. How well do I understand the strengths and challenges of my team members, both more experienced and less experienced? What am I doing or what more could I do to learn from their strengths and support them in their challenges?

RESOURCE

Patterson K, Grenny J, McMillan R, et al: Crucial Conversations: Tools for Talking When the Stakes Are High, 3rd Edition. New York, McGraw-Hill Contemporary, 2022

REFERENCES

Nancarrow SA, Booth A, Ariss S, et al: Ten principles of good interdisciplinary team work. Hum Resour Health 11:19, 2013 23663329
Patterson K, Grenny J, McMillan R, et al: Crucial Conversations: Tools for Talking When the Stakes Are High, 3rd Edition. New York, McGraw-Hill Contemporary, 2022
White BAA, Eklund A, McNeal T, et al: Facilitators and barriers to ad hoc team performance. Proc Bayl Univ Med Cent 31(3):380–384, 2018 29904320
Zuber TJ, James EH: Managing your boss. Fam Pract Manag 8(6):33–36, 2001 11547394

CHAPTER 15

Outpatient Services

Tram Nguyen, M.D.
Melissa Martinez, M.D.
Natalie Maples, Dr.P.H.

Compared with short-term inpatient work, outpatient work is focused on establishing a diagnosis, promoting and maintaining stability, and building relationships with patients. It provides opportunities to engage patients in shared decision-making and to see improvement over time. Although the transition from inpatient to outpatient clinical practice can initially be accompanied by insecurity and doubt, eventually these feelings are replaced with acquisition of new skills and confidence. Some of you may find that you prefer the routine and structure of an outpatient clinical setting, whereas others may learn that you enjoy the intensity and unpredictability of the hospital environment. Learning which environment is a better fit for you as an individual is an important part of your training. In this chapter we discuss common challenges that accompany outpatient work and strategies to overcome them.

KEY POINTS

- An essential part of outpatient treatment is to engage patients in a shared decision-making process.

- Outpatient treatment provides you the opportunity to hone your independent clinical decision-making skills with indirect supervision.

- It is important to navigate holding boundaries while maintaining rapport with your patients.

- Learning effective time management helps preserve work-life balance.

PATIENT AUTONOMY AND SHARED DECISION-MAKING

As you transition to outpatient work, the focus shifts from acute symptom stabilization to recovery, which is defined as "a process of change through which individuals improve their health and wellness, live self-directed lives, and strive to reach their full potential" (Substance Abuse and Mental Health Services Administration 2018). Discuss with your patient what recovery looks like for them and invite them into a shared decision-making (SDM) process. SDM is critical because patient engagement improves clinical outcomes and fosters safety. Patients whose preferences are respected are more likely to feel empowered, adhere to treatment, and trust their doctors (Butterworth and Campbell 2014; Parchman et al. 2010; Stacey et al. 2014; Weiner et al. 2013; Wilson et al. 2010). Taking a patient's cultural identity and structural experiences into consideration can help guide your approach (see Chapter 8, "Working With Historically Oppressed Patient Populations"). SDM also implicitly acknowledges that there is increased patient autonomy in outpatient work. Patients may disagree with your diagnosis and treatment plan, miss appointments, and misunderstand how to take their medications. Although this may be frustrating at times, remembering that patients are partners in SDM is helpful. Discuss concerns about medications with your patients. Maintain a stance of curiosity, a technique often used in psychotherapy, to help you learn about the patient. Ask in a nonjudgmental way what factors contributed to their decisions to understand relevant barriers to care. To maintain rapport, align with the patient—let them know that you share a common goal to improve their mental health, even if you disagree with their decisions about treatment.

Many times, there is no one clear "right" answer. Although using FDA-approved, evidence-based recommendations is advisable, the "best" option may be the one with which your patient is willing to engage. For example, you may want to maximize their fluoxetine dosage to address residual anxiety symptoms, whereas they want to try an alternative medication to minimize sexual side effects. Engaging in comprehensive formulation of your patient's symptoms and experience can help guide your treatment (see Chapter 7, "Learning to Develop a Case Formulation").

INDIRECT SUPERVISION

Both you and your patient will have less supervision in the outpatient setting. The idea of not having immediate feedback from an attending physician can feel daunting. Approach this as an opportunity to practice your self-directed learning skills, enhance independent clinical decision-making abilities, and learn when to consult your attending. If you feel unsure about a treatment plan but your patient is not presenting with acute symptoms or an emergency, you can continue to monitor the patient and formalize a plan at the next visit after discussing the case with your attending. Caring for patients hovering between stable and unstable, such as a passively suicidal or actively psychotic patient who is not under 24-hour supervision, can feel uncomfortable at first. Over time, you will become comfortable with the concept of *stable instability*, in which patients live meaningful lives while managing chronic psychiatric symptoms. It is important to seek guidance from your attending when learning how to manage these challenging circumstances. Discuss with your attending what to do if an acute concern arises and your attending is not immediately available. Anticipate this possibility and have a plan in place. Can you reach the attending by phone? Is another attending or a senior resident available?

You may fear loss of rapport if you do not know the answer to a patient's knowledge-based question. However, evidence has shown that a doctor's consultation skills—appearing interested, listening well, explaining clearly, demonstrating a willingness to discuss topics, and involving the patient in the decision-making process—factor strongly into building trust with the patient (Ridd et al. 2009). It is all right to say, "That's a great question. I'll get back to you." If the patient has a question about a medication, it can be helpful to pull out a psychopharmacology book and review the side effects alongside your patient. You can also create tip sheets for yourself of common psychiatric conditions and treatment recommendations.

NAVIGATING RELATIONSHIP BUILDING WHILE MAINTAINING BOUNDARIES

A perk to outpatient work is the opportunity to build long-term relationships with your patients. As such, it is important for you to establish your boundaries early. Boundaries can come in both tangible and intangible forms, ranging from how often and when to respond to messages to setting limits on self-disclosures.

As with any long-term relationship, times of conflict inevitably will arise. This is another area where SDM can be helpful. Discuss your patient's goals with them and decide with the help of your attending which treatment approach is the best fit. For example, your patient wishes to stop an antipsychotic medication, whereas you feel that the medication is needed to manage his psychosis. In discussion, your patient reveals that he is too sedated on the current regimen. You may agree together to reduce the dosage or change the medication to meet the patient's needs as well as the treatment goals.

Another potential conflict with patients can arise if you disagree with the patient's request for disability or leave of absence. These situations can be challenging and have an impact on the therapeutic alliance you have worked hard to craft. Read these request forms carefully and explain to your patient that you are required to fill out the forms honestly. Decide which parts you can and will fill out and which parts you cannot or will not. If there are parts you cannot complete, explain why. For example, explain to the patient that because you did not do a physical examination, you cannot comment on sections regarding physical limitations. You can work with the patient to navigate the situation together, such as directing the patient back to their primary care provider for a physical examination. It is also helpful to let your patient know that the final decision (i.e., how the form is interpreted) is up to the disability agency or the patient's employer.

For you as an outpatient provider, boundaries around direct clinical care hours are often part of clinic policy, meaning that your patients are not monitored 24 hours a day, with immediate access to a physician. It is prudent to create a safety net for yourself and your patients. Know who will cover direct clinical care when you are not available, such as after hours and when you are on vacation. Be sure to coordinate with clinic staff so that everyone is aware of the coverage plan. Share this information with your patient verbally and in writing, such as in an "After Visit Summary." It can be reassuring for you and your patients to know how they can receive help when you are not around. Share the number for local crisis lines and the National Suicide Hotline, which are available 24 hours a day. In addition, you may leave an "out of office" message on your voice mail or email so that patients are reminded of your plans and the available resources.

TIME MANAGEMENT

A large portion of outpatient work is indirect patient care—a substantial amount of time is spent answering messages, refilling medications, completing paperwork, and finishing documentation. Discuss with your attending the expected turnaround time for responding to patient messages.

Most clinics have a policy for how often to check and respond to messages, but if not, check with your clinical director or supervisor for guidance. For example, you may be responsible for checking messages intermittently until the clinic closes or just twice a day (e.g., at the beginning of and halfway through the day). Clinics often have standard practices for whether messages received after a certain time can wait until the next morning or should be forwarded to an answering service or on-call clinician. Inform your patients about the clinic structure and your availability and what to do in an emergency. It is not a realistic expectation from your patient or yourself that you will answer any message immediately. If your patient is leaving you multiple urgent messages, ask why. Do they need a higher level of care? What other services are they underutilizing (e.g., nursing, pharmacy, or front desk staff) that you can direct them to? You may share care for your patient with a therapist and collaborate to address your patient's additional needs.

One of the most time-consuming activities is documentation. Unfortunately, the use of electronic health records (EHRs) has increased the likelihood of burnout rather than reducing it (Tajirian et al. 2020). Take advantage of features within the EHR, including templates, shortcuts, and autofill functions, to save time. Consider the purpose and audience of your notes. In general, consider the following when writing notes:

1. *Clinical communication to other providers*—Would a colleague understand your clinical reasoning? Consider what information a provider in the emergency department might need to understand the clinical picture if they were quickly scanning the patient's most recent outpatient note.
2. *Rationale for medical decision-making*—Have you documented the options considered, the rationale behind choices made, the potential risks and benefits of the medications discussed, and the risks and benefits of not moving forward with the recommended treatment plan (Gutheil 2004)? Be familiar with the legal requirements for prescribing controlled substances, such as checking your local controlled substance monitoring program, and document that you fulfilled the requirements.
3. *Billing and insurance purposes*—Did you document enough to support your billing level?

Remember that per the 21st Century Cures Act (Pub. L. No. 114-255), patients have immediate access to your notes unless you indicate in the EHR specifically why the notes are blocked, such as to protect the safety of your patient or at the patient's request (patients can still request these blocked notes by going through medical records). As such, keep the language professional and relevant to clinical decision-making and avoid unnecessary commentaries. Consider what it would be like to read your notes through the lens of your patient and be ready to discuss your notes if your patient asks you about them. With this being said, *writing more does not necessarily equate to writing better notes.* For example, a medication visit note should focus on information relevant to diagnosis and treatment choices as well as positive and adverse responses to treatment. On the other hand, psychotherapy notes in the EHR can be kept brief, noting general trends (e.g., "processed marital discord") and psychotherapeutic intervention techniques used. You can keep separate, more detailed psychotherapy process notes that can be used for discussion in supervision. The rule of thumb for notes in the EHR is to write the least number of words that supports your assessment and plan.

SAFETY IN THE OUTPATIENT SETTING

Similar to work on an inpatient unit, it is prudent to be mindful of your patient's safety as well as your own in the outpatient setting. Consider the layout of your office. Ideally, both you and your patient should be able to see one another and have unobstructed access to the exit. A patient can feel threatened if their access to the door is blocked or doors are shut completely. Having your back to the patient while documenting can discourage dialogue and also be a safety risk. In addition, be aware of your clinic's emergency procedures and whether your office has a panic button. Unfortunately, 72%–96% of residents report being verbally threatened, and another 36%–56% report being physically threatened during residency training (Antonius et al. 2010). These interactions can occur in any setting, highlighting that safety is always a consideration.

Consider the decor within your office and be mindful of personal items that can affect the patient's experience. For example, putting up your credentials can seem pretentious, but it can also assure your patient that you are a qualified provider. Items such as personal photos can be a safety issue and a transference issue in psychotherapy. As a resident, you may not have complete control over your office space, but it is important to keep these details in mind.

DETERMINING LEVEL OF CARE

Be familiar with the legal requirements for placing a psychiatric hold in the area where you practice. If you decide to place a patient on a psychiatric hold (i.e., an involuntary or emergency evaluation) after completing a risk assessment, know the clinic protocol for who you need to contact and the fastest way to do so. You likely will need to contact your supervisor, the front desk, and perhaps even security for assistance. If you provide telepsychiatry services, you may need to have a welfare check performed on patients who are not physically in your office. It is prudent to ask your patient at the beginning of the session where they are located so that you can share this information with those performing the welfare check. Some counties have police officers or first responders who are specifically trained to respond to welfare checks. If possible, request these services for your patients.

KNOWING YOUR RESOURCES

In many cases, your patient may not need acute hospitalization but can benefit from additional support. Approach your patient holistically—consider what they need in order to function in their daily lives and who their other care providers are. Many patients taking long-term medications can develop significant metabolic side effects and drug-drug interactions. It is important to collaborate with their primary care doctors and other medical specialties to ensure safety and minimize medical errors. Likewise, it is important to consider psychiatric comorbidities. For example, substance use can have significant impacts on a patient's response to medications and ability to adhere to treatment. Consider medication-assisted treatment and connecting patients to support groups such as Alcoholics Anonymous or the National Alliance on Mental Illness, as indicated. You may write letters to support your patient's access to resources such as disability benefits, emotional support animals, supportive housing, and residential or sober living environments.

If your patient needs more intensive medication management and psychotherapy than what you can offer, consider referring them to a higher level of care such as an intensive outpatient program or a partial hospitalization where they can be seen multiple times a week. Sometimes being connected to these higher levels of care is enough to stabilize the patient and prevent hospitalization. Likewise, these programs can serve as an important step-down option for patients after an acute hospitalization so that they have longer symptom stability before returning to a regular outpatient schedule. Similarly, you also may refer your patient for neuropsychological testing or somatic treatments such as electroconvulsive therapy or repetitive transcranial magnetic stimulation if their symptoms persist.

Psychosocial components also can have great impacts on your patient's mental health. Becoming unemployed or living in chronic unstable housing can affect a patient's ability to engage in treatment. Talk with the case managers, the social workers, or your attending about resources that may be available to your patients, such as referrals for job rehabilitation, bus or meal vouchers, and housing vouchers. Being aware of these resources and understanding the referral process help you guide your patients, even if you do not directly make the referral yourself.

PREPARING FOR TERMINATION

Outpatient work provides physicians with the opportunity to develop longitudinal working relationships with patients. This is true for medication management and especially true for psychotherapy. However, residency is unique because any therapeutic relationship you develop has an inevitable end date. As a resident, you must anticipate that your entire caseload will need to be transferred at the end of your training (or end of rotation). Termination within residency can feel especially jarring because it is predetermined and not dictated by completion of therapeutic treatment or by mutual agreement between you and your patient. It can be an anxiety-inducing experience for you and your patient, but with preparation and planning, it may be a meaningful opportunity to reflect on the work you have done together. Have conversations with your medication and psychotherapy supervisors to consider how far in advance you should discuss termination with your patient. Typically, it can be shorter for medication patients and should be longer for therapy patients to allow time for them to process the transition with you. It is not unusual for a patient to offer you gifts, especially around termination. Be familiar with your institution's policy around accepting gifts. As a rule of thumb, it is usually ethical to accept gifts of low monetary value or homemade gifts. Regardless of the monetary value, gifts often represent a meaningful gesture from your patient. As such, it is advisable to acknowledge and discuss the gift with your patient.

HAND-OFFS

Hand-offs are an essential part of ensuring smooth clinical care between providers. Hand-offs can be in the form of shift change summaries where you sign out pertinent information to the on-call provider or overnight staff. In the outpatient setting, hand-offs are often part of the termination process in the form of transfer summaries to the patient's next provider after you complete the rotation or at the end of your residency. Include relevant information in the hand-off to help the next provider make informed decisions about the patient, such as prior treatment trials and responses, current active issues, and considerations for next steps in care. Likewise, ensure that your patient understands their follow-up plan, such as who the next provider will be, when they can expect a follow-up visit, and who they can contact if urgent issues arise during the transition.

SPECIFIC CHALLENGES AND STRATEGIES

⌘ **My patient is not taking their medications.** Poor insight, side effects, transference issues, and structural barriers often play a role in patients' decisions to not take medications. For example, a patient with schizophrenia may not take their medication because they do not believe they have psychosis. Involving family support, prescribing a medication formulation that increases adherence (e.g., a long-acting injectable), using tools that facilitate a structured routine for medication administration (e.g., weekly pill containers, alarms on personal phones) can help. Similarly, a patient will not take a medication if they perceive that the side effects outweigh the benefits or because of what the medication represents to them. Furthermore, patients will not take medications they cannot afford. Many commonly prescribed medications have generic forms available. If your patient has insurance, you (or your attending) might be asked to justify your medication choice by filling out a medication prior authorization. Fill out the authorization as quickly as possible because your patient will not get their medication until insurance approves this form. Delays in the process can delay your patient's treatment. GoodRx (www.goodrx.com) is a website that provides coupons for medications not covered by insurance. Ultimately, you will find greater success in your patient's treatment if you collaborate with your patient, design a treatment regimen that meets their real-world needs, and discuss fears or concerns related to medication openly.

⌘ **My patient frequently does not show up for appointments.** A patient may miss appointments because of a variety of factors, such as a lack of rapport, a rupture in the therapeutic relationship, lack of transportation, scheduling conflicts, or lack of childcare. Regardless, discuss missed appointments with the patient openly and without judgment. Problem-solve together. Can a case manager assist with transportation needs with a voucher? Would telepsychiatry suit the patient's needs better? Additionally, it is helpful to know institutional policy around cancellations and follow-ups. Who reaches out to the patient to reschedule? How often? If the patient will be charged or terminated for missing appointments, communicate this information early on.

⌘ **My patients wonder why I am prescribing medications that are different from what they read as FDA indications.** Although commonly done, off-label use can trigger a patient's anxiety. It is important to be up-front and honest with your patient when discussing treatment options. Explain your rationale for off-label use and, if necessary, share clinical data to support your recommendation. Always document your rationale and your discussion with the patient in the EHR as well.

SELF-REFLECTIVE QUESTIONS

1. Is there a way to incorporate more shared decision-making into my clinical care?
2. What goals do I have for indirect clinical supervision, and how can I communicate this with my supervisor?
3. What boundaries are important for me to establish in order to provide appropriate clinical care and also support work-life balance?

RESOURCES

Clarivate: www.fingertipformulary.com—website check to see if a patient's insurance will cover a prescription drug

Clozapine REMS: www.newclozapinerems.com/home—national registry for providers and patients taking clozapine; it also has guidelines for prescribing parameters for clozapine

Epocrates: www.epocrates.com—website to check for possible drug-drug interactions along with contraindications, black box warnings, and adverse effects

GoodRx: www.goodrx.com—website with free coupons for patients if a medication is not covered by insurance

MedlinePlus: https://medlineplus.gov—website by the National Library of Medicine and the National Institutes of Health for reliable information on medications

National Institute on Drug Abuse: https://nida.nih.gov—patient-friendly medication information in multiple languages

REFERENCES

Antonius D, Fuchs L, Herbert F, et al: Psychiatric assessment of aggressive patients: a violent attack on a resident. Am J Psychiatry 167(3):253–259, 2010 20194488

Butterworth JE, Campbell JL: Older patients and their GPs: shared decision making in enhancing trust. Br J Gen Pract 64(628):e709–e718, 2014 25348995

Gutheil TG: Fundamentals of medical record documentation. Psychiatry (Edgmont) 1(3):26–28, 2004 21191523

Parchman ML, Zeber JE, Palmer RF: Participatory decision making, patient activation, medication adherence, and intermediate clinical outcomes in type 2 diabetes: a STARNet study. Ann Fam Med 8(5):410–417, 2010 20843882

Ridd M, Shaw A, Lewis G, et al: The patient-doctor relationship: a synthesis of the qualitative literature on patients' perspectives. Br J Gen Pract 59(561):e116–e133, 2009 19341547

Stacey D, Légaré F, Col NF, et al: Decision aids for people facing health treatment or screening decisions. Cochrane Database Syst Rev 1(1):CD001431, 2014 24470076

Substance Abuse and Mental Health Services Administration: Recovery support tools and resources. Rockville, MD, Substance Abuse and Mental Health Services Administration, October 12, 2018. Available at: www.samhsa.gov/brss-tacs/recovery-support-tools-resources. Accessed May 8, 2021.

Tajirian T, Stergiopoulos V, Strudwick G, et al: The influence of electronic health record use on physician burnout: cross-sectional survey. J Med Internet Res 22(7):e19274, 2020 32673234

Weiner SJ, Schwartz A, Sharma G, et al: Patient-centered decision making and health care outcomes: an observational study. Ann Intern Med 158(8):573–579, 2013 23588745

Wilson SR, Strub P, Buist AS, et al: Shared treatment decision making improves adherence and outcomes in poorly controlled asthma. Am J Respir Crit Care Med 181(6):566–577, 2010 20019345

CHAPTER 16

Best Practices in Prescribing Medications

Nekisa Haghighat, M.D., M.P.H.

Phuong Vo, M.D., M.S.

Harika Reddy, M.D.

Takesha Cooper, M.D., M.S.

When should I prescribe medications for my patient? This is not a simple question, and even seasoned psychiatrists find themselves pondering this issue. Although medications can indeed be lifesaving, prescribing requires that you know your patient, the clinical situation, and the treatment options available to you. The best psychiatrists remain curious and inquisitive, with an element of humility and an ongoing interest in learning about and from their patient. In this chapter we aim to help you answer the question of "When to prescribe?" by addressing such topics as therapeutic alliance, agency, ambivalence, and nonadherence in addition to practical logistics surrounding prescribing medication for patients with mental illness.

KEY POINTS

- Developing a strong therapeutic alliance is key to an effective doctor-patient relationship.

- It is important to help the patient maintain agency and autonomy, involving them in decision-making about treatment,

- Identify the best treatment using all available information, including current symptoms, diagnosis, prior treatment, and evidence-based practices.

- Consider logistical barriers to medications and work with your patient to resolve them.

DEVELOPING A THERAPEUTIC ALLIANCE

Building an effective treatment plan undoubtedly starts with—and ultimately depends on—the strength and quality of the doctor-patient relationship. The therapeutic alliance has been shown to contribute more to the clinical outcome of pharmacological treatment than does the actual medication used (Krupnick et al. 1996). In order for this partnership to be effective and meaningful, however, it must be built on a foundation of mutual respect—with the provider seeking to earn the patient's trust while simultaneously acknowledging the patient's agency, autonomy, and treatment goals.

Establishing the therapeutic alliance begins with getting to know the patient. DSM-5-TR (American Psychiatric Association 2022) provides guidelines for identifying the specific traits of various psychiatric illnesses; however, it does very little to help characterize the unique attributes of the patient—characteristics that can, in fact, affect treatment outcomes. The DSM-5-TR Outline for Cultural Formulation and Cultural Formulation Interview help inform how ever-changing cultural constructs can help physicians avoid overgeneralizing or stereotyping patients with different backgrounds and life experiences, adding context to the patient's symptomatology and potentially affecting whether and what we prescribe. Viewing a patient through the lens of their illness alone aligns with a biologically reductionist model, in which the prescriber is concerned primarily with the discrete characteristics of the clinical diagnosis rather than focusing on the whole patient. It may seem instinctual to center a clinical conversation on the presenting problem, the so-called *chief complaint*; however, focusing entirely on the illness without considering the patient's personal characteristics (e.g., gender and gender identity, race/ethnicity, sexual orientation, socioeconomic environment, ability, veteran status), motivation for seeking treatment, and treatment goals may box the provider into using a one-size-fits-all approach that relies heavily on medications and leaves little room to explore other therapeutic modalities that may be better suited for their particular patient. One can avoid the one-size-fits-all approach by understanding the concepts of autonomy and agency and their importance in therapeutic relationships.

ENHANCING AUTONOMY AND AGENCY

Autonomy refers to a person's self-efficacy, or their "investment in persevering and increasing [their] independence, mobility, and personal rights" (Beck 1983, p. 265). A highly autonomous person derives gratification from directing their own activities to attain meaningful goals. The term *agency* refers to the thoughts and actions taken by people that express their individual power. Many providers may be inclined to use a biologically reductionistic framework to discuss psychiatric illnesses because this approach appears to relieve the patient of the burden of self-blame. In fact, comparing psychiatric disorders with more biologically rooted medical disorders is a common tactic used to battle the stigma associated with mental illness. This line of reasoning is a powerful tool that can be used effectively to motivate and engage the patient in treatment. However, you must be careful not to overemphasize the biological etiology of mental illness to a point that it causes the patient to feel helpless or entrapped by a disease beyond their control. Such a patient may surrender their personal agency to you, their psychiatrist, passively waiting for an equally biologically oriented treatment to cure their disease (Krupnick et al. 1996).

In the inpatient psychiatric setting, many psychiatric patients make their first contact with treatment teams against their will, and by definition appear (and may feel) as though they have little agency or autonomy. Strategies for establishing a therapeutic alliance must therefore consider the environment in which care is being delivered. Admittedly, in the inpatient setting, offering medications may be the most instinctual approach. This mentality, however, overlooks the beneficial impact that the unit's therapeutic milieu often has on the patient. Furthermore, it discounts the enormously therapeutic work that our colleagues, including occupational therapists, social workers, and other interdisciplinary teammates, diligently and regularly perform in both the inpatient and outpatient settings. A patient who voluntarily seeks outpatient psychiatric care is likely to approach the therapeutic alliance from a different perspective than a patient who is admitted to the psychiatric hospital on an involuntary hold. Regardless of the setting in which a patient is encountered, it is important to respect their agency and autonomy, involve them in decision-making, educate them about treatment options, and consider their preferences for treatment type. Just because a patient is on an involuntary hold does not mean that they lose their right to make known their preferences for their desired treatment plan.

Discussing treatment plans is a balancing act because you must be careful to set reasonable expectations and encourage the patient to take an active role in their recovery without diminishing hope or implying blame. One study found that patients with depression who felt that their providers were supportive of their autonomy were more intrinsically motivated during treatment. The patients felt that they had freely chosen their own goals and that these choices emanated from within, which was in turn a significant predictor of treatment outcome (Zuroff et al. 2007). Other studies have theorized that patients with high autonomous motivation adhere more closely to prescribed treatments; carry out therapies more carefully, persistently, and effectively; and even demonstrate stronger perseverance when treatment becomes difficult or discouraging (Markland et al. 2005).

One of the most common decisions a patient must make is whether they prefer a psychotherapeutic approach, medications, or a combination of the two. One study found that depressed patients who received their preferred treatment type achieved remission nearly 50% of the time, whereas remission rates among those who received their nonpreferred treatment type were 22.2% and 7.7% in patients who were treated with psychotherapy or medications, respectively (Kocsis et al. 2009). Another study found that patients who received their preferred treatment modality also saw improvements in mood more rapidly than did patients receiving nonpreferred treatments (Lin et al. 2005).

Overall, the patient's willingness to accept treatment depends on many factors; the transtheoretical or stages of change model is a helpful framework for gauging the patient's capacity to actively participate in treatment and contribute to the therapeutic alliance (Prochaska and DiClemente 2005). Patients who have been prompted by external or intrinsic factors to voluntarily seek help may be traversing the *contemplation* or *determination* stages of change and therefore may be more likely to engage in treatment planning or alliance building. Patients on an involuntary hold, on the other hand, are more likely to be *precontemplative* and thus unaware of the presence of a mental illness or need for treatment. Assessing the stage of change your patient is in can help guide your approach to the patient and can lead to deeper understanding (and empathy) when your patient is ambivalent about or nonadherent with treatment.

ADDRESSING AMBIVALENCE

Another important consideration when attempting to establish a strong therapeutic alliance is the patient's level of motivation to engage in psychiatric treatment. This can fall anywhere on a spectrum, ranging from outright refusal to participate to immediate acceptance of any offered treatment. Most patients, however, fall somewhere between these two extremes and are thus considered to be ambivalent about, or to have mixed feelings toward, treatment. Patients who are ambivalent about psychiatric medications in particular often weigh the benefit of treatment against the risks of side effects and the perceived stigma associated with taking psychiatric medications (Pound et al. 2005). It is important to seek to understand—and therefore address—a patient's ambivalence as soon as it is identified. Patients who express early ambivalence have been found to be twice as likely to discontinue medications prematurely in general and three times more likely to discontinue because of medication side effects in particular (Warden et al. 2009).

Strategies for adapting your approach to ambivalent patients rely on clearly assessing the patient's attitude toward medications and the reasons behind any reservations. What does it mean to or about the patient that they are being prescribed medication for mental health? Do they associate any stigma with taking medications? What specific concerns do they have about side effects? How likely are they to discontinue medications if side effects arise? Addressing these questions from the beginning helps validate the patient's thought process and involve them in shared decision-making.

In a study of patients' beliefs about antidepressant medications, Aikens et al. (2008) divided attitudes toward medication into four different camps and suggested prescribing strategies for each. Depressed patients who viewed antidepressants as necessary and who were not particularly concerned about side effects were found to be likely to adhere to medications, regardless of the treatment approach. On the opposite end of the spectrum, skeptical patients harbored low expectations of medication efficacy and high degrees of concern. In these patients, it is best to exhaust nonpharmacological approaches to treatment unless the severity of their illness necessitates intervention. Indifferent patients had low expectations about medication efficacy but similarly low concerns about negative consequences. These patients may need to see re-sults of medication efficacy before they are convinced to continue medications, and thus would benefit from a more aggressive escalation of treatment. Finally, ambivalent patients' reasonable expectations of treatment are counterbalanced by their concerns about negative effects of medications. In these cases, medications should be started at low doses and uptitrated slowly in order to minimize the risk of side effects while gradually achieving treatment goals (Mintz and Flynn 2012).

TAKING A GOOD HISTORY

Once the therapeutic alliance begins to take shape, attention can be shifted to the first step of designing a treatment plan: obtaining a thor-ough and relevant history, including an extensive medication history that includes past medications taken, dosages, side effects, duration, and why the medication was discontinued. Different providers have different styles for progressing through the history. Remember to be thorough in your assessment, to not neglect the patient's social history, and to obtain a full history of prior psychiatric treatments. It can be help-ful to preemptively discuss stigma regarding taking psychiatric medi-cations and gauge your patient's understanding of their illness.

IDENTIFYING A TREATMENT

After gathering a thorough history, the next step is to identify an appro-priate treatment regimen for the patient. This requires the consideration of many factors, as detailed in the following subsections.

Evidence-Based Treatments

It is important to examine evidence-based treatments in guiding treat-ment decision-making. When deciding between two different classes of medications or within a class of medications, review the literature to help shed light on which treatment you will recommend to your patient. Sometimes, studies focus on different populations (different patholo-gies and diagnoses) and often include a demographic breakdown of the subjects studied, such as gender and age. Looking at all of these differ-ing factors can be relevant in helping guide your treatment options.

Drug-Drug Interactions

After determining readiness for a patient to start medication treatment, it is important to first examine what medications a patient is already taking. Assessing any drug-drug interactions is important to avoid adverse outcomes. In addition, assessing the likelihood of a patient becoming pregnant or having plans to do so should be considered in guiding an appropriate treatment choice.

Side Effects

It also is important to use side effects of a medication to potentially treat more than one symptom. For example, if a patient is struggling with symptoms of depression and insomnia, rather than starting with an antidepressant and a separate sleep medication, you may consider starting an antidepressant that is more likely to be sedating. On the flip side, if a patient is already struggling with daytime sedation, a medication that is more activating could be more beneficial. Limiting polypharmacy, particularly in elderly people, children, and patients with multiple medical comorbidities, is extremely important in reducing the risk of side effects and improving quality of life while still treating symptoms.

Long-Term Planning

Another consideration is the long-term plan for the patient. For example, in an inpatient setting, the goal is often to stabilize a patient in an efficient manner so that they can be discharged to an outpatient level of care. However, when weighing risks versus benefits, the duration that a patient may need to be treated with medication and the feasibility of taking it long term should be considered. For example, olanzapine is often used on an inpatient basis for acutely psychotic symptoms; however, this medication is known to cause weight gain over time, and as a result, many outpatient providers change to a different medication for maintenance treatment—a process that might put the patient at risk of decompensation during a cross-titration. In some cases, it may be beneficial to start a medication acutely with plans to change treatment on an outpatient basis when the patient is stabilized, whereas in other cases initiating a medication with a more favorable long-term side effect profile from the start may be a better option.

Unique Patient Needs

A patient's daily routine and ability to remember to take medications also can play a role in deciding on a treatment choice. Some patients struggle with taking medication more than one time a day or remember only if it is dosed in the morning. Meeting the patient where they are and finding a plan to cater to what works for them are crucial for medication adherence and are more likely to lead to treatment effect. For patients taking an antipsychotic, choosing a medication with a long-acting injectable option can be particularly useful for improving adherence.

Psychotherapy

The utility of therapy should be considered in every patient's treatment plan either as their primary treatment or as an adjunctive treatment. In a recent meta-analysis of randomized controlled trials that compared psychotherapy alone and a combination of psychotherapy and pharmacotherapy, the combination was seen to be more efficacious in moderate chronic depression (de Maat et al. 2007). In a patient with borderline personality disorder, dialectical behavior therapy should be pursued if the patient is open to it, ideally before considering adjunctive pharmacological options (May et al. 2016). Physicians should review the literature for other evidence-based therapies showing efficacy for specific psychiatric disorders, remembering that comorbidities are common and should also be treated with approaches supported by the literature.

INITIATING TREATMENT AND MONITORING SYMPTOMS

When starting a medication, it is important to obtain informed consent, which involves having and documenting a detailed discussion between physician and patient regarding the purpose of the treatment, benefits and risks, and reasonable alternatives (Neilson and Chaimowitz 2015). You should consider starting low and going slow with certain populations (children, elderly patients, or those who are anxious about taking medication).

After starting a particular treatment, the next step is to determine if it is actually working. Clinical follow-up on the progress of your patients' symptoms as well as the use of evidence-based clinical scales such as the nine-item Patient Heath Questionnaire (PHQ-9) for depression (Kroenke et al. 2001) or Generalized Anxiety Disorder 7-item (GAD-7) for anxiety (Kertz et al. 2013) can help you and your patient determine the efficacy of the chosen treatment approach. When a medication is not working, consider whether the patient is actually taking the medicine consistently and, if so, whether the medication was trialed for an appropriate duration. With this information, you and your patient can then work together to decide to increase the medication dose or consider other alternatives.

Treatment resistance in depression, anxiety, and schizophrenia can be defined as "an inadequate response to at least two adequate (appropriate dose and lasting for at least 6 weeks) treatment episodes with different drugs" (Demyttenaere 2019, p. 354). By these criteria, if a patient's symptoms are considered to be treatment resistant, adjunctive medications can be considered as well as nonpharmacological options such as transcranial magnetic stimulation or electroconvulsive therapy.

Inviting the patient to talk with you about side effects is crucial to building an alliance and can prevent patients stopping medicine prematurely on their own, particularly because many side effects resolve with time and reassurance. Another challenge in the treatment plan is that patients cannot always tolerate side effects of medications. Working with a patient to validate these side effects while also trying to address their symptoms can be challenging. Strategies include lowering the dosage, adjusting the timing of the dose, and changing medications altogether.

ADDRESSING MEDICATION NONADHERENCE

Multiple components may affect medication trials, including how practitioners approach prescribing the medication, the route of administration, the cost of prescriptions, the color or appearance of the medication, and the dosage used (Mintz and Flynn 2012). As discussed in the section "Developing a Therapeutic Alliance," establishing a strong therapeutic alliance is tantamount to treatment efficacy and continued adherence. Obvious factors that may lead to nonadherence can include sedation, complicated dosing regimens, weight gain, sexual side effects, and involuntary movements. Also use caution with patients planning to become pregnant. Reviewing the variety of medication formulations with your patient, such as pill, liquid, sublingual, and long-acting injectable formulations or even valproic acid "sprinkles," can help you decide how best to meet your patient's needs and promote adherence to treatment. It can be challenging when a patient with severe mental illness has paranoia or delusions about their medications that may contribute to nonadherence. In these cases, you can only try your best to meet the patient where they are within the stages of change model (Prochaska and Velicer 1997). Leaning into the therapeutic alliance and listening to your patient's concerns will allow you to respect their autonomy and offer more welcome options.

ATTENDING TO ACCESS AND LOGISTICAL BARRIERS

Affordability of medication is a challenge for many patients. Resources can be given to patients for obtaining medications at a cheaper price, including websites that compare prices (see "Resources" at the end of the chapter). Local universities and schools specific to training health care professionals may also have affiliations with local free clinics that can provide free or reduced-cost medications for patients. Medicaid is funded jointly by states and the federal government and provides health care and prescription coverage to low-income adults, children, pregnant women, elderly adults, and individuals with disabilities.

If patients report to you that they are undocumented, reassure them that their immigration status is confidential and will not affect their care and that you will not record their immigration status in the chart. Working with social workers to learn more about community-based resources and communicating that knowledge is a preemptive way to help patients adhere to treatment recommendations.

When patients have complicated psychiatric problems, it is imperative to also consider logistical barriers to medication management. For example, some medications (e.g., clozapine) have significant resource requirements and demand strong social support for patients to continue treatment safely because of required weekly laboratory draws and side-effect monitoring. If patients are unhoused or have little access to health care, you first may have to adjust doses of medications other than clozapine or place the patient in a residential treatment program so that they receive the appropriate level of care. Similar concerns may be applied to starting patients on lithium or valproic acid. If the patient has a history of difficulty navigating the health care system, it may be beneficial to ensure a therapeutic blood level prior to discharge from a hospitalization. This minimizes safety concerns of toxic levels or subtherapeutic treatment that can precipitate symptom relapse. Recruiting family into patient care is paramount because family members can share the burden with the patient to help them get blood work, track side effects with the patient, and support treatment adherence and other management concerns.

SPECIFIC CHALLENGES AND STRATEGIES

⌘ **I'm concerned my patient may not continue to take the new medication I'm prescribing.** Anticipated nonadherence can be mitigated by having frank discussions in advance about potential side effects. You can gauge patient comfort in advance and discuss alternatives as concerns arise. Discussion and consistent psychotherapy using the therapeutic alliance you have built can be helpful (Munro and Mok 1995). An example to consider is acamprosate, which comes in a 666 mg formulation. This can be disconcerting to some patients, particularly those with strong religious beliefs. If your patient has discomfort with such a medication, discussing this concern ahead of time and discussing potential alternative medications such as naltrexone or disulfiram can mitigate future nonadherence.

⌘ **I am so frustrated that my patient is repeatedly nonadherent to their medication.** The constructive approach is to maintain professionalism, refrain from judgment, and remain mindful about approaching the patient from a place of concern and empathy. Meet the patient where they are. Even with adherence, keep in mind that some patients may achieve only partial recovery or decrease in symptoms but not necessarily be "cured" even with the optimum effort and treatment (Bhui 2017). The goal is to help the patient maintain or return to an adequate level of functionality despite their mental illness and be able to navigate their life journey with tools that include medication and therapy. You may also consider using supervision with your attending physician to express your frustration and receive additional support and guidance.

⌘ **My patient refuses to take any medication, but I know that their depression is only worsening despite psychotherapy.** Patients may decline to take medication for a variety of reasons, such as stigma, concerns about side effects, or cost. It is important to take some time to listen to your patient in a nonjudgmental way and uncover some of the barriers to their accepting medication as a treatment option. In this case, you and the therapist may be able to work together to understand the patient's concerns as well as their goals for treatment. Providing clear information about medication efficacy and side effects and debunking any misconceptions may be helpful. In addition, it is important to acknowledge and address any logistical barriers, including cost. Finally, aligning the treatment goals with your patient's personal goals may be motivating—for example, adding another treatment option might improve the patient's depression enough for them to reengage in employment. Providing your patient with some antidepressant options to choose from and prioritizing their goals will allow them to exercise their own agency and autonomy in the treatment plan.

SELF-REFLECTIVE QUESTIONS

1. How can I further improve my therapeutic alliance with my patients?
2. How can I involve my patients more in treatment decision-making?
3. How can I better anticipate future obstacles when starting a medication?

RESOURCES

Cooper T, Maguire G, Stahl SM: Stahl's Essential Psychopharmacology Case Studies, Vol 3. New York, Cambridge University Press, 2021

GoodRx: www.goodrx.com

Walmart $4 prescriptions: www.walmart.com/cp/4-prescriptions/1078664

REFERENCES

Aikens JE, Nease DE Jr, Klinkman MS: Explaining patients' beliefs about the necessity and harmfulness of antidepressants. Ann Fam Med 6(1):23–29, 2008 18195311

American Psychiatric Association: Diagnostic and Statistical Manual of Mental Disorders, 5th Edition, Text Revision. Washington, DC, American Psychiatric Association, 2022

Beck AT: Cognitive therapy of depression: new perspectives, in Treatment of Depression: Old Controversies and New Approaches. Edited by Clayton PJ, Barett JE. New York, Raven Press, 1983, pp 265–284

Bhui K: Treatment resistant mental illnesses. Br J Psychiatry 210(6):443–444, 2017

de Maat SM, Dekker J, Schoevers RA, et al: Relative efficacy of psychotherapy and combined therapy in the treatment of depression: a meta-analysis. Eur Psychiatry 22(1):1–8, 2007 17194571

Demyttenaere K: What is treatment resistance in psychiatry? A "difficult to treat" concept. World Psychiatry 18(3):354–355, 2019 31496099

Kertz S, Bigda-Peyton J, Bjorgvinsson T: Validity of the Generalized Anxiety Disorder-7 scale in an acute psychiatric sample. Clin Psychol Psychother 20(5):456–464, 2013 22593009

Kocsis JH, Leon AC, Markowitz JC, et al: Patient preference as a moderator of outcome for chronic forms of major depressive disorder treated with nefazodone, cognitive behavioral analysis system of psychotherapy, or their combination. J Clin Psychiatry 70(3):354–361, 2009 19192474

Kroenke K, Spitzer RL, Williams JB: The PHQ-9: validity of a brief depression severity measure. J Gen Intern Med 16(9):606–613, 2001 11556941

Krupnick JL, Sotsky SM, Simmens S, et al: The role of the therapeutic alliance in psychotherapy and pharmacotherapy outcome: findings in the National Institute of Mental Health Treatment of Depression Collaborative Research Program. J Consult Clin Psychol 64(3):532–539, 1996 8698947

Lin P, Campbell DG, Chaney EF, et al: The influence of patient preference on depression treatment in primary care. Ann Behav Med 30(2):164–173, 2005 16173913

Markland D, Ryan RM, Tobin VJ, et al: Motivational interviewing and self-determination theory. J Soc Clin Psychol 24(6):811–831, 2005

May JM, Richardi TM, Barth KS: Dialectical behavior therapy as treatment for borderline personality disorder. Ment Health Clin 6(2):62–67, 2016 29955449

Mintz DL, Flynn DF: How (not what) to prescribe: nonpharmacologic aspects of psychopharmacology. Psychiatr Clin North Am 35(1):143–163, 2012 22370496

Munro A, Mok H: An overview of treatment in paranoia/delusional disorder. Can J Psychiatry 40(10):616–622, 1995 8681259

Neilson G, Chaimowitz G: Informed consent to treatment in psychiatry. Can J Psychiatry 60(4):1–11, 2015

Pound P, Britten N, Morgan M, et al: Resisting medicines: a synthesis of qualitative studies of medicine taking. Soc Sci Med 61(1):133–155, 2005 15847968

Prochaska JO, DiClemente CC: The transtheoretical approach, in Handbook of Psychotherapy Integration. Edited by Norcross JC, Goldfried MR. New York, Oxford University Press, 2005, pp 147–171

Prochaska JO, Velicer WF: The transtheoretical model of health behavior change. Am J Health Promot 12(1):38–48, 1997 10170434

Warden D, Trivedi MH, Wisniewski SR, et al: Identifying risk for attrition during treatment for depression. Psychother Psychosom 78(6):372–379, 2009 19738403

Zuroff DC, Koestner R, Moskowitz D, et al: Autonomous motivation for therapy: a new common factor in brief treatments for depression. Psychother Res 17(2):137–147, 2007

CHAPTER 17

Best Practices in Providing Psychotherapy

Anne E. Ruble, M.D., M.P.H.

Sarah C. Collica, M.D.

Sallie G. De Golia, M.D., M.P.H.

Raziya S. Wang, M.D.

Erin M. Crocker, M.D.

More than any other aspect of psychiatry residency training, practicing psychotherapy can feel unclear and confusing. How do you know what to say and how to say it? How is talking to your patient in psychotherapy different from talking to a friend? How can you make sure that your practice of psychotherapy is effective for your patient when you are so new at it? Unlike most interventions in medicine, psychotherapy provides psychiatry residents few opportunities to watch skilled psychotherapists in action, but you are expected to learn psychotherapy and offer it to your patients. Indeed, the Accreditation Council for Graduate Medical Education (2021) Program Requirements for Graduate Medical Education in Psychiatry, section IV.B.1.b).(1).(b).(ix), requires psychiatry residents to become competent in three different modalities of psychotherapy: supportive, cognitive-behavioral, and psychodynamic. Residents have a number of resources for learning about the theoretical model and application of each of these modalities (see "Resources" at the end of the chapter), but we focus here on best practices for psychotherapy regardless of modality. We start with preparing to meet your patient; move on to building a therapeutic alliance, setting the frame and boundaries, using supervision, and navigating ruptures in the alliance; and conclude with best practices in termination.

KEY POINTS

- Creating a clear and consistent therapeutic frame helps enable treatment.

- You should document only what is medically necessary as well as themes of discussions.

- Termination requires careful consideration and guidance from a supervisor.

- Supervision in psychotherapy is where you learn about the modality and interpersonal dynamics of therapy and is a place where you can sort through your own responses to the therapy.

PRIOR TO STARTING THERAPY

Before you meet your first psychotherapy patient, it is important to consider how you will create a safe space where the patient may reveal their innermost concerns. This process is called developing the therapeutic frame, those aspects of treatment within the therapy space (e.g., confidential, predictable) and relationship (e.g., nonjudgmental, empathic) that allow a patient to work effectively within the therapy. In psychotherapy practice, the frame includes all the expectations and guidelines that you and your patient will attend to in psychotherapy, such as confidentiality, expected frequency of sessions, timing and duration of meetings, and communication outside the therapy appointments. Your clinic policies may already set some of these general guidelines, and you and your psychotherapy supervisor can further clarify the frame for the particular modality you will offer your patient. Most commonly, you will offer your patient psychotherapy weekly at a designated and reliable time for about 45–60 minutes' duration.

Part of sustaining a frame is carefully attending to boundaries, defined as "the limit to personal or social contact between clinician and patient" (Bender and Messner 2022, p. 433). Boundaries help patients understand the difference between a friendship and psychotherapy and typically include limited personal disclosures on the part of the therapist and a curious, attentive, and nonjudgmental approach to the patient's concerns. Boundaries also typically include not meeting the patient outside set appointments and refraining from social interactions. A well-known boundary prohibits romantic relationships between therapists and patients. By developing a clear frame and attending to boundaries, patients are able to more readily divulge troubling worries, symptoms, and life situations as well as hopes and goals, which eventually allows for change.

Prepare Your Therapy Space

The physical space of your office contributes to the frame and boundaries of your psychotherapy practice. If you have an individual office, it is important to consider the privacy and comfort of your space. If your office is located in a busy area of the hospital, obtain a white noise machine from your department so patients are reassured of confidentiality. To prevent interruptions, you also may want to place a sign on your door that indicates you are in session. The comfort of your space may be enhanced by a setup where you and the patient sit face to face and you each have a view of a clock to keep track of the time remaining in session. If you need to use your computer during sessions, try to arrange your computer in a place where you can alternate between documenting and making eye contact with the patient.

Finally, adequate lighting, neutral artwork, and a box of tissues within the patient's reach can all make the patient feel more comfortable. Although it is common for physicians in other fields to display personal photos in their offices, psychiatrists must carefully consider the impact of such items. Personal photos can be a form of self-disclosure to your patient, which is often more limited in psychotherapy, distinguishing therapy from other friendly social interactions. This limited self-disclosure is in the service of enhancing your patient's sense of safety and providing a nonjudgmental space for their concerns. For example, a patient seeking therapy for infertility support may feel uncomfortable seeing pictures of your children. A patient who is estranged from their own family may feel uncomfortable or less open if your office is lined with family photos. When the patient has access to your "real" life, they may more often make assumptions about who you are and whether you can be helpful to them.

Prepare Your Method of Communication

The frame also includes creating safe and predictable ways of communicating with your patient. It is good practice to use a work email that is different from your personal email and a phone number different from your personal number. These practices continue to reinforce the boundary between the therapeutic relationship and a friendship. If your therapy space does not have a phone, consider setting up a phone number through an internet phone dialer to share with your patients. Some hospital systems also allow you to contact the patient through the hospital operator to protect your personal phone number.

You should set up a confidential voice mail that includes the following information: your name, your affiliated institution, what information you would like the patient to leave in their message, when the patient can expect a response from you, and to call 911 or proceed to the nearest emergency department if the patient is experiencing an emergency and cannot wait for a return call. Different clinics have different policies regarding time frames expected for callbacks, whether the patient should contact your direct extension or a central clinic number, and whether you will be responsible for returning patient calls directly or if a clinic staff member will call back on your behalf. Regardless of your clinic policies, it is important that you inform your patient in advance so that they know what to expect.

THE FIRST FEW SESSIONS

The first couple of sessions with a new patient are critical. Your patient will use this time to decide whether they feel safe enough to engage in psychotherapy and feel that the setting is a "good fit" for them. You need to focus on creating a safe space for the patient, assessing their needs, developing a formulation to determine a treatment plan, and obtaining consent for the treatment to follow.

Establish the Alliance

As an intern, you likely became comfortable with gathering all of the information for a history and physical during the first session. However, this may not be the best approach when meeting a psychotherapy patient for the first time. Collecting a structured history may allow you to arrive at recommendations for treatment more quickly, but open-ended time allows you to provide support and build trust with a patient who may be anxious about entering therapy. Remember, you will likely have many sessions to get to know this person. However, you should always perform a risk assessment even if you do not complete a full structured intake.

The goal of the first few sessions is typically to establish an alliance so that the patient will feel comfortable returning for ongoing care (Bender and Messner 2022). The alliance is the partnership you and your patient will develop as you work together and is built on a foundation of trust. You can foster an alliance by listening empathically and without judgment (a skill you have been practicing since medical school) and by providing validation for your patient's concerns. The trust and partnership you establish early with your patient will help sustain the psychotherapy in the face of inevitable challenges in the work ahead.

Articulate the Frame

It is important to share the basic guidelines for treatment early on in psychotherapy. You may review confidentiality policies of your clinic and expectations about timing and duration for appointments as well as logistics for communication. If you have prepared these guidelines in advance, you may even consider giving them to your patient as a handout that they can refer to later. You also may discuss and develop some shared expectations with your patient. For example, establish how much notice you require if a patient wants to reschedule their appointment and how long you will wait until you need to reschedule if a patient is late for their appointment. If you will be carrying a pager or may, at times, be interrupted with an emergency, it is important to alert your patient to this possibility.

Discuss Reading of Clinic Notes

Discuss with your patient the fact that they have open access to clinic notes through the electronic medical record system, a requirement of the 21st Century Cures Act (American Psychiatric Association 2022). It is important to discuss with the patient your thought process when writing the note so they understand why you documented in a certain way, and you should encourage questions. It also can be helpful to review your notes with your supervisor to see if they have any suggestions about your level of detail or phrasing.

Agree on Goals and Tasks

After gathering information over the first few sessions and discussing with your supervisor, ask the patient to suggest some goals for their psychotherapy. Validate these goals, add goals you have developed with your supervisor, and then prioritize the goals with the patient. Consider starting with a goal that is not so simple that a patient can solve it on their own without need for processing or support. On the other hand, try to avoid starting with a goal so challenging that your patient feels overwhelmed, which may lead to them discontinuing therapy prematurely (Bender and Messner 2022).

Develop a Formulation and Decide on a Modality

Forming a clear understanding of the factors influencing the patient's symptoms and current presentation and selecting the appropriate modality of therapy are vitally important and should be discussed with your supervisor. For therapy to be successful, the chosen approach needs to align with the patient's needs, the treatment goals, and available resources for therapy. The differential psychotherapeutics cycle provides a framework for systematically approaching treatment-matching decisions (Cabaniss and Holoshitz 2019). The differential psychotherapeutics cycle is a four-step rubric in which the provider learns about the patient and their needs, then thinks about what is going wrong and what needs to change before matching the patient with a particular type of treatment. The provider then discusses the recommendation with the patient (see also Chapter 7, "Learning to Develop a Case Formulation"). Integrate information about the selected modality into your informed consent discussion (see bulleted item below).

The specific modalities required to be taught in residency include the following:

- *Supportive psychotherapy.* Supportive therapy emphasizes the collaborative relationship between therapist and patient and focuses heavily on the therapeutic alliance, including the establishment of agreed-on goals and tasks of the therapy work itself. The supportive therapist not only learns about the patient's current problems and challenges but also listens for areas of strength (such as adaptive coping skills or potential sources of social support) and then works with the patient to mobilize these available strengths in order to reduce distress and improve functioning in the here and now (Welton and Crocker 2021). Supportive therapy is the foundation on which you will build work in psychodynamic or cognitive-behavioral therapy (CBT) approaches. One way to visualize this relationship between supportive, psychodynamic, and CBT therapies is with the Y model (Goldberg and Plakun 2013). In the stem of the Y, supportive therapy provides the elements that become the foundation for the other therapy branches.
- *Psychodynamic psychotherapy.* Psychodynamic therapy focuses on helping the patient gain insight into their internal experience. Conversation between the therapist and patient is often open-ended, driven by what is on the patient's mind and what might be troubling them at that time. The therapist's role is both to listen deeply to what is being said and to pay close attention to what is not said. As a new psychodynamic therapy practitioner, you might feel pressure to make astute detailed "interpretations" about what is going on for a patient, but most often, a gentle observation or expression of curiosity will be enough for the patient to reflect and consider. The nature of psychodynamic work has been described as "exploring those as-

pects of self that are not fully known, especially as they are manifested and potentially influenced in the therapy relationship" (Shedler 2010, p. 98). Ultimately, the goal is for the patient to live a healthier life as they understand more about themselves.

- *Cognitive-behavioral therapy.* CBT assumes an interactive relationship between a patient's thoughts, emotions, and behaviors that leads to their symptoms. For example, a patient's thought "No one cares for me" might interact with their depressed mood, leading to a behavior of withdrawal from a social group, which in turn leads to further isolation and depressed mood. CBT therapists use a variety of tools and a coaching approach to help patients identify and change these maladaptive interactions. With modified thoughts and behaviors, patients often experience improved mood and symptoms as well.

- *Informed consent for therapy.* Once you have selected a modality, it is important to obtain informed consent for therapy just as you would with any other therapeutic intervention. If your clinic has a psychotherapy consent form, review and sign it with the patient. If this is not the case, walk the patient through what they may expect from therapy and the benefits, including symptom relief, behavioral change, and insight. Also, review possible risks, including the possibility of feeling worse before feeling better as the therapy progresses (a common experience of patients in therapy) or of the therapy potentially not being successful for them. Once your patient has consented to a particular modality of therapy, discuss the evidence and expected structure of the modality chosen, including the expected length and frequency of treatment (see "Resources").

ONGOING THERAPY

When establishing an ongoing relationship with a new patient, it is often helpful to meet weekly to start. This active working phase will build on your initial therapeutic alliance to help your patient reflect on and change their perspectives, hopefully helping them to ultimately experience relief from their symptoms as well. As you and your patient engage in this longitudinal work, you often will refer to your ever-expanding formulation to inform the interventions you make throughout the therapy.

Tracking Progress

Many residents struggle with how to track the progress of their patient in psychotherapy. Although psychiatric symptoms can be tracked with evidence-based measures such as the nine-item Patient Health Questionnaire (PHQ-9; Kroenke et al. 2002) or Generalized Anxiety Disorder

7-item (GAD-7; Spitzer et al. 2006) scale, psychotherapy may not lead neatly and efficiently to measurable symptom improvement right away. Other ways to measure your patient's progress might be to consider their engagement in the modality and their likely growing capacity for self-reflection and change based on their trusted relationship with you. These observations are evidence of progress, and deepened work often leads to symptom improvement as well. Notably, it is inevitable that conflicts or misunderstandings will arise in therapy, and you must not view them as failures or setbacks in the psychotherapy work. The intimacy and intensity of talking about one's emotional experience with a therapist is often challenging for both the patient and the therapist. Despite your best intentions, you will likely say something that is upsetting or distressing to the patient. If this happens, help the patient explore their reactions to what transpired, validate the patient's feelings, and consider offering a genuine apology if needed (Bender and Messner 2022).

Conducting Psychotherapy via Telehealth

If you are performing psychotherapy via telehealth, you may need to engage in additional conversations with the patient about the therapeutic alliance and incorporate periodic check-ins about the patient's comfort with this frame for therapy. As an advantage to the therapeutic alliance, if masking requirements are in effect for in-person appointments, the virtual session format allows the provider to visualize the patient's entire face (Ruble et al. 2021).

Combining Medication With Therapy

As your patient progresses in therapy, you may decide they would benefit from medication. Explain your reasons for considering a medication and help your patient process any feelings about introducing a medication to the treatment. Patients may feel that taking a medication means that they have "failed" or are "weak," so it may be helpful to review the evidence for combining medications and therapy for symptom reduction. Discuss who might be the best provider of medication, either yourself or the patient's primary care physician. If the patient is already receiving a medication from another source, make sure to keep in close contact with the prescribing physician. Reasons for you to consider prescribing a medication or taking over prescribing include the frequency of your visits, your ability to tease out the complex effects of interpersonal or life events on symptom exacerbation, and/or the nature of the medications being prescribed (some primary care physicians may not be comfortable with medications beyond a selective serotonin reuptake inhibitor). If prescribing takes away from the therapy process, then it might be worthwhile having another provider prescribe. Discuss with the patient issues related to prescribing, and, if appropriate, confirm that changes to prescribing are acceptable to the other provider. Ensure that the patient understands who is responsible for managing psychiatric medication; multiple physicians making medication changes can create problems and may result in issues with medication safety. Do not hesitate to consult often with your psychotherapy supervisor, who will be able to help you navigate some of these issues and offer advice on how to proceed. See Chapter 16, "Best Practices in Prescribing Medications," for additional guidance around prescribing.

Documenting Psychotherapy

Documentation of psychotherapy interventions differs slightly from other clinical documentation in psychiatry. When writing a psychotherapy note, it is often best to write as little information as necessary. Remember, your patient may share intimate details about their lives that have no place in the medical record. Potentially, they also will be reading their notes, so if they find that what they tell you ends up in the records, they may be more hesitant to share in the future. Document only what is medically necessary: session start and stop times, modalities and frequency of treatment, test results, medication, diagnosis, functional status, treatment plan, symptoms, prognosis, and progress. As a rule of thumb, you may document themes of discussions (e.g., "discussed marital issues"). The Health Insurance Portability and Accountability Act of 1996 includes a privacy rule that provides additional confidentiality protection to any personal psychotherapy notes (optional clinician notes with personal analysis of sessions) about your patient that you may keep outside the medical record (Office of Civil Rights 2017). If you are considering keeping any notes outside the medical record for supervision, it is important to consult with your supervisor about how to ensure that you comply with the additional confidentiality protections for these notes and secure them according to your institution's policies and procedures. However, psychotherapy notes are not completely confidential. They can be subpoenaed, and a patient can authorize their release to others.

TERMINATION

Termination refers to the conclusion of psychotherapy work with your patient. There are two types of terminations: mature termination, which has an agreed-on end of treatment, and leaving treatment prematurely, when a patient terminates therapy prior to reaching agreed-on goals (Bender and Messner 2022). In a mature termination, you and the patient agree that they have resolved the distressing situation or goals that brought them to psychotherapy. A mature termination may provide a satisfying ending to work that you and your patient accomplished together. In contrast, a premature ending of therapy by the patient can be distressing and may lead you to wonder whether you made a mistake or did not help the patient enough. No matter the type of termination, difficult feelings often arise for the patient and therapist alike when it comes to saying goodbye. It is important to seek supervision because this phase is potentially difficult and also extremely important to the ultimate success of the therapy.

The reality in residency training is that many residents do not reach the mature termination phase with their patients. Instead, residents must "force" a termination by transferring their patients to another resident after a clinic block or when completing residency. Even if this type of forced termination is not your "fault," it is still important to address the termination directly with the patient. Explain the reasons for the end of your work together and provide as much information as you have about their next therapist. In some training settings, patients may be transferred several times between residents, leading to disruptive therapeutic work. Discuss with your supervisor whether your patient would be better served by being referred to a therapist outside the program where they might have care without interruptions. Whenever you transfer a psychotherapy patient, it is important to do a *warm handoff*, taking particular care to give both the new therapist and the patient information about each other and even setting up an introductory meeting if possible. If you are the receiving resident psychotherapist, anticipate and plan to address the likely effects of forced termination with the previous therapist. Some common issues may involve idealization of the former or new therapist, frustration at the former therapist for leaving, and/or triggering issues of loss or abandonment.

USE OF SUPERVISION

Supervision is where you will learn about the modality of psychotherapy you are practicing and how to effectively work with your patient. To optimize these learning experiences, meet with your supervisor regularly for support and guidance. As a psychotherapy practitioner, you will experience your own emotional responses to the psychotherapy work. Sometimes you will feel embarrassed or worried about sharing these responses or concerns about psychotherapy. As a good rule of thumb, if at any time you wonder whether you need to talk with your supervisor, go ahead and talk to your supervisor. Remember that your supervisor likely has vast experience with a variety of psychotherapy situations and that sharing your embarrassing experience can lead to a great learning opportunity. See Chapter 22, "Supervision," for additional information on how to use supervision effectively when practicing psychotherapy.

Come Prepared

Come to supervision on time and be prepared. Try to be clear about your learning needs and bring clinical questions or questions from psychotherapy didactics to supervision. Be prepared to show a video of your session or discuss your process notes in supervision. When you provide objective data through audio or video recordings, your supervisor will be better informed about the therapy work being done and will be able to provide more specific feedback and guidance (Crocker and Sudak 2017).

Be Receptive

Be open to your supervisor's observations. They usually have a great deal of experience working within the modality and may see things that you do not immediately pick up. Other times, your supervisor's comments may not resonate with you. If you do not understand why your supervisor interprets something the way they did or suggests a particular intervention that does not quite seem right, ask them. Remember, you are the person in the room with the patient, and that makes a difference. Your supervisor does not have the same vantage point. It is OK to disagree, but process the disagreement so you both learn from the moment.

Process Your Countertransference

Your emotional experience in the room with the patient is critical, particularly in psychodynamic therapy. Your patient's interpersonal dynamics will push and pull you, and you will have a reaction—just as others in the patient's life may react. Your patient may also bring up issues within yourself that either resonate with you or trigger something from your past. This is all appropriate to process within supervision as long as it is relevant to the care of your patient. However, supervision is *not* psychotherapy. If there are experiences in your past that you do not feel comfortable sharing or if the emotions you experience with your patient affect your ability to intervene appropriately, you might want to consider starting or continuing your own individual therapy.

Manage Multiple Supervisors

At times, it can be helpful to seek help from more than one supervisor on a single case. At other times, you might report to two supervisors at once—one who signs off on the case and one who has more expertise in the psychotherapy modality at hand. In either of these cases, residents may wonder how to integrate supervision from more than one supervisor, particularly if the different supervisions conflict. There is not one single way to provide care, so learning about different perspectives and approaches can be enriching. However, if you find yourself confused or caught in a conflict between two supervisors that cannot be mediated by speaking with them, you might reach out to your director of psychotherapy training or program director for guidance.

SPECIFIC CHALLENGES AND STRATEGIES

⌘ **My patient is upset about something I said during psychotherapy. Am I a bad therapist?** Know that psychotherapy is a great opportunity for a patient to learn about expressing feelings in a safe space, where they can learn that their hurt feelings are accepted and met with compassion. If a patient responds to something you said with hurt, anger, or another strong emotion, encouraging them to speak about their feelings is important. This is an opportunity to strengthen the therapeutic relationship. Validation of the patient's feelings and openness to their anger, frustration, or upset may deepen the alliance and elucidate what the underlying issue is. If there has been a misstep on your part as the therapist, a sincere apology can go a long way. The ruptures and repairs are a core part of any psychotherapy modality and should not be viewed as a mistake or evidence of novice-level skills. Indeed, a psychotherapy alliance that never has any conflict or strong emotions may not be doing much therapeutic work. The goal is not to always get along with your patient but to try to understand, validate, and create a space where your patient can share challenges and ultimately find healing and recovery. This will always be a bumpy road. Discuss this process in supervision, including the underlying causes of the patient's feelings, which can include misinterpretation of one of the patient's cues or a countertransference reaction. It has happened to every experienced therapist.

⌘ **My patient keeps arriving late and then wanting to go over time.** If a patient is having difficulty with the boundaries you set, address the issue promptly without avoiding it. Begin with curiosity because there may be many reasons behind the behaviors. Your patient may have anxiety about sessions, reactions to a prior intervention, or childcare or transportation issues preventing them from arriving on time. Help the patient problem-solve these concerns. If your initial attempts at these conversations feel awkward or fail to resolve the issue, involve your supervisor. Your supervisor will help you explore these issues, which can be complex and have a greater meaning that can help the patient if addressed in therapy.

⌘ **I'm so frustrated because I just "inherited" a new psychotherapy patient who spends all of our sessions talking about how much she misses the graduating resident who used to be her therapist.** With the frequent forced psychotherapy terminations that occur during residency training, it is common for residents to receive transferred cases from residents who are graduating or changing rotations. Although it is understandably frustrating to hear only about how amazing your resident colleague (their former therapist) is, try to take the perspective of your patient, who was obligated to change therapists partway through the work. Approach with compassion, validate the patient's feelings, and create a safe space for them to share what's on their mind. This is the foundation of building your therapeutic alliance and will serve you and your patient well as you progress in your work together. Engaging in your own psychotherapy also can help you reflect on your own emotional experience and increase your capacity to observe and manage your feelings toward your patients.

SELF-REFLECTIVE QUESTIONS

1. Have I articulated a clear frame for my patient and myself?
2. How does my patient formulation inform which psychotherapy modality I might suggest?
3. What is my own internal emotional experience during my psychotherapy sessions with my patient? What factors might contribute to my feelings?

RESOURCES

General

Brenner AM, Howe-Martin LS: Psychotherapy: A Practical Introduction. Philadelphia, PA, Wolters Kluwer, 2021

Crocker EM, Brenner AM: Teaching psychotherapy. Psychiatr Clin North Am 44(2):207–216, 2021

Wampold BE: The Basics of Psychotherapy: An Introduction to Theory and Practice, 2nd Edition. Theories of Psychotherapy Series. Washington, DC, American Psychological Association, 2018 (Theories of Psychotherapy is a 31-book series covering many evidence-based psychotherapies.)

Wampold BE, Imel ZE: The Great Psychotherapy Debate: The Evidence for What Makes Psychotherapy Work. New York, Routledge, 2015

Beginning Therapists

Bender S, Messner E. Becoming a Therapist: What Do I Say, and Why? 2nd Edition. New York, Guilford, 2022

Consenting for Psychotherapy

Patel S, Brenner AM: Fitting the therapy and therapist to the patient, in Psychotherapy: A Practical Introduction. Edited by Brenner AM, Howe-Martin LS. Philadelphia, PA, Wolters Kluwer, 2021, pp 43–68 (page 60 offers a helpful guide)

Managing Suicide in Psychotherapy

Suicide Prevention Resource Center: Stanley-Brown Safety Plan Template. National Suicide Prevention Lifeline, 2021. Available at: https://bgg.11b.myftpupload.com/wp-content/uploads/2021/08/Stanley-Brown-Safety-Plan-8-6-21.pdf. Accessed April 19, 2022.

Differential Psychotherapies

Cabaniss DL, Holoshitz Y: Different Patients, Different Therapies: Optimizing Treatment Using Differential Psychotherapeutics. New York, WW Norton, 2019

Prescribing Medications in Psychotherapy

Mintz DL, Flynn DF: How (not what) to prescribe: nonpharmacologic aspects of psychopharmacology. Psychiatr Clin North Am 35(1):143–163, 2012

Managing Microaggressions in Psychotherapy

Williams MT: Managing Microaggressions: Addressing Everyday Racism in Therapeutic Spaces. New York, Oxford University Press, 2020

Using Psychotherapy Supervision

De Golia SG, Tan ME: Using psychotherapy supervision in training and beyond, in Psychotherapy: A Practical Introduction. Edited by Brenner AM, Howe-Martin LS. Philadelphia, PA, Wolters Kluwer, 2021, pp 363–390

REFERENCES

Accreditation Council for Graduate Medical Education: ACGME program requirements for graduate medical education in psychiatry. ACGME-approved focused revision, June 13, 2021; effective July 1, 2021. Available at: www.acgme.org/globalassets/pfassets/programrequirements/400_psychiatry_2021.pdf. Accessed April 19, 2021.

American Psychiatric Association: 21st Century Cures Act. Washington, DC, American Psychiatric Association, 2022. Available at: www.psychiatry.org/psychiatrists/practice/practice-management/health-information-technology/interoperability-and-information-blocking. Accessed May 30, 2022.

Bender S, Messner E: Becoming a Therapist: What Do I Say, and Why? 2nd Edition. New York, Guilford, 2022

Cabaniss DL, Holoshitz Y: Different Patients, Different Therapies: Optimizing Treatment Using Differential Psychotherapeutics. New York, WW Norton, 2019

Crocker EM, Sudak DM: Making the most of psychotherapy supervision: a guide for psychiatry residents. Acad Psychiatry 41(1):35–39, 2017 27909977

Goldberg DA, Plakun EM: Teaching psychodynamic psychotherapy with the Y model. Psychodyn Psychiatry 41(1):111–126, 2013 23480163

Kroenke K, Spitzer RL: The PHQ-9: A new depression and diagnostic severity measure. Psychiatr Ann 32:509–521 2002

Office of Civil Rights: Does HIPAA provide extra protections for mental health information compared with other health information? Washington, DC, U.S. Department of Health and Human Services, September 12, 2017. Available at: www.hhs.gov/hipaa/for-professionals/faq/2088/does-hipaa-provide-extra-protections-mental-health-information-compared-other-health.html. Accessed May 31, 2022.

Ruble AE, Romanowicz M, Bhatt-Mackin S, et al: Teaching the fundamentals of remote psychotherapy to psychiatry residents in the COVID-19 pandemic. Acad Psychiatry 45(5):629–635, 2021 34405385

Shedler J: The efficacy of psychodynamic psychotherapy. Am Psychol 65(2):98–109, 2010 20141265

Spitzer RL, Kroenke K, Williams JBW, Löwe B: A brief measure for assessing generalized anxiety disorder: the GAD-7. Arch Intern Med 166(10):1092–1097, 2006 16717171

Welton RS, Crocker EM: Supportive therapy in the medically ill: using psychiatric skills to enhance primary care. Prim Care Companion CNS Disord 23(1):e1–e5, 2021 34000137

CHAPTER 18

Telehealth Services

Alka Mathur, M.D.

Neal D. Amin, M.D., Ph.D.

In the past several years, we have witnessed a rapid and widespread adoption of telehealth, followed by an exponential increase in its use during the COVID-19 pandemic as health care systems transitioned to virtual visits en masse. Although numerous medical specialties use telehealth, psychiatry is particularly amenable to the platform given the conversational nature of appointments and the reduced need for a physical examination. Telepsychiatry overcomes many impediments to care and addresses in a cost-effective manner the uneven geographic distribution and shortage of psychiatrists both within the United States and internationally. As more residency programs incorporate telehealth into their training, it is our goal to provide a foundation of practical knowledge that allows residents to be well equipped when seeing patients virtually.

KEY POINTS

- Practicing telepsychiatry can overcome geographic inequities and is comparable in efficacy to in-person visits.

- Discussing risks and benefits of telehealth and obtaining consent are important first steps when introducing telehealth to new patients.

- Proper camera positioning and provider familiarity with technology strengthens rapport with patients and enhances patient satisfaction.

- Routinely obtaining a patient's phone number and location and planning ahead with your attending physician are important aspects of preparedness in managing unanticipated psychiatric emergencies.

EFFICACY AND BENEFITS OF TELEHEALTH

Historically, rural and underserved communities have struggled with access to specialty mental health services. Because of provider shortages and difficulty in recruiting mental health specialists, there are often long wait lists for psychiatrists serving those populations. This results in detrimental delays in care and frequently requires patients to travel great distances to attend their appointments. Even more concerning, non–mental health providers may be left to care for these patients with limited training and resources. This results in poorer quality care, particularly for patients who require a higher level of services.

Telehealth can be an extremely effective way to overcome these barriers and offers multiple benefits for patients, clinicians, and communities. It is a cost-effective tool that improves access to mental health services by narrowing gaps caused by provider shortages. Additionally, telehealth allows patients greater flexibility to attend their appointments by cutting out numerous inconveniences associated with in-person appointments (e.g., need for childcare and time off from work, transportation limitations, travel and parking time and cost, privacy concerns in waiting rooms). Many patients greatly appreciate attending appointments during the workday without having to take off extra time for travel. Virtual contact has been particularly important during the COVID-19 pandemic, allowing both physicians and patients to reduce viral spread, particularly in vulnerable populations.

Another advantage can be found when working with patients who find it difficult to express their emotions more freely, such as patients with PTSD or social anxiety disorder. These populations can struggle with avoidance symptoms and have great difficulty opening up to others. The combination of being physically alone but still emotionally connected and aligned with their doctor may allow these patients to share their experiences more openly during telehealth appointments than in-person appointments. Being seen in their home or other "safe" space can facilitate greater feelings of safety, security, and privacy (Shore et al. 2014).

Numerous randomized controlled trials and other studies have demonstrated the effectiveness of telepsychiatry, showing equivalence and, in some cases, superiority to in-person visits (Guaiana et al. 2021). Additionally, no studies have found any negative impact on general mental health patient populations. Regarding specific subgroups, a literature review found equal efficacy of videoconferencing compared with in-person visits for patients with psychotic disorders (Sharp et al. 2011). A randomized trial demonstrated that the addition of telehealth monitoring was related to decreased number and length of medical hospitalizations in veterans with schizophrenia and schizoaffective disorder (Flaherty et al. 2017).

As psychiatrists, we often gain many benefits by providing telehealth as well, such as reduced commute times when working from home and decreased turnaround time between virtual patients compared with retrieving patients from waiting rooms. Multitasking by typing notes, entering orders, or reviewing the chart can be less disruptive in televisits than during in-person visits because we can more easily maintain eye contact and attention on the patient while also using the computer. Psychiatric supervision can be provided effectively in training settings by having a supervisor join you as a third participant for part or all of the video session. Alternatively, many video platforms allow high-quality recording of sessions and automatically generated verbal transcripts for psychotherapy sessions. If your institution has Health Insurance Portability and Accountability Act of 1996 (HIPAA)–compliant access to these transcripts, you or your supervisor can view them later to improve care. Video recording in telehealth, as with in-person visits, requires explicit permission from patients and protocols for data security.

It is important to note that telehealth visits may not always be appropriate when you are thoroughly assessing for medication side effects (e.g., to track changes in vitals or when performing physical examinations), when making standardized assessments (e.g., cognitive testing), or in situations when clinical staff must be present to administer treatment (e.g., long-acting injectable antipsychotics, ketamine for depression). Review these cases with your attending to determine the best plan of action.

HOW TO BE AN EFFECTIVE TELEPSYCHIATRIST

Before embarking on your telehealth journey, it is important to familiarize yourself with the basics of being an effective telepsychiatrist, including patient consent, legal regulations, technology, the treatment framework, and rapport with the patient.

Obtain and Document Patient Consent

Prior to or at the very beginning of the appointment, you should review a consent form with the patient and obtain their signature on completion. Document verbal consent and, if possible, obtain an electronic signature or have the patient send back the physical form. Remember to include documentation in your note reflecting this conversation and your review of risks, benefits, and alternatives, as well as patient consent to proceeding with telehealth. The elements of consent forms specific to telehealth are provided in Table 18–1.

TABLE 18–1.   Components of effective telehealth consent forms

Description of telehealth and the specific videoconferencing modality

Limitations to the specific video platform being used
• Presence of end-to-end encryption
• Concerns about privacy breaches

Benefits of telehealth
• Easier access to care
• Greater flexibility in scheduling and patient location at time of appointment

Risks of telehealth
• Technical difficulties on patient or provider side
• Interruptions
• Unauthorized access

Notice of ability for patient to discontinue telehealth modality at any time

Suitable alternatives
• In-person visits
• Telephone visits
• Transferring care

Patient's agreement to do a telehealth consultation

Source.   Adapted from U.S. Department of Veterans Affairs 2018.

Be Aware of the Most Current Legal Regulations Surrounding Psychiatric Telehealth Visits

During the COVID-19 pandemic, many regulations, including interstate prescribing and interstate video visits, were temporarily lifted, and there may be ongoing changes to regulations. Review the following information with your attending:

• Your state medical board's regulations at the time you are practicing to determine the exact legislation surrounding medical appointments

- Your medical board's stance on prescribing medications, particularly controlled substances, which may have stipulations such as requiring annual in-person visits
- Billing codes used for reimbursement, which may differ between virtual and in-person visits and can vary with insurance carriers

Establish the Framework for Treatment

Because telehealth enables greater flexibility in care delivery, patients can be located in a wide variety of physical sites. Certain settings can increase the likelihood of unintended distractions that may significantly interfere with the delivery of care. A basic checklist of expectations for patients includes the following:

- The patient should be stationary, in a quiet confidential area with no distractions (e.g., grocery shopping, socializing, driving, simultaneously using other electronic devices, running errands) to avoid interruptions and to ensure privacy
- The patient should have a strong, stable internet or cellular connection
- The patient must provide the exact address of their physical location at the time of the appointment for emergency purposes
- The patient should present themselves in the same manner they would in an in-person visit (fully clothed, sitting upright, focused on the appointment)

Build Rapport With Sight and Sound

Whereas much of psychiatry training focuses on in-person rapport building, this art has different nuances when it comes to telehealth. Spend time reviewing basic functionalities of the system, including using audiovisual tools, sharing your screen, and sending patients documentation or other resources. With regard to your appearance, try to use a neutral background and wear solid, nondistracting clothes, such that your appearance does not detract from the session. If there are additional aspects of your attire that you normally wear to reflect your role as a psychiatrist, include them in your ensemble. For example, you can wear your work badge, as you would for in-person visits, to further establish the frame of the video visit. Place yourself in a well-lit area, where the light source comes from behind your camera and in front of you, so that your face is illuminated and easy to see. You can achieve this by having a window or lamp set up behind your camera source or using commercially available lighting kits designed for videoconferencing. If instead the light source is behind you, you will appear shadowy and unclear to the patient.

Regarding audio settings, ensure that your computer microphone and speakers or headphones are set at appropriate volumes and sensitivities. Some teleconferencing software includes features that automatically reduce background noise so that patients can hear you more clearly. Ensure that you are speaking at a pace and frequency that the patient can understand, which you can confirm by asking them directly. Audio delays can make it seem as though you are interrupting the patient, so be mindful of allowing ample time for patients to complete their thoughts.

No matter the modality of care delivery, good eye contact is an integral component of making a patient feel both seen and heard. Look directly at the camera when speaking to the patient *so that they feel that you are looking directly at them.* If you are looking at their image on the computer screen, it appears to patients that you are looking downward instead of at them. With experience, you will become very efficient at maintaining your gaze at the camera, while also periodically looking at the screen to assess the patient and their presentation. An additional and important consideration is camera location. If your camera is too low, it will appear as if you are looming over the patient. To ensure that your camera sits at eye level, you may need to elevate your desktop screen or laptop by placing books, a small table, or other sturdy objects underneath it. These seemingly small actions go a long way in conveying professionalism, building alliances, and increasing patient comfort levels.

EMERGENCY PLANNING

Telehealth visits may involve psychiatric emergencies such as patients presenting with acute suicidal or homicidal risk. Prepare for these situations in advance by routinely confirming and documenting a patient's precise location and address at the start of every visit as well as the number for the local police department in the patient's county. Keep this number available in advance in the chart. This is the fastest and most effective way to direct first responders to the patient's location and is more effective than dialing 911 because your local 911 operators will be unable to transfer your call to another county. In case of a psychiatric emergency, use a second phone or place the patient on hold and call the 10-digit phone number for the police department in the patient's county. You should engage in more extensive emergency planning with at-risk patients by being aware of the nearest emergency department, crisis stabilization unit, or emergency services available at the patient's location.

If a patient is unable to provide this information to you for any reason, you should ascertain the reasons why and discuss with your supervisor the risks of delivering care.

For moderate- and high-risk patients, make it a regular practice to preemptively go through safety plans with the patient in greater detail with your attending present. This might include obtaining permission to contact family or friends who are local to the patient if they are feeling distressed and in need of in-person support. Check with your attending whether verbal consent or written consent is needed. Furthermore, always consider transitioning a patient to in-person visits for closer medical or psychiatric monitoring when clinically warranted.

PRIVACY CONCERNS

Privacy facilitates patients' comfort with discussing sensitive issues during a psychiatric visit. Confidentiality fosters a deeper therapeutic alliance and accurate data collection, which are bedrocks of clinical decision-making. Unlike in office settings, you cannot directly control the physical space available to a patient during telehealth encounters. A patient may face logistical barriers to finding a private location for a session. At the outset of care, you should initiate a discussion and help navigate privacy-related issues that might arise during telehealth visits. A useful starting point can be for you to directly ask the patient if there are any particular relationships or sensitive topics that they might feel uncomfortable discussing in their current location. If the patient shares significant concerns, help brainstorm alternative locations that might afford a greater level of privacy and openness. It is not uncommon for patients to sequester themselves in sometimes physically uncomfortable places such as a bathroom or parked car for the sake of greater confidentiality. Use of headphones by the patient can facilitate more discreet communication with you.

Some patients may not fully appreciate the extent to which they might self-censor themselves when other people are around, so you need to be aware of the patient's setting and how it influences body language and the content of telehealth encounters. For example, patients may have strong conscious or subconscious reservations about recollecting trauma, sharing suicidal thoughts, or displaying raw emotions that make them feel intensely vulnerable in a suboptimal setting. When unexpected events occur that abruptly jeopardize privacy (e.g., a partner interrupting a session), it is helpful to debrief with the patient at a later time to understand how the session was affected.

COUNSELING PATIENTS WHO DISLIKE TECHNOLOGY

Navigating video platforms, internet accessibility, and general technical issues may cause significant stress for certain patients whose familiarity and comfort with technology are low. These issues are frequently observed in geriatric populations but can occur with any patient (or even providers) at one time or another. You should directly address concerns about telehealth technology and its perceived negative effects on clinical care so that the patient's struggles are understood, validated, and addressed. Clinicians, support staff, or patients' caregivers may need to provide technical support in order to have the patient successfully engage with telehealth providers, especially with patients who have cognitive deficits. Furthermore, you should be able to explain the potential benefits of telehealth so patients understand why this nontraditional model of care is being implemented.

TECHNOLOGY FAILURES

When teleconferencing technology acutely fails, a patient may not know whether this was intentional (i.e., the session is over) or whether their own device has contributed to a connectivity problem. Unanticipated technology issues can cause confusion and stress for patients and can contribute to decreased satisfaction with telepsychiatry and potentially adverse outcomes. To ensure that the delivery of your care is both effective and reliable, preemptively make contingency plans and communicate them with the patient prior to or at the outset of an appointment. For example, you can attempt to reconnect or troubleshoot technology issues for a reasonable amount of time (and ask the patient to do the same if the issue is suspected to be on their end). If the problem remains unresolved after several minutes, you should notify the patient that you will call them via telephone. It is important to verify the accuracy of patients' listed phone numbers for this reason. Coordinating these plans with your attending (via a predetermined method such as text, paging, or phone call) is also crucial during technology disruptions and more generally during particularly challenging clinical encounters in which support is needed.

TELEPSYCHIATRY FOR CHILDREN

Play therapy is an important therapeutic modality for child psychiatry patients because it can help you obtain information from the patient's perspective and observe their behavior and responses to challenges. The use of toys can be challenging in telepsychiatry; providers may have toys on their side to engage patients in pretend play or use toys provided to the patient by caregivers. Furthermore, the inherent distractions of a computer can reduce the quality of a child's attention to the telepsychiatrist. Nevertheless, there are many ways to engage in play via the screen. Having a whiteboard in your room visible to the camera can be helpful for drawing engaging images. You can ask parents to give the child pencils and paper or other play items ahead of an appointment. Some video software allows for patients and providers to draw on the same virtual whiteboard, which can result in more direct interaction and a shared experience that can enhance alliance and trust. Providers have also engaged with pediatric patients by joining popular online gaming platforms to co-build virtual worlds.

Setting boundaries on disruptive behavior can also be a challenge in virtual visits with children, and greater reliance on caregivers in the room to set limits may be necessary. In general, the way child psychiatry patients interact with you in the virtual setting (even if they are disruptive or avoidant) can be representative of how they interact in school or other settings. Thus, challenging sessions can still meaningfully guide treatment.

One potential benefit of telepsychiatry visits for child psychiatry patients is the opportunity for caregivers in multiple locations to join in on the visit. For example, a parent at a work location or separated parents can join the televisit as third-party participants while another caregiver assists the child at home. Thus, telepsychiatry can facilitate greater and more direct interaction with multiple caregivers.

SPECIFIC CHALLENGES AND STRATEGIES

⌘ **While I was interviewing a new patient with manic symptoms who was telling me about their suicide plan, my internet disconnected and I wasn't able to reconnect.** It is important to be prepared for emergencies by confirming a patient's telephone number at the outset of your appointments. Stay connected to the patient by calling them while you simultaneously attempt to troubleshoot the technology issue. Because several aspects of this patient's psychiatric condition are concerning, you should facilitate their being evaluated at an emergency department. Involve your attending in high-risk cases by texting or paging the attending or placing the patient on a brief hold to call them. You might identify the emergency department closest to the patient's location and direct the patient there if they are in agreement and have a safe means of transportation. In the face of an acutely suicidal patient who is not willing to go to the hospital, you should continue to engage the patient in dialogue while you ask your attending to notify the police of the emergency and request a welfare check.

⌘ **My 88-year-old patient with depression and age-related cognitive decline logged into his video appointment 20 minutes late for a 30-minute appointment. He was frustrated about being unfamiliar with the computer software. After he yelled directly into the microphone while trying to adjust his computer (I could see only the top of his head), we only had 5 minutes remaining to discuss his psychiatric issues.** Patient discomfort and technical issues most commonly occur during the first telehealth appointment. To best assist with the transition from in-person to telehealth care, don't shy away from a direct discussion about the issues patients face and the reasons why you think telehealth care is effective. To start such a discussion, you might say the following:

Technical issues with video chat software are frustrating and happen to many of my patients—and clinicians like myself, too. I'm sorry you experienced these issues today, and I hope our staff will help you successfully navigate these challenges before our next appointment. However, my patients have really appreciated the flexibility of telehealth and its ease of use once it becomes routine. I know finding transportation to psychiatric clinics has been an issue for you in the past, and my hope is that our telehealth visits will be more convenient and may save you time since they can be done from the comfort of your home. Finally, I want to acknowledge that a telehealth visit may not be the same experience as seeing each other in person, but I do believe I can provide you with excellent care remotely. I'd like to hear more about how we can work together to address your needs.

⌘ **During today's telepsychiatry visit, my patient's parents placed my 7-year-old patient in front of the camera as usual. This time, however, she was downcast and did not engage with me, despite cajoling from her parents. When her parents left the room, she appeared to be opening a video game on the computer rather than talking with me.** If you are not able to engage with a young patient or provide effective care, ask the patient to call their parents back into the room. Have a discussion with the parents around possible reasons for this change in behavior, such as a potential mood disorder, conduct issues, or recent stressors. If this avoidant interaction persists, help brainstorm potential behavioral strategies to promote more engaged patient behavior, such as reward systems. You may also consider thinking about new ways to engage the patient, such as introducing age-appropriate games consistent with the patient's interests.

⌘ **Sitting at the dining room table of her apartment, my 24-year-old patient spoke in hushed tones when she recounted a recent altercation with her live-in partner but then became increasingly anxious and hesitant. I heard footsteps and then briefly saw her partner in the frame of the video, at which point the patient abruptly changed the topic. She clearly felt unsafe to discuss her relationship in her present location.** In this type of situation, it can be helpful to start a discussion about privacy at a later point in the session (after the patient's partner has left the area) or after the appointment via secure messaging. You might say, "I want to be sure that you feel as comfortable as possible to discuss sensitive topics. Having a private space to talk is important to make sure that you feel safe enough to share your personal thoughts and feelings. Can you think of other locations where you can be sure our conversation won't be overheard?" You might also reschedule her appointments to another time when her partner will be out and she will have the apartment to herself.

SELF-REFLECTIVE QUESTIONS

1. Have I spent enough time familiarizing myself with the particular telehealth software and technology my clinic uses?
2. Can I comfortably discuss the risks of, benefits of, and alternatives to telepsychiatric care with my patients?
3. Am I aware of the medicolegal aspects of telepsychiatry in my particular state and region?
4. Have I developed a comprehensive plan with my supervisors to address telepsychiatric emergencies?

RESOURCES

American Medical Association: Telehealth Implementation Playbook. Chicago, IL, American Medical Association, 2020. Available at: www.ama-assn.org/system/files/2020-04/ama-telehealth-implementation-playbook.pdf. Accessed October 4, 2022.

American Psychiatric Association: Telepsychiatry toolkit. Washington, DC, American Psychiatric Association, 2022. Available at: www.psychiatry.org/psychiatrists/practice/telepsychiatry/toolkit. Accessed October 4, 2022.

American Psychological Association: Telehealth continuing education resources. Washington, DC, American Psychological Association, 2020. Available at: www.apa.org/ed/ce/telehealth. Accessed October 4, 2022.

Centers for Disease Control and Prevention: The use of telehealth and telemedicine in public health. Atlanta, GA, Centers for Disease Control and Prevention, 2020. Available at: www.cdc.gov/phlp/publications/topic/telehealth.html. Accessed October 4, 2022.

Stanford Mental Health Tech and Innovation Hub: Reset: a resource toolkit. Stanford, CA, Stanford Mental Health Tech and Innovation Hub, 2021. Available at: www.stanfordmhtech.com/covid19-resources. Accessed October 4, 2022.

U.S. Department of Health and Human Services: Telehealth: health care from the safety of our homes. Rockville, MD, Health Resources and Services Administration, 2022. Available at: www.telehealth.hhs.gov. Accessed October 4, 2022.

VA Telehealth: https://telehealth.va.gov

REFERENCES

Flaherty LR, Daniels K, Luther J, et al: Reduction of medical hospitalizations in veterans with schizophrenia using home telehealth. Psychiatry Res 255:153–155, 2017 28550756

Guaiana G, Mastrangelo J, Hendrikx S, et al: A systematic review of the use of telepsychiatry in depression. Community Ment Health J 57(1):93–100, 2021 33040191

Sharp IR, Kobak KA, Osman DA: The use of videoconferencing with patients with psychosis: a review of the literature. Ann Gen Psychiatry 10(1):14, 2011 21501496

Shore JH, Mishkind MC, Bernard J, et al: A lexicon of assessment and outcome measures for telemental health. Telemed J E Health 20(3):282–292, 2014 24476192

U.S. Department of Veterans Affairs: National Center for Ethics in Health Care. VHA Directive 1004. Washington, DC, Veterans Health Administration, October 31, 2018. Available at: www.ethics.va.gov/docs/policy/VHA_Handbook_1004_NCEHC.pdf. Accessed February 2, 2022.

CHAPTER 19

Legal Issues

Michael Kelly, M.D.
Zachary Lenane, M.D., M.P.H.

Residency training is difficult, and for good reason. It is a time of rapid professional growth marked by new and often unforeseen challenges. Psychiatry training cannot be completed in a classroom, and it necessitates degrees of "trial by fire" learning to develop the skills required of an excellent psychiatrist. Psychiatry residents routinely make decisions that have major impacts on the lives of patients and their loved ones. Thus, it is no surprise that the power, privilege, and accountability that come with becoming a psychiatrist can feel daunting. For instance, helping patients with severe and persistent mental illness decide on the best medication for themselves can have major impacts on their safety, mental health, and overall well-being. Additionally, anyone who has worked in a psychiatric emergency department knows that the decision to involuntarily commit someone is a high-stakes situation for patients and their loved ones. Therefore, it is not enough for psychiatrists to be skilled at psychotherapy and prescribing medication. Our work requires a fundamental grasp of medical ethics, professionalism, and the legal framework of psychiatric practice.

This chapter is designed to be a practical introduction to some of the legal and ethical challenges encountered during training. Although it is beyond the scope of this chapter to cover all the legal and ethical issues you will face, the content within provides a conceptual foundation for thinking critically about such matters in clinical settings.

KEY POINTS

- Competent persons have the right to decide what happens to their bodies, and, with few exceptions, ethical psychiatric care requires informed consent.

- Psychiatrists are ethically bound to maintain patient confidentiality except when patients waive their doctor-patient privilege.

- In most states, physicians are mandated to report abuse and/or neglect of vulnerable populations (e.g., children, elderly persons, persons with developmental disabilities).

INFORMED CONSENT AND DECISIONAL CAPACITY

The three core elements of informed consent are 1) information sharing, 2) decisional capacity, and 3) volunteerism. In other words, informed consent relates to providing patients or their guardians with information (e.g., potential risks, benefits, prognosis with and without treatment, alternatives) they need to voluntarily make informed health care decisions. In some states, nonnegligent medical care mandates that physicians obtain informed consent in a manner consistent with what a "reasonable medical practitioner" would disclose to patients. However, most states necessitate that physicians provide patients with the level of detail that a "reasonable person" would want to know, including information about potential serious associated risks and benefits, when deciding whether to engage in treatment.

With regard to the practice of psychiatry, two legal cases that underscore the importance of informed consent are *Clites v. Iowa* (1982) and *Zinermon v. Burch* (1990). In the case of *Clites v. Iowa*, a doctor was sued for prescribing antipsychotic medication for an institutionalized man with developmental disability for many years without proper monitoring or informed consent from his legal guardians. The patient eventually developed tardive dyskinesia (an irreversible side effect), and the doctor was sued for negligence. The Iowa Court of Appeals ultimately ruled that prescribing antipsychotics without informing patients and/or their guardians about potential risks, benefits, and side effects constitutes malpractice.

In the case of *Zinermon v. Burch* (1990), a floridly psychotic and injured Mr. Burch was found wandering on a Florida highway and taken to a psychiatric hospital, where he was voluntarily admitted and treated with antipsychotic medication. After 3 days, the patient remained psychotic and was transferred to a state hospital, where he voluntarily signed the admission forms. Mr. Burch eventually sought release from the hospital and sued the state of Florida for allowing him to consent to voluntary treatment despite the fact that he was psychotic and lacked the decisional capacity required for informed consent. The U.S. Supreme Court agreed with Mr. Burch and ruled that the state's actions violated his civil liberties. These cases, and others like them, underscore the importance of respecting our patients' autonomy and obtaining informed consent before initiating treatment.

In psychiatry, determining *capacity* or *decisional capacity* involves a clinical appraisal of an individual's ability to function in relation to specific demands or situations (Mishkin 1989). For example, a psychotic individual may possess the decisional capacity requisite to make decisions about whether to take antihypertensive medication. That same individual could simultaneously lack decisional capacity to consent to urgently needed heart surgery because of a delusional belief that doctors merely want to implant an electronic monitoring device in his body. Dr. Paul Appelbaum (2007) succinctly described decisional capacity as follows:

> Legal standards for decision-making capacity for consent to treatment vary somewhat across jurisdictions, but generally they embody the abilities to communicate a choice, to understand the relevant information, to appreciate the medical consequences of the situation, and to reason about treatment choices. (p. 1835)

In summary, decisional capacity is requisite for informed consent. That said, decisional capacity can fluctuate within the same person depending on the situation. For instance, an elderly woman with mild dementia may display changes in her decisional capacity over the course of a few days due to mental status changes associated with a urinary tract infection. Therefore, it is important to be familiar with these concepts so that you can apply them flexibly in a variety of situations, rather than developing a "script" for various types of patient encounters.

CIVIL COMMITMENT

There are numerous examples, past and present, of the medical establishment abusing its privilege and power at the expense of innocent people. For instance, in the Tuskegee Experiment, the Centers for Disease Control and Prevention and the U.S. Public Health Service systematically and surreptitiously denied treatment for syphilis to impoverished Black American sharecroppers from Macon County, Alabama, for 40 years, through 1972 (Centers for Disease Control and Prevention 2021). Lapses in the integrity of scientific research and/or fraud, recently exemplified by reviews suggesting that between 10% and 20% of published medical literature may be based on untrustworthy data, are an important reminder that the medical establishment and associated institutions are not entitled to society's unquestioning trust (Horton 2015; Smith 2021). Regarding psychiatry, many people are familiar with the fictionalized real-life account of the authoritarian abuse of psychiatric patients in the book and film *One Flew Over the Cuckoo's Nest.* Less well known, yet equally compelling, is the story behind the U.S. Supreme Court case *O'Connor v. Donaldson* (1975).

Kenneth Donaldson drove from his home in Pennsylvania to Florida to visit his parents in 1956. After arrival, Mr. Donaldson told his father that his neighbor in Philadelphia had been poisoning him. Mr. Donaldson's father filed a petition for a sanity hearing that led to Mr. Donaldson being diagnosed with schizophrenia and being civilly committed to a state hospital. Mr. Donaldson refused to take antipsychotic medication in the hospital, which was consistent with his being a member of the Christian Science faith. Mr. Donaldson spent 15 years inside a Florida state hospital for his psychosis despite the fact that he was not dangerous to himself or others, was able to care for himself adequately, and received only milieu therapy. Mr. Donaldson eventually sued the superintendent, Dr. J.B. O'Connor, for taking away his liberty. The U.S. Supreme Court agreed in its ruling that "a State cannot constitutionally confine, without more, a non-dangerous individual who is capable of surviving safely in freedom by himself or with the help of willing and responsible family members or friends" (*O'Connor v. Donaldson* 1975, pp. 573–576). The Court added the following:

> May the State fence in the harmless mentally ill solely to save its citizens from exposure to those whose ways are different? One might as well ask if the State, to avoid public unease, could incarcerate all who are physically unattractive or socially eccentric. (*O'Connor v. Donaldson* 1975)

The ruling in *O'Connor v. Donaldson* sparked shifts in civil commitment standards around the country from a paternalistic treatment model to one that prioritizes patient autonomy by necessitating that persons who are involuntarily committed must pose acute danger to self or others or be incapable of caring for themselves safely in the community. Despite the gains the field of psychiatry has made since the 1970s, the potential for abuses of power still exist. Such examples are not meant to discourage you but instead underscore the importance of remaining cognizant of our values, our duty as physicians, and how we can maintain both while working in flawed and sometimes violent (e.g., Tuskegee Experiment) systems of care.

MANDATED REPORTING AND DUTY TO PROTECT

Psychiatrists are usually required to make an official report when they learn of abuse or neglect of vulnerable persons, such as children, elderly people, and adults with developmental disabilities (American Bar Association Commission on Law and Aging 2020; Child Welfare Information Gateway 2019). Some states also require psychiatrists to report domestic violence. Most states mandate reporting when the psychiatrist reasonably suspects that a vulnerable person has been abused and/or neglected.

In most states, mental health therapists and physicians also have a legal duty to protect (or warn) third parties about dangerous patients who intend to harm them. This duty to protect is a common exception to confidentiality that you are likely to encounter. These laws are often referred to as Tarasoff statutes, referencing the *Tarasoff v. Regents of the University of California* (1976) California Supreme Court ruling that found that therapists have a duty to protect individuals credibly threatened by their patients. Consistent with this ruling, duty-to-protect statutes generally require a therapist to contact the intended victim(s) and/or law enforcement regarding their patient or client's threat of violence, although there is significant variation by state. In 29 states and Puerto Rico, this duty to report is mandatory; in 16 states it is "permissive," meaning they allow reporting without risk of civil liability but do not strictly require it; and in 4 states there is no duty to protect. It is important to know the specific requirements in your state of practice, which can be found through the National Conference of State Legislatures' Database of State Tarasoff Laws, last revised in 2022 (National Conference of State Legislatures 2022).

Psychiatrists should discuss the duty to protect or the mandated reporting of suspected abuse in detail during the initial patient meeting as a means of setting the treatment frame. In order to respect patient autonomy and promote beneficence, you should describe in advance the circumstances in which you may be required to break confidentiality, no matter how unlikely. Reporting your patient or their guardian can rupture the therapeutic alliance, sometimes irreparably, even if they are aware of your duty to report. However, if you wait to disclose your duty to report until you are in a situation where you *must* report, your patient likely will be surprised, leading to both a potential rupture in the therapeutic alliance and, possibly, an unwillingness to seek care from the broader mental health system in the future.

NEGLIGENCE

Simply put, negligence is a "dereliction of duty directly causing damages" (Sadoff 1975). That is, a negligent physician is one who abandons their duty of care in a manner that directly leads to personal injury or other damages to the patient. Psychiatrists are the least likely medical specialty to be sued for negligence (Jena et al. 2011). When psychiatrists are sued, the leading causes of malpractice claims are often related to patient suicide. For example, prescribing antidepressant medication to a depressed patient, then failing to respond to reports of side effects and/or worsening symptoms leading to patient injury or death would be considered negligent care.

SPECIFIC CHALLENGES AND STRATEGIES

⌘ **My vulnerable patient reported abuse in the presence of their legal guardian, who is also the alleged abuser.** This is a scenario that many psychiatrists have or will encounter at some point in their careers. Because you are a mandated reporter in these circumstances, it is important to have already alerted the patient and legal guardian of this possibility when setting the treatment frame. Referring back to your previous conversation will communicate that this is your duty and that you are not "pulling the rug out" from under patients whose trust you have gained. Maintaining the therapeutic alliance in these situations is difficult. That said, even if the therapeutic relationship is damaged beyond repair, being honest and up-front about your mandated reporting duties at the start of treatment may enable the patient and/or legal guardian to consider the prospect of continuing treatment more easily with another provider, at a later time. If you did not disclose your duty to report at the beginning of your work with the patient, approach with transparency at this point and consider bringing in your supervisor for support.

⌘ **My patient wants to spend time with me outside treatment.** Although it may seem obvious that crossing boundaries with patients in and outside the treatment setting is a "no go," these situations can be awkward and are not uncommon. Setting the treatment frame with appropriate expectations in the beginning of treatment will provide you with a solid foundation for declining such requests while maintaining the therapeutic alliance. Also, do not be afraid to explain to patients the reasons why meeting outside the therapy setting is counterproductive to their treatment and your ability to remain professional in these circumstances. Most often, issues like this one can be resolved and may even be an important segue to discussing topics and ideas that are quite useful in treatment.

⌘ **I'm not sure how to obtain informed consent from my psychotic patient.** Mental illness, including psychosis, does not in and of itself negate a patient's decisional capacity. For instance, persons who are psychotic and delusional may be capable of weighing the risks and benefits of psychiatric medications. Thus, it is essential that we do not assume that mentally ill persons, including psychotic individuals dealing with schizophrenia, lack capacity simply because of their symptoms or apparent resistance to treatment.

SELF-REFLECTIVE QUESTIONS

1. How do I determine whether a patient should be placed on a legal hold and involuntarily admitted? How do I consider patient autonomy, safety, and decisional capacity in this case?
2. How will I respond to patients with genuine distrust of the medical and/or mental health profession who resist the course of treatment I am recommending?
3. Although I have less power to make change in my institution as a trainee, how can I still approach clinical work in a manner that is consistent with my values?

RESOURCES

American Bar Association Commission on Law and Aging: Adult protective services reporting laws. Chicago, IL, American Bar Association, 2020. Available at: www.americanbar.org/content/dam/aba/administrative/law_aging/2020-elder-abuse-reporting-chart.pdf. Accessed August 19, 2021.

Child Welfare Information Gateway: Mandatory reporters of child abuse and neglect. Washington, DC, Children's Bureau, U.S. Department of Health and Human Services, 2019. Available at: www.childwelfare.gov/topics/systemwide/laws-policies/statutes/manda. Accessed August 19, 2021.

National Conference of State Legislatures: Mental health professionals' duty to warn. Washington, DC, National Conference of State Legis-

latures, March 16, 2022. Available at: www.ncsl.org/research/
health/mental-health-professionals-duty-to-warn.aspx. Accessed
May 17, 2022.

REFERENCES

American Bar Association Commission on Law and Aging: Adult protective
services reporting laws. Chicago, IL, American Bar Association, 2020.
Available at: www.americanbar.org/content/dam/aba/administrative/
law_aging/2020-elder-abuse-reporting-chart.pdf. Accessed August 29,
2021.

Appelbaum PS: Clinical practice: assessment of patients' competence to consent
to treatment. N Engl J Med 357(18):1834–1840, 2007 17978292

Centers for Disease Control and Prevention: The Tuskegee timeline. Atlanta,
GA, Centers for Disease Control and Prevention, April 22, 2021. Available
at: www.cdc.gov/tuskegee/timeline.htm. Accessed September 7, 2021.

Child Welfare Information Gateway: Mandatory reporters of child abuse and
neglect. Washington, DC, Children's Bureau, U.S. Department of Health
and Human Services, 2019. Available at: www.childwelfare.gov/topics/
systemwide/laws-policies/statutes/manda. Accessed August 29, 2021.

Clites v. State, 322 N.W.2d 917 (Iowa Ct. App. 1982)

Horton R: Offline: what is medicine's 5 sigma? Lancet 385(9976):1380, 2015

Jena AB, Seabury S, Lakdawalla D, et al: Malpractice risk according to physician
specialty. N Engl J Med 365(7):629–636, 2011 21848463

Mishkin B: Determining the capacity for making health care decisions. Adv Psychosom Med 19:151–166, 1989 2686360

National Conference of State Legislatures: Mental health professionals' duty to
warn. Washington, DC, National Conference of State Legislatures, March
16, 2022. Available at: www.ncsl.org/research/health/mental-health-
professionals-duty-to-warn.aspx. Accessed August 29, 2021.

O'Connor v. Donaldson, 422 U.S. 563, 95 S. Ct. 2486, 45 L. Ed. 2d 396 (1975)

Sadoff RL: Forensic Psychiatry: A Practical Guide for Lawyers and Psychiatrists. Springfield, IL, Charles C Thomas, 1975

Smith R: Time to assume health research is fraudulent until proven otherwise?
BMJ Opinion, July 5, 2021. Available at: blogs.bmj.com/bmj/2021/07/05/
time-to-assume-that-health-research-is-fraudulent-until-proved-otherwise.
Accessed July 14, 2021.

Tarasoff v. Regents of the University of California, 17 Cal. 3d 425, 551 P.2d 334,
131 Cal. Rptr. 14 (Cal. 1976)

Zinermon v. Burch, 494 U.S. 113, 110 S. Ct. 975, 108 L. Ed. 2d 100 (1990)

CHAPTER 20

Managing Patient Suicide

Zheala Qayyum, M.D., M.M.Sc.

Rachel Conrad, M.D.

Jeffrey Hunt, M.D.

About 30%–60% of general psychiatry residents will experience the suicide of a patient during their training years (Ruskin et al. 2004). Suicide brings with it a suddenness and lack of closure that has impacts on the friends, family, and professionals involved in the care of the individual, becoming a significant and notable event in their lives. Unfortunately, most psychiatrists experience the suicide of a patient at some point in their careers. Because patient suicide can significantly affect trainees in their personal and professional lives, in this chapter we provide guidance for self-care and seeking support within institutions.

KEY POINTS

- Most systems of care do not respond adequately to the deep emotional impact of a patient suicide.

- Institutions, together with the help of trainees, can develop planful responses to support individuals affected by patient suicide.

- There is a great need for physicians to recognize the importance of self-care and to model wellness and openness to talking with vulnerable peers.

STARTING WITH PREVENTION

Ideally, programs should offer training early in residency on managing and coping with patient suicide. By modeling discussions of difficult moments that can occur in professional careers, program directors and faculty can foster a safe and trusting environment where trainees may feel more comfortable to express their needs and seek support. Unfortunately, this training often does not occur soon enough, and the program response to a patient suicide tends more often to be a reactive one. However, setting up a culture that normalizes and rewards seeking help and support as a part of training can help trainees more readily identify their needs and reduce the risk of burnout, and as a result, fewer trainees may suffer silently.

RECEIVING NOTIFICATION

If you have not already been informed, your direct supervisor, medical director, or training director ideally will notify you in the event of a suicide and provide you support and guidance. However, given how many people within a system have contact with a patient, this does not always happen. It can be very challenging to get this news from someone with whom you do not have an established relationship. If you hear from other sources, such as indirectly on social media, phone calls from the patient's family, other staff members, or general department emails, reach out to your supervisor of record, medical director of the service, and program director as soon as possible (Qayyum et al. 2021b). They may not be aware of the event, and it can be challenging to navigate the next steps or know how to respond to these notifications without support or guidance. Ensuring that the right people know and can support you during this entire process can help alleviate the anxiety associated with conversations with the family and subsequent meetings with risk management. Finally, when you receive the notification of a patient's death from suicide, it may be helpful to surround yourself with trusted family or friends.

GATHERING FACTS

The medical director or the attending physician who treated the patient is often the one who gathers as much accurate information about the event as possible to minimize speculation and confusion (American Foundation for Suicide Prevention 2022). Gathering this information in a timely manner is important to mitigate the spreading of incorrect information and reduce common (and *normal)* trainee feelings that they missed something or did something wrong.

RESPONDING EMOTIONALLY TO A SUICIDE

Death is one of the most stressful experiences for residents across specialties (Firth-Cozens 1989), and residents often feel unprepared for its intense emotional impact (Qayyum et al. 2021a; Sullivan et al. 2003; Vallurupalli 2013). The death of a patient from suicide may be accompanied by further complexities and may have a unique emotional impact on trainees, given its suddenness and the trainees' perceived sense of responsibility. You may have heard from supervisors that the patient is at high risk of suicide on the basis of the suicide risk assessment, but the moment that it actually happens can feel devastating. These feelings of shock often are followed by sadness for the patient and their family. You also may experience shame and guilt, which may lead to hesitation in accessing support. In addition, you may experience feelings of anger, betrayal, disappointment, or even traumatization, which are expected and normal. It is important to recognize these feelings as they arise.

In the immediate aftermath, ensure that you prioritize taking care of yourself and allow your supervisors to provide that space for you. Step away and go for a walk, connect with your supervisor, or ask to speak with someone in your program who has had this experience. You may desire frequent and transparent communication with your colleagues or may not be comfortable overtly sharing your emotional experience and prefer privacy. However, reaching out to loved ones or friends for support or asking to go home early can help you make space for your emotional response. In addition, programs are required to offer you 24/7 access to mental health support, and you may want to reach out to a crisis counselor at this time. Even if you are not immediately ready to process the event with others, it can be helpful to leave the door open to have these conversations once you feel ready for them.

Suicide of a patient affects everyone differently; the grief and mourning process will look different for each person, takes different amounts of time, and can evolve over time. After the immediate crisis response, some individuals continue to experience the emotional impact of patient suicide in a cyclical way or as an ebb and flow over time, making ongoing supports necessary.

The suicide of a patient can also shake your confidence as a psychiatry resident and result in self-doubt, especially around clinical decision-making or even your choice of career. You may hesitate to discharge patients and focus excessively on risk assessments and documentation. Although these are normal responses, supervision and support can help you regain confidence and a sense of competence in your clinical practice (Qayyum et al. 2021a).

ACCESSING SUPPORT

Be honest and open about what you need and make sure to check in with yourself to access the supports that would be best for you. Unfortunately, clinical demands persist even while many physicians are simultaneously grieving a loss. Creating space for emotional reactions while minimizing potential disruptions to patient care may become challenging. You may find that you need to remove yourself from clinical obligations for a few days, or you might find that staying occupied and being around peers is more comforting.

By finding an effective way to cope with this experience, you can reduce the risk of your own burnout and provide effective and safe medical care (Papadatou 2000). Prioritize self-care and ensure that you receive adequate sleep and rest. Take time for yourself and engage in activities that are relaxing and meaningful and help reduce stress.

Internal programmatic supports may include workload modification, time off to take care of yourself, changes in on-call schedules, and supervision around processing this event (Qayyum et al. 2021b). Often, your supervising attending physician on record can be a partner during this challenging time. They can support you in both the grieving and meaning-making processes, as well as guide you during the departmental formal reviews, meetings with risk management, and contact with the family. If you already have a good relationship with your supervisor, then this supervisory relationship can have a positive impact on your experience (Qayyum et al. 2021b).

Supervisors and peers who have experienced a patient suicide may help you cope with such a death through their modeling and support (Curtis and Levy 2014; Kelly and Nisker 2010; Ratanawongsa et al. 2005; Qayyum et al. 2021b). Other residents are often the most helpful source of emotional support for trainees (Eldridge et al. 2021; Redinbaugh et al. 2003). Additional support such as counsel from chaplains; legal guidance; and assistance from the human resources office, employee health office, or public relations office may be helpful to you as well.

Furthermore, many trainees find comfort and spiritual support within their communities. If you feel you would like support outside the program, ask for external referrals for psychotherapy, from which many trainees benefit.

MEETING WITH RISK MANAGEMENT

A meeting with risk management or the legal department is important for gaining more guidance about the next steps on the basis of state laws and the statute of limitations. Risk management may discourage the clinicians involved from discussing the specifics of the case with others. In such instances, trainees may feel that they have no recourse to discuss their experience. It is important to note that clinicians and trainees involved may still seek out supervision support to process their own emotional and psychological response to the patient suicide without discussing the details of the case (Qayyum et al. 2021b).

The patient's family may file a malpractice lawsuit in which the members of the clinical team are named. It is important to remember that the institution will provide legal support and that the burden of responsibility lies on the attending and the institution, not as much on the trainee. If you ever find yourself in this situation, recruit the support of your supervisor and reach out to risk management for further guidance. Often, the institution will work with legal counsel to have the trainee dismissed from the case. In rare situations, a trainee may have acted without the knowledge or approval of their supervisor or failed to share information with them. In such cases, the trainee might be pulled into the litigation; however, even in these instances, the institution bears the burden of responsibility. The loss of a patient must be owned by everyone and must not be placed on a few individuals alone.

TALKING TO THE PATIENT'S FAMILY

The trainee should be supported and guided in how to contact the family or return the family's call. This is best done as a team with consultation from risk management and after discussion with the supervisors and other members involved in caring for the patient within the institution. Prepare yourself ahead of time because the family, who is no doubt devastated, may displace their anger onto you and your team. Sometimes, families just need a space to process. It is important to acknowledge the family's distress, offer condolences, and allow them to ask questions, which should be answered to the best of your ability while maintaining an appropriate level of confidentiality. The patient may have given permission for the family to be involved and contacted as part of their care, which may facilitate this process (Qayyum et al. 2021b). If the patient had not allowed permission for the family to be contacted, the concerns of the family can still be heard, condolences offered, and their anxieties or questions answered to the best of your ability without the release of the patient's confidential and privileged information. Providing compassion and support to the family can be a meaningful experience for you as a resident and aid in your own emotional processing as well.

PARTICIPATING IN INSTITUTIONAL REVIEWS

Ideally, institutions have structured policies to follow in the event of a patient suicide. It is important for programmatic leadership to connect directly with faculty, trainees, and nonphysician colleagues to alert them of the event and assess the most appropriate forum for processing the information. Institutional internal reviews for patient suicide may range from informal reviews such as the involvement of a crisis response team for the clinicians and staff involved in the care of the patient to more formal reviews. These informal debriefings are meant to create a safe space for staff members to process such a difficult event. Formal reviews can take several forms within an institution (Table 20–1).

MAKING MEANING OF A SUICIDE

Grief and loss take time. Healing from a patient suicide is a process, and it is important to share this experience with people who can be supportive. It is helpful to understand what this event means in your personal and professional life and what you will take with you moving forward without self-blame.

Try to engage in any case discussions that take place in the event of a patient suicide, even if the individual was not your own patient, because they may help you process and learn from the event and/or prepare you for navigating a future loss. Making meaning of a suicide is a unique journey. A suicide may ignite fervor for mental health advocacy, clinical work, or research. A suicide may inspire efforts to create a more supportive culture and promote well-being. Finally, a healthy grieving process can deepen connections between colleagues, create a culture of trust, and promote resilience.

TABLE 20–1.   Examples of institutional reviews

Type of review	Description	Trainee involvement
Peer review	Usually held with the medical directors, departmental leadership, and the attendings on the case	Trainees who are involved in the case may be asked to attend, but often trainees rotate off rotations and may not be aware of these proceedings when they occur.
Departmental mortality and morbidity conferences or root cause analysis meetings	Venues where the suicide of a patient may be discussed; these formal debriefings and reviews are more analytical, with less attention on emotionally supporting the team involved	Trainees need supervisor and/or clinical team support and presence at these formal proceedings. Trainees may request to not have the responsibility of presenting at such conferences in order to focus more on processing and learning from the event (Qayyum et al. 2021b).
Case conferences	A thorough review of the case more focused on understanding the patient; often invites an open discussion of diverse perspectives	The trainee involved and chief residents or supervisor present the case and facilitate a discussion. The case conference can be limited to trainees or involve participation from a multidisciplinary team.

SPECIFIC CHALLENGES AND STRATEGIES

⌘ **I just was informed of my patient's death from suicide in the middle of my workday and feel paralyzed.** You may feel torn between the obligation toward taking care of your patients and the obligation toward taking care of yourself. It's OK to ask your supervisor or team to step away and take some time for yourself. Take a walk or speak to a trusted supervisor or peer. If you need to take the afternoon or the following day off, ask for some time. You may want to keep busy and not think about the patient, but keep the option open for taking time off to regroup and take care of yourself. Consider accommodations if offered proactively by chief residents or the program. Set up time to debrief with the attending of record or a trusted supervisor with whom you have a good relationship. It is helpful to hear from someone who has had this experience. Make sure you have family or friends who can support you when you go home. If you are having difficulty performing your duties or focusing on work, make sure you let the program directors know and seek support and guidance.

⌘ **I'm not sure whether I should go to the funeral.** Going to a patient's funeral can provide closure and support for the family. It also allows for the training team to come together and mourn the loss. In outpatient or longer treatment relationships, attendance of the clinical team at the funeral is often appreciated by families. However, it is always advised to check with risk management first. It is helpful to gauge where the family is and if it would be acceptable to them. At times, the family may manifest their grief as anger directed toward the team.

SELF-REFLECTIVE QUESTIONS

1. Who are the people within my program and community from whom I can seek supervision and support in the event of a patient dying from suicide?
2. What will I carry from this experience moving forward?
3. What are the things I can do to take care of myself?

RESOURCES

American Foundation for Suicide Prevention: After a suicide: a toolkit for physician residency/fellowship programs. New York, American Foundation for Suicide Prevention, 2022. Available at: www.acgme.org/globalassets/PDFs/13287_AFSP_After_Suicide_Clinician_Toolkit_Final_2.pdf. Accessed October 1, 2022.

American Psychiatric Association: Helping residents cope with a patient suicide. Washington, DC, American Psychiatric Association, 2022. Available at: www.psychiatry.org/residents-medical-students/residents/coping-with-patient-suicide. Accessed October 1, 2022.

Seize the Awkward: https://seizetheawkward.org

UC San Diego Healer Education Assessment and Referral (HEAR) Program: https://medschool.ucsd.edu/som/hear/resources/Pages/links.aspx

UPMC WELL toolkit: https://gmewellness.upmc.com

REFERENCES

American Foundation for Suicide Prevention: After a suicide: a toolkit for physician residency/fellowship programs. New York, American Foundation for Suicide Prevention, 2022. Available at: www.acgme.org/Portals/0/PDFs/13287_AFSP_After_Suicide_Clinician_Toolkit_Final_2.pdf. Accessed June 13, 2022.

Curtis JR, Levy MM: Our responsibility for training physicians to understand the effect patient death has on them: the role of the intensivist. Chest 145(5):932–934, 2014 24798827

Eldridge A, Chen J, Furnari M, et al: Adopting a peer-to-peer approach to trainee suicide prevention. Acad Psychiatry 45(3):306–307, 2021 32696427

Firth-Cozens J: Stress in medical undergraduates and house officers. Br J Hosp Med 41(2):161–164, 1989 2653534

Kelly E, Nisker J: Medical students' first clinical experiences of death. Med Educ 44(4):421–428, 2010 20236239

Papadatou D: A proposed model of health professionals' grieving process. Omega (Westport) 41(1):59–77, 2000

Qayyum Z, AhnAllen CG, Van Schalkwyk GI, et al: "You really never forget it!" Psychiatry trainee supervision needs and supervisor experiences following the suicide of a patient. Acad Psychiatry 45(3):279–287, 2021a 33575964

Qayyum Z, Luff D, Van Schalkwyk GI, et al: Recommendations for effectively supporting psychiatry trainees following a patient suicide. Acad Psychiatry 45(3):301–305, 2021b 33532917

Ratanawongsa N, Teherani A, Hauer KE: Third-year medical students' experiences with dying patients during the internal medicine clerkship: a qualitative study of the informal curriculum. Acad Med 80(7):641–647, 2005 15980080

Redinbaugh EM, Sullivan AM, Block SD, et al: Doctors' emotional reactions to recent death of a patient: cross sectional study of hospital doctors. BMJ 327(7408):185, 2003 12881257

Ruskin R, Sakinofsky I, Bagby RM, et al: Impact of patient suicide on psychiatrists and psychiatric trainees. Acad Psychiatry 28(2):104–110, 2004 15298861

Sullivan AM, Lakoma MD, Block SD: The status of medical education in end-of-life care: a national report. J Gen Intern Med 18(9):685–695, 2003 12950476

Vallurupalli M: Mourning on morning rounds. N Engl J Med 369(5):404–405, 2013 23902480

CHAPTER 21

Public Mental Health

Jonathan Tsang, M.D.

Kristoffer Strauss, M.D., M.B.A.

Janet Baek, M.D.

Vanessa de la Cruz, M.D.

You may ask, what is public psychiatry? Public psychiatry is mental health care financed by state or federal funding sources such as Medicaid or Medicare. It is the area of U.S. health care offering safety net services to low-income individuals with serious mental illness (SMI) and substance use disorders (Jacobs and Steiner 2016). As a psychiatry resident rotating in a public hospital or in a community mental health center, you will encounter a unique set of treatment challenges. You will provide care to a population burdened with chronic mental illness often exacerbated by psychosocial stressors. You will need to be mindful of the clinical, cultural, and structural challenges these patients face. You have the opportunity and privilege to provide care to those patients suffering from the most significant mental health disorders while also helping the system of care become more integrated, equitable, and accessible. In this chapter we outline the history of public psychiatry, as well as challenges and opportunities you will face as a resident working in public mental health systems.

KEY POINTS

- Historical legislative context is essential to understanding how and where public psychiatry is delivered to patients in the United States.

- Care delivery should incorporate a recovery-oriented approach to treatment that includes evidence-based psychosocial interventions beyond medication management.

- Structural competency and advocacy are critical to improving the care of patients seeking care in public psychiatry settings.

HISTORICAL CONTEXT

SMI is a diagnosable mental disorder in an adult that causes functional impairment that substantially interferes with or limits one or more major life activities (Jacobs and Steiner 2016). Typical diagnoses include schizophrenia, bipolar disorder, treatment-resistant depression and anxiety, and personality disorders. Individuals with SMI often experience homelessness, substance use, and incarceration due to loss of social support and challenges with access to care.

Legislation and political movements have long shaped public psychiatry and the level of care available to the SMI population. The past 70 years witnessed a dramatic change in the delivery of public psychiatric care in the United States. In the 1950s, more than 500,000 Americans were institutionalized in overcrowded state psychiatric hospitals; today, that number is approximately 50,000 (Sharfstein 2000). New advances in psychotropic medications offered the promise of treatment in the community. A complicated confluence of public backlash, the enactment of entitlement programs, the approval of new medications, and changing funding sources led to deinstitutionalization. Numerous federal laws subsequently reshaped how mental health care is paid for and delivered. These historical developments have persistent impacts on the role you will have as a clinician delivering mental health care to patients with SMI during your residency training.

The inflection point for U.S. mental health policy occurred in 1963, when President John F. Kennedy signed the Community Mental Health Centers Construction Act (CMHCA; Feldman 2012). The goal of this legislation was to support treatment of patients in community mental health clinics (as opposed to state psychiatric hospitals) by providing federal block grant funding for more than 1,500 clinics across the country. The Medicare and Medicaid Act of 1965 provided federal reimbursement for Medicaid-funded community mental health treatment but not for state psychiatric hospitals, contributing to the patient exodus from state hospitals (Smith 2013). However, the federal funding to support the CMHCA was ultimately inadequate, and poorly defined clinic intake criteria meant that the clinics could not meet the needs of formerly institutionalized patients once they were discharged to the community (Sharfstein 2000). With nowhere to live, nowhere to receive psychiatric care, and limited social support, many individuals ended up in homeless shelters, jails, and prisons. In the past three decades, correctional facilities have surpassed state psychiatric hospitals in institutionalizing seriously mentally ill individuals.

However, there is cause for optimism as you embark on your training. Access to mental health care for patients with SMI has increased substantially in the past 30 years. As a result of legislation from the 1980s and 1990s, Medicaid coverage expanded to include clinic-based services, case management, rehabilitation, and assertive community treatment (ACT). Recent legislative efforts, such as passage of the Mental Health Parity and Addiction Equity Act of 2008, the Patient Protection and Affordable Care Act of 2010, and the Protecting Access to Medicare Act of 2014, increased access to mental health services nationally by ensuring that mental health treatment is covered by insurance at the same level as other medical conditions. Current trends are focused on integrating mental health into primary care, promoting harm reduction, improving housing availability, and focusing treatment on the recovery model. Challenges with access remain, particularly among the most vulnerable patients with SMI. For a summary of key legislation in public mental health, see Table 21–1.

CHALLENGES FACED BY PSYCHIATRY RESIDENTS WORKING IN PUBLIC PSYCHIATRY SETTINGS

Psychiatric care for people with SMI in a public mental health setting is challenging. You will often encounter complex clinical scenarios that are not covered by reference materials or residency didactics. You may feel overwhelmed by your patients' traumatic experiences and by how difficult it can be to overcome the structural barriers to care they face. You may feel as if your patients' challenges are so significant that they may never recover. However, it is important to keep in mind that although you may rarely see short-term improvements, many patients experience

TABLE 21–1.   Key legislation impacting public psychiatry,
                  1963–2021

Year	Legislation	Summary	Impacts and Results
1963	Mental Retardation Facilities and Community Mental Health Centers Construction Act of 1963	Provided federal block grant funding to 1,500+ community mental health clinics	• The legislation contributed to deinstitutionalization. • Population in state psychiatric hospitals plummeted. • No long-term federal funding source was established (Smith 2013). • Over time, Congress added numerous amendments that restricted funding (Sharfstein 2000). • Only half of community clinics were built (Ornstein 2016).
1965	Medicare and Medicaid Act	Provided national health insurance for the elderly (Medicare: 100% federally funded) and the poor (Medicaid: 50% federal, 50% state)	• States were incentivized to shift patients from state-funded psychiatric hospitals to Medicaid (states+federal) funded community hospitals and nursing homes (Geller 2000; Grob 2005). • Restrictions kept Medicaid patients from inpatient psychiatric hospital beds. • State mental health funding fluctuated and was not prioritized similar to other public initiatives (Elpers 1989).

TABLE 21–1. Key legislation impacting public psychiatry, 1963–2021 *(continued)*

Year	Legislation	Summary	Impacts and Results
1980	National Mental Health Service Systems Act (NMHSSA)	Sought to support underserved SMI populations by funding community mental health centers, including psychiatric care, primary care, and case management, to address fallout of deinstitutionalization; based on the results of the 1978 Commission on Mental Health (Grob 2005; Sharfstein 2000)	• Impacts were minimal because NMHSSA was defunded the following year.
1981	Omnibus Budget Reconciliation Act	Repealed 1980 NMHSSA; provided federal block grant funding to states to pay for mental health services at 75%–80% of level advocated by NMHSSA (Grob 2005)	• Significant reduction in availability of services to SMI population resulted. • States were made responsible for payments for nursing homes for patients with SMI (which were grossly underfunded). • Reduced federal spending on mental health by as much as 30% (Yohanna 2013).

TABLE 21–1.   Key legislation impacting public psychiatry,
                  1963–2021 (continued)

Year	Legislation	Summary	Impacts and Results
1996	Mental Health Parity Act (MHPA)	Required large-group private insurers that provided mental health care coverage to have no annual or lifetime dollar limits lower than medical or surgical services (Goodell 2014); did not mandate mental health coverage	• Numerous legal loopholes prevented the legislation from being effective. • Insurers charged higher copayments and deductibles for mental health services, and the limit and frequency of services were capped.
2008	Mental Health Parity and Addiction Equity Act (MHPAEA)	Required payment for mental health services to have parity with other medical payments (Goodell 2014) and mandated treatment for substance use disorders	• Loopholes from the 1996 MHPA were closed, and insurers were required to provide parity in mental health coverage, which could be no more restrictive than coverage for other medical services. • MHPAEA expanded the number of individuals, including those with SMI, who could afford to receive mental health treatment.

TABLE 21–1. Key legislation impacting public psychiatry,
1963–2021 *(continued)*

Year	Legislation	Summary	Impacts and Results
2010	Patient Protection and Affordable Care Act	Mandated universal coverage, including for mental health care, as one of 10 essential health benefits (Goodell 2014); expanded Medicaid by removing criteria that limited who could qualify; required MHPAEA mandates to apply to individual plans offered on individual market	• Access to care was increased (20 million more people were covered). • The share of people going without mental health care because of cost fell by one-third. • Private insurance premiums went down, and coverage for young adults increased. • Coverage could no longer be denied to individuals with preexisting conditions such as mental illness (National Alliance on Mental Illness 2020).
2014	Protecting Access to Medicare Act (PAMA)	Required that certified community behavioral health clinics offer a specific set of services, including 24-hour psychiatric care and substance use treatment regardless of ability to pay or insurer, reimbursed by Medicaid (Ornstein 2016; U.S. Department of Health and Human Services 2019)	• Piloted in eight states over 2 years (subsequently funded through SAMHSA and the American Rescue Plan), PAMA increased clinic staffing levels and mandatory trainings, paid for clinic expansions and renovations, increased access by as much as 50%, and improved care coordination between providers (U.S. Department of Health and Human Services 2019). • Currently, U.S. senators are working to expand PAMA through the proposed Excellence in Mental Health and Addiction Treatment Act of 2021.

Note. SAMHSA = Substance Abuse and Mental Health Services Administration; SMI = severe mental illness.

improved quality of life over time. Longitudinal care relationships with your patients with SMI can provide the anchor that allows them to experience recovery. Prioritizing your patients' own perspectives and treatment goals will help them achieve recovery. Ultimately, you are providing care to those who need it most, which can be meaningful and inspiring work. Taking care of yourself and your own well-being will provide the foundation for you to take care of others.

Patients With Complex Medication Regimens

Many of the patients you will treat in a community mental health clinic will be on a polypharmacy medication regimen. Some patients may not be candidates for traditional first-line treatment options for their conditions because of contraindications and practical challenges to taking those medications. For example, lithium or divalproex is the first-line recommended treatment for a patient with bipolar disorder, but barriers to recommended blood draws and challenges patients face in obtaining and taking medications consistently can make these medications less desirable treatment choices. Thus, you may need to consider an atypical antipsychotic with fewer monitoring requirements and less risk of adverse outcomes if patients accidentally or intentionally overdose. It is important for you to carefully weigh the risks and benefits of your treatment recommendations and consult your supervisor to navigate these situations to maximize safety, adherence, and quality of clinical care. Always document the clinical reasoning behind your recommendations to justify your clinical rationale and ensure appropriate care transitions.

Certain medications are used more commonly in the community mental health setting, including depot antipsychotics and clozapine. Depot antipsychotics, or long-acting injectables, have been shown to reduce rehospitalization rates, particularly if the patient has difficulty with medication adherence (Kane et al. 2013; Maestri et al. 2018). This is an excellent option for patients with severe mental illness requiring long-term antipsychotic treatment. Clozapine is the gold standard for treatment-refractory schizophrenia, but it is underutilized in the United States, partly because of rigorous monitoring requirements (Kelly et al. 2018). You should work closely with your supervisors to ensure that your patients are receiving the treatment that is indicated, tolerated, and achievable.

Patients With Chronic Comorbid Medical Conditions

You should be mindful of the medical complexity of your patients and collaborate closely with their primary care doctors. Patients with SMI die 10–20 years earlier when compared with the general population, with an elevated risk of death due to cardiovascular, respiratory, and infectious disease (Liu et al. 2017). Medical and social impairments affect the disease trajectory for patients with SMI and vice versa. A variety of factors contribute to this reality, including environmental stressors (e.g., homelessness), poor health habits (e.g., smoking), side effects from psychotropics taken for SMI (e.g., metabolic syndrome), and systematic obstacles such as stigma by the medical community and structural inequities. You should be aware of barriers to care faced by your patients because you can help address them. For example, you can help ensure that patients are reminded about their clinic appointments and have appropriate transportation. You are an essential advocate not just for your patient's psychiatric treatment but for their medical treatment as well.

Patients Who Are Unhoused

You will encounter numerous patients who experience homelessness and housing instability. According to the U.S. Department of Housing and Urban Development report in 2021 (U.S. Department of Housing and Urban Development 2020), on a given night, about 580,000 people experience homelessness in the United States, out of which about 120,000 are severely mentally ill. Homelessness can significantly limit a patient's ability to engage in treatment. Be mindful that medication compliance and appointment attendance are often affected by lack of housing. Potential solutions include being flexible with your appointment schedules, offering drop-in hours, using telehealth, and engaging the patient in the community through ACT or homeless outreach teams. Because housing instability poses significant challenges, consider a *housing-first model* in your treatment planning. In this approach, housing is prioritized without requiring sobriety or treatment compliance. This has been shown to be effective in improving outcomes and reducing costs in the SMI population (Larimer et al. 2009; Parker 2010).

Patients Who Have Been or Are Currently Incarcerated

Because of the historical context of deinstitutionalization and mass incarceration, the public psychiatric and criminal justice systems have become intertwined. Treating a public mental health population often requires you to work with individuals who are currently or were formerly incarcerated. You might find it helpful to seek out a correctional psychiatry rotation at county jails, state prisons, diversion programs, or probation departments to gain further experience. Treating a patient in a correctional setting requires that you be mindful of the inherent powerlessness of being an inmate, the potential for misuse or diversion of psychotropic medications in jail (sometimes for therapeutic reasons such as suboxone for addiction when this option is not available from treatment providers), and the limited treatment options in this setting. You may also need to be aware of probation requirements and help patients get assistance navigating the legal system.

Patients With Co-occurring Substance Use and Mental Health Disorders

Individuals who seek care in the public setting often have both substance use and mental health disorders. These patients will benefit from integrated outpatient or residential treatment settings that address both mental health and substance use treatments. Interventions should be appropriate to each patient's readiness to change. Treatment approaches such as motivational interviewing and medication-assisted treatment (MAT) are important for you to consider when treating this population. The current standard of care involves harm reduction. You may be expected to use MAT as part of your residency training, and an understanding of these treatments is essential.

RECOVERY MODEL AND PSYCHOSOCIAL INTERVENTIONS

The current focus of treatment has shifted from symptom reduction toward a recovery-based model. The core tenet of this model is the assertion that even people with SMI can live meaningful and productive lives. Numerous guidelines and resources now incorporate such principles, including the American Psychiatric Association (APA) practice guidelines on the treatment of patients with schizophrenia (American Psychiatric Association 2021) and the 2009 Schizophrenia Patient Outcomes Research Team recommendations (Dixon et al. 2010). Many of the recovery model approaches involve patient-centered care and collaborative team-based treatment.

Patient and Family Psychoeducation

You should be aware of who the primary social supports and caregivers are for your patients and involve them in treatment planning. This approach can help manage family concerns and make the patient more likely to engage with treatment. It has been demonstrated that psychoeducation for patients and families can reduce relapse and rehospitalization rates in patients with SMI as well as the burden and stress level of caregivers (McFarlane et al. 2003).

Trauma-Informed Practice

It is important for you to consider the traumatic and structural roots that often affect the development of SMI. Patients in the public mental health system carry a significant trauma burden and face psychosocial stressors that often exacerbate their symptoms and lead to unhealthy coping mechanisms. Adopting trauma-informed care principles can enable a supportive, nonjudgmental attitude crucial to building a therapeutic relationship with your patients (see "Resources" section for link).

Working With Community Partners

While working in a clinic or hospital delivering public psychiatric care, you will have the opportunity to interface with numerous community partners in support of patient care. These partners could include representatives from community-based organizations, such as housing support agencies, food pantries, and employment support organizations. You should develop awareness of resources in your community to help patients stay housed, employed, and fed.

Examples of work with community partners could include the following:

- Your clinic receives access to applications for subsidized housing vouchers, which you offer to one of your housing-disadvantaged patients.
- You connect a patient with food insecurity to a supplemental nutrition assistance program or provide contact information for community food pantries.
- After a patient is stabilized on a long-acting injectable antipsychotic, you refer them to a club house or vocational work program.

Assertive Community Treatment

ACT is an evidence-based treatment model using a multidisciplinary team that provides care to patients in the community wherever they reside (e.g., shelter, encampment). ACT has been demonstrated to reduce hospitalization and homelessness and improve quality of life among those with SMI (Bond et al. 1995; Scott and Dixon 1995). The key elements of ACT include a multidisciplinary team, a shared caseload among team members, direct service provision by team members, a high frequency of patient contact, low patient-to-staff ratios, frequent outreach to patients in the community, and a commitment to providing services as long as patients need them. Participating as a resident in an elective with an ACT team can provide you experience with an effective team-based model of care that might counter the emotional fatigue from the chronic challenges in clinical work.

Supported Employment

Supported employment programs have been shown to be effective in helping mentally ill individuals procure and maintain employment to ensure financial independence in the community (Kinoshita et al. 2013). Consider referring patients to supportive employment programs or collaborating with case managers in these referrals as part of a comprehensive recovery-oriented treatment plan.

PUBLIC PSYCHIATRY WORK BEYOND THE INDIVIDUAL PATIENT

Given the psychosocial and systemic challenges faced by public psychiatry patients, educating yourself regarding structural inequities is essential (Metzl and Hansen 2014). Patients from historically oppressed or marginalized communities experience tremendous additional health inequities, and it is of paramount importance that you are both ready to advocate for your patients in the public psychiatry setting (see Chapter 8, "Working With Historically Oppressed Patient Populations"). Structural competency allows you to see opportunities for advocating for your patients on individual, clinical care, organizational, community, and government levels (See Chapter 32, "Advocacy"). On an individual patient level, you might collaborate with a case manager to refer your patient to a supportive housing program. On a clinical level, you might advocate for your clinic to hire providers with language proficiency that matches the needs of the communities served. On an institutional level, you might advocate for integration of medication-assisted therapy for substance use disorders in correctional settings or for a review of potential racial inequities in prescribing practices.

Advocacy at the community and government levels helps to influence public mental health policies that can improve availability of services that have direct impacts on the quality of care that patients receive in the public sector. As a resident, you can explore community and government advocacy efforts through the APA and its district branches. The APA offers fellowships for residents to engage in various projects and committees to gain experience and foster local and national advocacy efforts. You may also connect with your local chapter of the National Alliance on Mental Illness and other patient rights advocacy groups.

A Career in Public Psychiatry

Public psychiatrists do meaningful, service-oriented work (Carpenter-Song and Torrey 2015). The challenges your patients face are great, but you have the opportunity to help people stabilize, recover, and lead meaningful lives. You can work for federal, state, and local governments or nonprofit organizations in a variety of clinical and administrative settings such as inpatient psychiatric units, emergency departments, and community clinics. Depending on your residency program's affiliations, you can have varying degrees of exposure to the public sector. If you are considering a career in the public sector, consider relevant elective rotations such as a community clinic or homeless outreach team. Residents at community psychiatry programs may gain additional experience through quality improvement projects, collaborative projects with community partners, and residency leadership opportunities. Getting involved in regional and national organizations can help you understand system issues that affect clinical care. The APA has a public psychiatry fellowship during residency that allows for networking and mentorship. If you want to pursue further public sector training after residency, numerous public psychiatry fellowships offer a mix of clinical and academic exposure supplemented by management and leadership training.

Specific Challenges and Strategies

⌘ **My patient is taking eight different medications, and she still has psychosis complicated by ongoing methamphetamine use.** Polypharmacy and comorbid substance use is common with patients who are chronically mentally ill. It is important for you to review the patient's medication regimen and consider an approach that reduces polypharmacy. Harm reduction is essential for patients with co-occurring substance use disorder, particularly when it interferes with their ability to take their medications consistently. Use motivational interviewing techniques to assess the patient's readiness and willingness to reduce or stop using methamphetamine. A referral to a substance treatment program may be indicated.

⌘ **I'm not sure how to help my patient who is currently unhoused. He often doesn't come to his appointments or take his medications.** Consider working with a case manager or peer counselor affiliated with your clinic to support the patient. They can check in with the patient between appointments to offer reminders, and they can also potentially connect the patient with available transportation services (e.g., bus tokens) to help them get to the appointments.

⌘ **My patient will not agree to tapering their benzodiazepines and/or other medications.** Employ a compassionate, nonpunitive approach—it may take many months to taper. Use motivational interviewing to help the patient identify how benzodiazepine use is negatively impacting their life as well as ways that stopping benzodiazepines will help them achieve their self identified goals. Review alternative medications and refer to behavioral therapy such as cognitive-behavioral therapy if appropriate. Offer choices when possible and slow down taper if needed, but never go backward (i.e., increasing the dose).

SELF-REFLECTION QUESTIONS

1. How is public mental health in my area funded?
2. What public mental health resources are available in my area to patients with no insurance or with public health insurance?
3. How would I explain what public psychiatry or community psychiatry is to a medical student interested in the field?

RESOURCES

American Association for Community Psychiatry: www.community psychiatry.org

American Psychiatric Association: The American Psychiatric Association Practice Guideline for the Treatment of Patients With Schizophrenia, 3rd Edition. 2021. Available at: https://psychiatryonline.org/doi/pdf/10.1176/appi.books.9780890424841. Accessed September 18, 2021.

American Psychiatric Association: The Mental Health Services Conference: www.psychiatry.org/psychiatrists/meetings/the-mental-health-services-conference

American Psychiatric Association: Treatment of patients with schizophrenia. Available at: http://eguideline.guidelinecentral.com/i/1303678-treatment-of-patients-with-schizophrenia/23?. Accessed September 18, 2021.

The Trauma Informed Care Project: www.traumainformedcareproject.org

REFERENCES

American Psychiatric Association: The American Psychiatric Association Practice Guideline for the Treatment of Patients With Schizophrenia, 3rd Edition. Washington, DC, American Psychiatric Association, 2021

Bond GR, McGrew JH, Fekete DM: Assertive outreach for frequent users of psychiatric hospitals: a meta-analysis. J Ment Health Adm 22(1):4–16, 1995 10141270

Carpenter-Song E, Torrey WC: "I always viewed this as the real psychiatry": provider perspectives on community psychiatry as a career of first choice. Community Ment Health J 51(3):258–266, 2015 24989962

Dixon LB, Dickerson F, Bellack AS, et al: The 2009 Schizophrenia PORT Psychosocial Treatment Recommendations and Summary Statements. Schizophr Bull 36(1):48–70, 2010 19955389

Elpers JR: Public mental health funding in California, 1959 to 1989. Hosp Community Psychiatry 40(8):799–804, 1989 2759568

Feldman JM: History of community psychiatry, in Handbook of Community Psychiatry. Edited by McQuistion HL. New York, Springer, 2012, pp 11–18

Geller JL: The last half-century of psychiatric services as reflected in psychiatric services. Psychiatr Serv 51(1):41–67, 2000 10647135

Goodell S: Mental health parity. Health Affairs Health Policy Brief, April 3, 2014. Available at: www.healthaffairs.org/do/10.1377/hpb20140403.871424/full. Accessed on September 16, 2021.

Grob GN: Public policy and mental illnesses: Jimmy Carter's Presidential Commission on Mental Health. Milbank Q 83(3):425–456, 2005 16201999

Jacobs SC, Steiner JL (eds): Yale Textbook of Public Psychiatry. New York, Oxford University Press, 2016

Kane JM, Kishimoto T, Correll CU: Assessing the comparative effectiveness of long-acting injectable vs. oral antipsychotic medications in the prevention of relapse provides a case study in comparative effectiveness research in psychiatry. J Clin Epidemiol 66(8)(suppl):S37–S41, 2013 23849151

Kelly DL, Freudenreich O, Sayer MA, et al: Addressing barriers to clozapine underutilization: a national effort. Psychiatr Serv 69(2):224–227, 2018 29032704

Kinoshita Y, Furukawa TA, Kinoshita K, et al: Supported employment for adults with severe mental illness. Cochrane Database Syst Rev (9):CD008297, 2013 24030739

Larimer ME, Malone DK, Garner MD, et al: Health care and public service use and costs before and after provision of housing for chronically homeless persons with severe alcohol problems. JAMA 301(13):1349–1357, 2009 19336710

Liu NH, Daumit GL, Dua T, et al: Excess mortality in persons with severe mental disorders: a multilevel intervention framework and priorities for clinical practice, policy and research agendas. World Psychiatry 16(1):30–40, 2017 28127922

Maestri TJ, Mican LM, Rozea H, et al: Do long-acting injectable antipsychotics prevent or delay hospital readmission? Psychopharmacol Bull 48(3):8–15, 2018 29713100

McFarlane WR, Dixon L, Lukens E, et al: Family psychoeducation and schizophrenia: a review of the literature. J Marital Fam Ther 29(2):223–245, 2003 12728780

Metzl JM, Hansen H: Structural competency: theorizing a new medical engagement with stigma and inequality. Soc Sci Med 103:126–133, 2014 24507917

National Alliance on Mental Illness: What the Affordable Care Act has meant for people with mental health conditions: and what could be lost. Arlington, VA, National Alliance on Mental Illness, November 2020. Available at: www.nami.org/Support-Education/Publications-Reports/Public-Policy-Reports/What-the-Affordable-Care-Act-Has-Meant-for-People-with-Mental-Health-Conditions-What-Could-Be-Lost/NAMI_IssueBrief_ACA_11-10-20. Accessed September 12, 2021.

Ornstein N: How to fix a broken mental health system. The Atlantic, June 8, 2016. Available at: www.theatlantic.com/politics/archive/2016/06/getting-mental-health-on-the-docket/485996. Accessed September 18, 2021

Parker D: Housing as an intervention on hospital use: access among chronically homeless persons with disabilities. J Urban Health 87(6):912–919, 2010 21125341

Scott JE, Dixon LB: Assertive community treatment and case management for schizophrenia. Schizophr Bull 21(4):657–668, 1995 8749892

Sharfstein SS: Whatever happened to community mental health? Psychiatr Serv 51(5):616–620, 2000 10783179

Smith MR: 50 years later, Kennedy's vision for mental health not realized. The Seattle Times, October 20, 2013. Available at: https://web.archive.org/web/20131023010233/http://seattletimes.com/html/nationworld/2022091710_mentalhealthxml.html. Accessed September 17, 2021.

U.S. Department of Health and Human Services: Certified community behavioral health clinics demonstration program: report to Congress 2018. Washington, DC, U.S. Department of Health and Human Services, September 2019. Available at: aspe.hhs.gov/sites/default/files/private/pdf/262266/CCBHRptCong.pdf. Accessed September 18, 2021.

U.S. Department of Housing and Urban Development: HUD 2020 continuum of care homeless assistance programs homeless populations and subpopulations. December 15, 2020. Available at: files.hudexchange.info/reports/published/CoC_PopSub_NatlTerrDC_2020.pdf. Accessed September 20, 2021.

World Health Organization: Information sheet: premature death among people with severe mental disorders. 2021. Available at: www.who.int/mental_health/management/info_sheet.pdf. Accessed September 12, 2021.

Yohanna D: Deinstitutionalization of people with mental illness: causes and consequences. Virtual Mentor 15(10):886–891, 2013 24152782

CHAPTER 22

Supervision

Csilla N. Lippert, M.D., Ph.D.
Sallie G. De Golia, M.D., M.P.H.

Supervision in psychiatry residency is very different from what you experienced in most of medical school or even in your nonpsychiatry rotations during intern year. In contrast with frequent shadowing experiences in medical school, you are now more directly responsible for patient care decisions. Depending on the venue and context, you may experience delays between those decisions and supervisor oversight, increasing the need to prepare for and actively engage in supervision. Early on, you may feel particularly dependent on your supervisors for goal setting, overall guidance, and help with important clinical decisions. As you progress in training, you will identify your own supervision goals, including areas of knowledge or skill sets you want to refine before you enter unsupervised clinical practice. In this chapter we aim to provide a framework for optimizing your supervision experience.

KEY POINTS

- To expand your growth and learning in supervision, you should be aware of supervision phases and your supervisor's multiple roles.

- It is important to optimize your relationship with your supervisor because it is the basis for effective supervision.

- How you approach supervision will vary depending on your stage of training and the clinical setting.

SUPERVISION FUNCTION AND DEFINITION

Supervision serves multiple clinical and training functions, ranging from promoting safe, effective patient care to providing essential skills for unsupervised practice and professional development. It will look and feel different depending on whether you are being supervised in the inpatient or outpatient setting and depending on the treatment modality for which you are being supervised (medication management or type of therapy). Learning about the supervision components and process can help you make the most of supervision (Crocker and Sudak 2017; Johnson 2017). Let's start with a definition of supervision:

> [T]he formal provision, by approved supervisors, of a relationship-based education and training that is work focused and which manages, supports, develops and evaluates the work of colleagues. (Milne 2009, p. 15)

SUPERVISION PHASES

Supervision can be broken down into four key phases: the preparatory, introductory, working, and termination phases. By understanding these phases, you will have a better sense of where you are in the process and what you can expect.

Preparatory Phase

Before you meet with your supervisor for the first time, come prepared in order to get the most out of the experience.

- Engage in a self-assessment by evaluating your strengths, areas for growth, motivation, and learning goals in the context of your training level. You could start by reviewing the Accreditation Council for Graduate Medical Education (2020) milestones and any prior evaluations or constructive feedback you have received as a starting point for internally reflecting about your current foundation and next steps.
- When reflecting on learning goals, consider expanding not only your knowledge base but also the skills and attitudes you would like to develop within the learning experience. For example, you might

want to become more sensitive to racial and cultural differences, including traumas, in your patients or to your countertransference.

- Review the evaluation tool used by your supervisor to better understand what you will be evaluated on.
- Consider the clinical setting where supervision will occur and be aware of possible benefits and challenges to supervision in that setting. For example, high-acuity inpatient psychiatry supervision may more easily support your safety, triaging, prescribing, and supportive psychotherapy learning goals than your psychoanalytic formulation learning goals.
- In some cases, such as psychotherapy supervision, you may be able to select your supervisor. If your program allows this, consider meeting with prospective supervisors to explore their background, theoretical orientation (e.g., cognitive-behavioral, Jungian), and supervision style, including preferred supervision techniques. You can also learn a lot from talking to prior trainees about their experiences with specific supervisors, with the caveat that one person's worst supervisor may be another's favorite.
- Before meeting with new supervisors, consider reviewing their professional websites for background on their research activities, career interests, special areas of training, and/or career goals (Berger and Graff 1995; Pearson and Students 2004). Having background on your supervisors may help you identify shared interests and guide some of your supervision questions, including questions related to your own career interests.

Introductory Phase

Arguably the most important aspect of the introductory phase, which occurs in the first few meetings of supervision, is establishing a strong relationship with your supervisor. This *working alliance* is foundational to supervision (Watkins and Callahan 2019). A lot of what you learn in psychiatry occurs through supervision, so investing early in this relationship is pivotal.

During this phase, your supervisor hopefully will discuss the *frame* of supervision—how they plan to create an environment and relationship that will allow you to feel safe and open. They may review logistics of when, where, and how long to meet for supervision, their preferred timing and methods for communication (e.g., phone, secure text or email, electronic medical record, paging) between supervision sessions and expectations and learning goals. Ideally, you might share your preliminary self-generated learning objectives, then be open to any comments or feedback from your supervisor, including their goals and expectations for you. If your supervisor has not offered any goals, logistics, or frame setting, ask what they expect from you within supervision. For example: What do they expect you to achieve by the end of your work together? How do they expect you to show up to supervision? Do they want you to consider them as consultants? Should you be prepared to present videos, transcripts, or process notes? Do they want you to call every time you enter an order or request a consultation? Having a clear understanding of expectations is important in establishing a more seamless working relationship.

Confidentiality is an important part of the frame; however, this is tricky because your supervisor also evaluates you and provides feedback to your program. It may be helpful to talk directly about this dual role early in the relationship. If possible, you might ask your supervisor what information they feel obligated to share with program leadership and how they determine what information remains confidential between the two of you. Recognizing the inherent limitations of confidentiality and being clear about what parts of your supervision relationship remain confidential is important.

Working Phase

The working phase accounts for the majority of supervision time, which "involves four major supervisory domains: oversight, mentorship, teaching, and evaluation and feedback activities" (De Golia 2019, p. 12) to ensure that supervision goals are being met. These approaches will help you optimize this time together.

- Come to supervision with specific questions (e.g., What else should I consider on my differential diagnosis? How else could I have responded to the patient's question about my training background? How might I deepen the emotions?).
- *Set an agenda that prioritizes your most immediate supervision needs.* Your supervisor will no doubt respond to your questions or needs through a variety of methods, including discussion, role-playing, and review of audio or video recordings, or direct you to (or encourage you to find) articles relevant to the discussion at hand.
- *Be as open as possible to feedback without becoming defensive.* Substantial learning comes from your supervisor's feedback based on watching you with a patient or through discussion of concepts. Try to inhabit a growth mindset in which you are capable of improving, embrace challenges, share your areas that need improvement, and recognize that setbacks or mistakes are opportunities from which you can learn and grow. It can be really tough and humbling to hear corrective

feedback, but this is how we learn. After all, you and your supervisor are not expected to know everything already.

- *Try to be as direct as possible with your supervisor when challenges arise in the relationship.* All relationships become strained at times. Working through the discomfort together allows you to restore the critical learning environment. At times, approaching your supervisor directly may seem too difficult. In these situations, you might seek advice from a peer, other supervisors, site director(s), and/or training director(s) on how to navigate your specific supervision challenge. It is important to try to regain the positive working alliance that allows for more learning opportunities.

- *Seek guidance from your supervisor about your future career, work-life integration, and how to navigate situations in residency.* Your supervisor may serve as an important mentor to you. Given your supervisor's dual role as an evaluator, you have to decide what information you are willing to reveal. For example, maybe you are in the early stages of family planning (or even in the first trimester of a pregnancy) and want to be able to brainstorm about work-life balance without the pressure of your program administration knowing before you are ready to make an announcement. Or maybe your program is hoping to recruit you after residency, but you hope to discuss other career options, including salary negotiations, with your supervisor. Before engaging in these sensitive conversations, ask whether this type of conversation can be held in confidence.

- *Engage in self-directed learning.* Your supervisor might direct you to articles, bring up topics you are not familiar with, or reveal some skills to be worked on during your meetings. Use time between supervisory sessions to read, engage in deliberate practice, reflect on your work, or review videos of your session to better formulate a question or clarify areas for improvement to discuss during the following session.

Termination Phase

The termination phase, often described in psychotherapy relationships but similarly important in all supervision contexts, marks the ending for supervision with a particular supervisor. However, rather than think of it as an ending, consider conceptualizing this phase as part of your transition to another supervisor or to unsupervised learning. Explicitly review key learning moments, discuss your current strengths and areas for improvement, define new goals for your work with future supervisors, plan steps for self-directed learning, and/or reflect on what you would like to incorporate from your supervisor's style into your own style as a supervisor. Remember that your supervisor is a learner as well, and your feedback can help them grow as an educator.

SUPERVISION FORMATS

Psychiatry residency supervision is most often provided individually or in group settings. Individual supervision has a significant benefit of personalized time with your supervisor to consider your patients and learning goals. Even so, it can be challenging to address differences between your and your supervisor's thoughts on patient care, especially if you are vulnerable to second-guessing yourself in a one-on-one setting with a more senior clinician. Group supervision, where you are in supervision with peers, allows you to learn from a broader array of patient presentations and provides more opportunity for feedback and insights from peers. Although it can be intimidating in the group setting to share vulnerable patient care challenges, support from your peers can sometimes make it easier to discuss differences between your and your supervisor's views on patient care.

SUPERVISION LEVELS

Supervision levels are divided into direct, indirect, or oversight supervision on the basis of a resident's graduated progression of competency development (Accreditation Council for Graduate Medical Education 2022). Details of these levels, including their benefits and drawbacks, are included in Table 22–1. As you progress through residency, you will become increasingly independent in your decision-making capabilities and will seek more autonomy, reflected in the different levels of feedback required throughout training. Knowing the different supervision levels could help you advocate for adjusting the supervision level that your supervisor is offering and help you reflect on the supervision level you want to provide for your own medical student supervisees.

SUPERVISION TECHNIQUES

Supervisors often have their preferred supervision techniques. Advocate for the ones tailored to your learning goals but be open to trying new approaches. You might not be keen on role-play, but despite any discomfort, you might find that you understand a concept or develop a skill better by being directly immersed in a scenario or by being observed practicing a technique. See Table 22–2 for sample techniques, in-

TABLE 22–1. Benefits and drawbacks of various supervision levels

Supervision type	Definition	Common sites	Benefits	Drawbacks
Direct—live	Supervisor is physically present with you and the patient	• Inpatient units • One-way mirror supervision during psychotherapy • Psychopharmacology clinics	• Directly observed performance • More accurate feedback on your clinical interactions • Easier for supervisor to model clinical approach • Easier access to supervisor—helps decrease clinical errors in your early training	• Anxiety provoking to be "watched" • Less autonomy if your supervisor takes over patient encounter (mitigated by use of one-way mirrors)
Direct—asynchronous	Supervisor watches video of your patient encounter after the encounter	• Psychotherapy supervision	• Minimizes reliance on your subjective report of patient encounters	• Feedback is delayed until after patient encounter • Requires patient consent, recording equipment, and secure storage

TABLE 22–1. Benefits and drawbacks of various supervision levels *(continued)*

Supervision type	Definition	Common sites	Benefits	Drawbacks
Indirect—with direct supervision immediately available vs. direct supervision available	Supervisor is not initially present during patient encounters but can be within the patient care setting (immediately available) or reachable by phone or electronic means (available) for potential to convert to direct supervision	• Psychopharmacology clinics • Inpatient "card" rounds or "running the list"	• Potential for greater independence than with direct supervision	• Relies on self-report of patient encounter, which may involve recall and implicit bias • Can have unexpected delays in supervision
Oversight	Supervisor reviews patient care after care is delivered	• End of a call shift or night float • Weekly outpatient case conference • Psychotherapy clinic	• High trainee independence • Potential for efficient review of large number of patient encounters with big picture perspective	• Relies on self-report of patient encounter, which may involve implicit bias and even more recall bias if longer delay between patient encounter and supervision • Feedback is delayed until after patient encounter

cluding their benefits and challenges. See "Resources" at the end of the chapter for more in-depth discussions of these techniques. If specific techniques resonate with you as a particularly useful way of learning, you might introduce them to your supervisor and request their use in supervision. You also may find that you want to practice these techniques in your supervision of medical students and other trainees.

SPECIFIC CHALLENGES AND STRATEGIES

⌘ **Supervision feels awkward—my supervisor jumped right into clinical work without really getting to know me.** If your supervisor doesn't take time to get to know you at the beginning of supervision (the introductory phase), consider modeling it for them to see if they respond in kind. You might begin a supervision session by asking how your supervisor became interested in the modality they are supervising, why they went into the field, what parts of psychiatry they find most compelling, or how they managed raising a family while working. This may break the ice a bit and create more back and forth exchange. You might ask how they view developing the frame in the patient-provider relationship and then express curiosity about the frame in supervision. You might say, "How do you see developing the frame in therapy differently from or similar to developing the frame of supervision?" Or you might reflect aloud on what you hope supervision might incorporate as part of the frame. For example, "I'm wondering if I could share my goals for supervision with you so that we can check in from time to time to see how I'm doing with them." Or you could say, "It is helpful for me if I can talk through my treatment plan or propose an intervention before you advise me so I can see if I understand it correctly."

⌘ **I disagree with my supervisor's patient care recommendations.** This can be particularly difficult when you are the one who has spent more time with the patient, which gives you an individualized, personalized perspective on next steps for patient care. It is helpful to take a step back and explore your supervisor's rationale for their recommendations in more detail as an opportunity to learn from your supervisor's years of experience. However, it is possible that even after such discussion, you still disagree with your supervisor in a way that negatively affects the work of supervision. Attempt to discuss conflicts with your supervisor directly and as soon as possible (Crocker and Sudak 2017). By doing this, you are practicing repairing a relationship, which is useful in your clinical work. If you need additional support working through alliance repair, consider consulting with peers, chief residents, other clinical mentors, rotation directors, and/or your training director(s). Finally, in the event that after discussion with your supervisor and consultation with others,

TABLE 22–2. Supervision techniques

Technique	Definition	Benefits	Challenges
Educational questioning ("pimping")	Supervisor assesses knowledge through asking test-like questions	• Similar format to medical school training • Provides quick knowledge assessment that your supervisor can use to guide teaching points	• Sometimes encourages awkward power dynamic • Can be tough to admit when you do not know the answer to a direct question
Role-play	Consists of • Modeling (you act as patient and supervisor acts as clinician) • Rehearsal (you act as clinician and supervisor acts as patient) • Feedback (reflection and correction)	• Supervisor directly observes you practicing skills and provides real-time feedback • Space to grow from missteps using time-outs and rewinding • Can easily vary the clinical scenarios	• Uncomfortable for many people • Can feel artificial or fake • You may need to remind your supervisor to provide space for all aspects of the role-play, including feedback
Deliberate practice	Steps: • Supervisor identifies a specific microskill to improve • Supervisor breaks down the skill into well-defined steps, models the skill, and practices role-play with you • You practice the skill multiple times before your next supervision, similar to practicing a sports or music drill	• Identifies microskill just beyond your skill level • Provides clear, incremental approach to improve microskill • Avoids overwhelming you with excessive expectation	• Requires you to spend time practicing the skill outside supervision • Can be frustrating if microskill is too advanced for you

TABLE 22–2. Supervision techniques (*continued*)

Technique	Definition	Benefits	Challenges
SNAPPS	Steps: • *Summarize* patient history and findings • *Narrow* differential diagnosis • *Analyze* differential • *Probe* preceptor (ask about challenges or alternatives) • *Plan* management for patient's medical issues • *Select* case-related issue for self-directed learning	• Case-based, detailed look at a learning topic • Organized approach for combining supervised and solo learning	• You will likely need to teach your supervisor about this technique before using it • Technique involves many steps

Source.   Adapted from De Golia and Corcoran 2019. See "Resources" for specific chapters.

it still feels as if you are unable to maintain the supervision relationship, it may be time to terminate supervision. If you are not allowed to terminate supervision, consider adding a second supervisor. If that is not possible, work with your supervisor as best you can while also giving yourself space to use other supports to cope with a tough supervisory relationship. Engage in self-care activities, make use of peer supports, or remind yourself that the supervision is time limited and may teach you what not to do when you are a supervisor.

⌘ **My supervisor is not always aware of the implications of what she is saying.** You are likely to work with supervisors with different cultural backgrounds, including your own and/or those of your patients. There may be instances in which you have more knowledge or direct experience with a particular diversity or equity issue. It is ideal for you to have a sufficiently comfortable and respectful working alliance to discuss sensitive cultural differences with your supervisor. However, it is not your responsibility to educate your supervisor or to tread carefully around white fragility. If you do not feel comfortable addressing your supervisor's unconscious bias(es) directly, you might ask for help from the clinic director, the training director, or a trusted colleague. If you experience retaliation, you should seek help from your training director to manage the situation (see Chapter 39, "Handling Mistreatment and Discrimination"). At other times, you and your supervisor may need to work together to seek out a cultural consultation with an experienced colleague or other resources in the field (Shah et al. 2019). If your supervisor is not receptive to learning from your cultural experience or to pursuing outside consultation, you may need to seek additional supervisors or trusted faculty or senior residents to process and discuss cultural differences that are coming up with your primary supervisor. It may feel vulnerable to admit unease in the supervision relationship, but it may be a starting point for working with your supervisor to provide better patient care. You may want to implement a structured approach for discussing culture in supervision, such as consistent consideration for the DSM-5-TR cultural formulation (American Psychiatric Association 2022) for all patients.

⌘ **My supervision is starting to feel like therapy.** Psychiatry supervision is a particularly vulnerable setting, where you are more likely to find boundary blurring, particularly within the psychodynamic therapy model. Discussions of countertransference are important because they relate to patient care, but you are not expected to share personal feelings and life experiences beyond their impact on patient care. Although supervision is not meant to be therapy, it can provide some helpful directions or guidance about what you may want to address offline in individual therapy.

SELF-REFLECTIVE QUESTIONS

1. What are my supervision goals?
2. What have been some of my biggest supervision challenges?
3. What have I found the most helpful in supervision?
4. Who have been my favorite supervisors and why?
5. How have my experiences with supervision informed what kind of supervisor I aspire to be?

RESOURCES

General

Bernard JM, Goodyear RK: Fundamentals of Clinical Supervision, 6th Edition. Upper Saddle River, NJ, Merrill, 2019

De Golia SG, Corcoran KM: Supervision in Psychiatric Practice: Practical Approaches Across Venues and Providers. Washington, DC, American Psychiatric Association Publishing, 2019

De Golia SG, Tan M: Using Psychotherapy Supervision, in Training and Beyond in Psychotherapy: A Comprehensive Introduction. Edited by Brenner A, Howe-Martin L. Philadelphia, PA, Wolters Kluwer, 2021, pp. 363–388

Techniques

Bullock KD: Role-play, in Supervision in Psychiatric Practice: Practical Approaches Across Venues and Providers. Edited by De Golia SG, Corcoran KM. Washington, DC, American Psychiatric Association Publishing, 2019, pp 69–77

Gold J, Bentzley J: Other supervisory techniques: before, during, and after the patient encounter, in Supervision in Psychiatric Practice: Practical Approaches Across Venues and Providers. Edited by De Golia SG, Corcoran KM. Washington, DC, American Psychiatric Association Publishing, 2019, pp 119–125

Rousmaniere T: Deliberate practice for clinical supervision and training, in Supervision in Psychiatric Practice: Practical Approaches Across Venues and Providers. Edited by De Golia SG, Corcoran KM. Washington, DC, American Psychiatric Association Publishing, 2019, pp 97–104

Rousmaniere T: Mastering the Inner Skills of Psychotherapy: A Deliberate Practice Manual. Seattle, WA, Golden Lantern Books, 2019

REFERENCES

Accreditation Council for Graduate Medical Education: Psychiatry milestones. March 2020. Available at: www.acgme.org/globalassets/pdfs/milestones/psychiatrymilestones.pdf. Accessed October 14, 2022.

Accreditation Council for Graduate Medical Education: ACEGME program requirements for graduate medical education in psychiatry, Section VI.A.2.c. July 1, 2022. Available at: www.acgme.org/globalassets/pfassets/programrequirements/400_psychiatry_2022v2.pdf. Accessed October 14, 2022.

American Psychiatric Association: Diagnostic and Statistical Manual of Mental Disorders, 5th Edition, Text Revision. Washington, DC, American Psychiatric Association, 2022

Berger N, Graff L: Making good use of supervision, in Basics of Clinical Practice: A Guidebook for Trainees in the Helping Profession. Edited by Martin DG, Moore AD. Prospect Heights, IL, Waveland Press, 1995, pp 408–432

Crocker EM, Sudak DM: Making the most of psychotherapy supervision: a guide for psychiatry residents. Acad Psychiatry 41(1):35–39, 2017 27909977

De Golia SG: Elements of supervision, in Supervision in Psychiatric Practice: Practical Approaches Across Venues and Providers. Edited by De Golia SG, Corcoran KM. Washington, DC, American Psychiatric Association Publishing, 2019, pp 3–24

De Golia SG, Corcoran KM: Supervision in Psychiatric Practice: Practical Approaches Across Venues and Providers. Washington, DC, American Psychiatric Association Publishing, 2019

Johnson EA: Working Together in Clinical Supervision. New York, Momentum, 2017, pp 19, 35–55

Milne DL: Evidence-Based Clinical Supervision: Principles and Practice. Malden, MA, BPS/Blackwell, 2009

Pearson QM, Students C: Getting the most out of clinical supervision: strategies for mental health. J Ment Health Couns 26(4):361–373, 2004

Shah R, Tan M, Bandstra BS: Supervising cross-cultural topics in a clinical setting, in Supervision in Psychiatric Practice: Practical Approaches Across Venues and Providers. Edited by De Golia SG, Corcoran KM. Washington, DC, American Psychiatric Association Publishing, 2019, pp 337–344

Watkins CE, Callahan JL: Psychotherapy supervision research: a status report and proposed model, in Supervision in Psychiatric Practice: Practical Approaches Across Venues and Providers. Edited by De Golia SG, Corcoran KM. Washington, DC, American Psychiatric Association Publishing, 2019, pp 25–34

PART 4

Building Skills

CHAPTER 23

Blue Ink Spots

Working Toward Accurate Self-Knowledge Through Self-Awareness

Seamus Bhatt-Mackin, M.D., FAPA,
   CGP, AGPA-F
Aaron Feiger, M.D.

As our circle of knowledge expands, so does the circumference of darkness surrounding it.

*Source unknown; misattributed to
Albert Einstein (Calaprice 2019)*

The fact is that we sometimes do not know our own minds. Our brains do a lot of work silently and quietly. We do not have access to all of it…. And our brains contain associations from the larger culture—a thumbprint of the culture—outside of our awareness.

Mahzarin Banaji

Imagine sitting down to talk with a patient and discovering—just as you retrieve it from your pocket—that your blue ballpoint pen has burst. After noticing some embarrassment, laughing together with your patient, excusing yourself to wash up, and returning to conduct an interview, you find yourself scratching your nose and rubbing your chin with hands that are still stained and sticky. At this point, you do not know whether you have blue ink on your face. How do you deal with the fact that this could happen—in this way or some other way—again and again?

You might be tempted to just start using pencils. You might also try accepting the fact that—as human beings—we all move through the world with some kind of "ink on our face" in the form of cognitive, emotional, and behavioral unawareness. You might also accept that because we change over time, it is not possible to ever become completely self-aware; the learning process is ongoing and never finished. In clinical work, self-knowledge through self-awareness is important for generating hypotheses about the patient using subjective experience, maintaining professional role boundaries, and appropriately attending to personal needs with regard to self-care and wellness. In this chapter we provide you with guidance by reviewing some relevant attitudes and concepts, general strategies, and specific advice for challenging situations.

KEY POINTS

- We all have habits of thoughts, emotion, and behavior outside our awareness; self-awareness is always incomplete.

- Increasing accurate self-knowledge through self-awareness takes work and requires experiential practices.

- Other people can help us with increasing self-awareness.

- It is vitally important to identify beliefs and attitudes about race, gender identity, sexual orientation, and social identity—those that are both in our awareness and outside it.

DEFINING SELF-AWARENESS

Self-awareness has been defined as "the capacity of becoming the object of one's own attention" (Morin 2011, p. 807). Eurich (2018) has described two broad categories: *internal self-awareness*, which represents "how clearly we see our own values, passions, aspirations, fit with our environment, reactions (including thoughts, feelings, behaviors, strengths, and weaknesses) and impact on others" (p. 4) and *external self-awareness*, which involves understanding how other people view us in terms of those same factors. Consider the following vignette:

Case Vignette

In the second month of residency, Dr. B, a busy intern, is paired with a senior medical student, Lauren, for 2 weeks on the inpatient ward. Dr. B remembers intentionally speaking with Lauren often and intentionally noting their similarities, with two goals in mind: decreasing hierarchy and empowering the student. Specifically, Dr. B frequently noted that they "weren't so far apart" with regard to development as physicians. Despite this effort, Dr. B was surprised, confused, and hurt to receive a lukewarm review from Lauren, who reported feeling overwhelmed and not an active member of the treatment team.

As a busy intern, Dr. B had spent a lot of time and energy communicating to Lauren that they were on the same level, assuming that she held the same view and assuming that assigning tasks and providing feedback would not make her feel upset or intimidated. However, Dr. B was not externally self-aware that Lauren had looked to him for more leadership, direction, and guidance. When this was not available, she felt overwhelmed. In addition, Dr. B was not internally self-aware of areas in need of improvement with regard to his teaching skills. He had routinely been top of the class throughout college and medical school and had not encountered areas that called for more practice and skill development.

Working to increase internal and external self-awareness is important for the professional development of trainees in psychiatry and for the ongoing clinical work of practicing psychiatrists.

Facilitating Self-Knowledge

Working to increase self-knowledge through self-awareness is a challenging task. Factors that facilitate self-knowledge include taking a self-compassionate attitude, inhabiting a growth mindset, and cultivating psychological safety.

Self-Compassion

Self-compassion, as defined by Neff (2009), includes three components: *self-kindness* (the tendency to be caring and understanding with oneself, rather than harshly critical or judgmental), *common humanity* (the recognition that all humans are imperfect, fail, and make mistakes), and *mindfulness* (the intentional focusing of awareness in the present momentary experience without attachment to it). Self-compassion is quite different from self-esteem, which often involves self-judgment, comparison with others, competition with them, and focus on positive outcomes.

Training in psychiatry is challenging work that requires the development of therapeutic attitudes, the integration of a wide range of theoretical and practical knowledge, and the acquisition of many different clinical skills. It is inevitable that mistakes will happen along the way. Using punitive self-criticism as motivation and linking self-esteem to positive outcomes are not viable long-term strategies. In fact, harsh self-criticism may make one less likely to notice areas in need of improvement, perpetuating unawareness and allowing them to grow in size. Similarly, focusing only on outcomes may make it more difficult to notice important process factors.

Growth Mindset

Dweck (2016) has identified and described two mindsets related to beliefs about learning. In the *fixed mindset,* intelligence is static and not affected by effort; appearance and performance are prioritized and challenges are avoided. Others' successes are viewed as threatening, and feedback is viewed as irrelevant and is often ignored. In the *growth mindset,* intelligence can be developed; learning and mastery are prioritized and challenges are embraced. Others' successes are viewed as inspirational and feedback is often used to aid learning.

A growth mindset is one way to respond to inevitable areas of unawareness. You do not know everything yet. This is one reason that residency is 4 years long. And the learning will not be completed even by the end of your residency—there are opportunities to learn throughout your career. This includes both the acquisition of new factual knowledge and increased amount and accuracy of self-knowledge.

Psychological Safety

Edmonson writes that "psychological safety describes perceptions of the consequences of taking interpersonal risks in a particular context such as a workplace" (Edmonson and Lei 2014, p. 24). In an environment with higher psychological safety, you may be more likely to share information that facilitates learning, even if that information may be perceived as negative in some way (e.g., unflattering, embarrassing, diminishing). In environments with lower psychological safety, you may be less likely to share this information and learning can be inhibited.

Although you and your coresidents contribute, it is your supervisors, teachers, and program and organization's leaders who have the most impact on psychological safety in your residency training program. Edmonson (2018) recommends that leaders be accessible and approachable, acknowledge the limits of their current knowledge, be willing to display fallibility, invite participation, highlight failures as learning opportunities, use direct language, set boundaries, and hold people accountable for boundary transgressions.

PRACTICING SELF-AWARENESS

Increasing self-knowledge through self-awareness requires focus and practice. Important areas of focus include openness to feedback and awareness of unconscious bias and social privilege. Experiential practices include mindfulness, personal psychotherapy, and T-groups.

Openness to Feedback From Clinical Supervisors

Residency is filled with feedback about professional practice in the day-to-day experience of clinical supervision. It is inevitable that some of this feedback will not be consistent with your prior experiences. Human minds are built to seek out evidence in support of current beliefs; this is known as *confirmation bias,* and it contributes to the persistence of unawareness. To counter confirmation bias, we need to actively seek out evidence that disconfirms our beliefs about ourselves. In addition, recall that the feedback offered by psychiatry attending physicians comes from people who have been trained to observe human behavior and respond to it sensitively. One recommendation is to imagine "In what way is this true?" when receiving feedback. It is always possible to set it aside as inaccurate after more reflection, but it is difficult to genuinely consider the feedback if a defensive stance is taken from the beginning.

Awareness of Unconscious Bias and Social Privilege

We are all formed by our social experiences. Throughout human history, and into the present, this experience has included inequality across social identity (racism, sexism, homophobia, transphobia) at the interpersonal and structural levels. It has also included positions of maximal social power and privilege for white heterosexual cisgender men and places of relative intersectional power and privilege for people with other social identities. As a result of these social experiences, we each hold what social psychologist Mahazarin Banaji and others have described as *implicit bias*: associations that are outside awareness that link attributes with members of a particular social identity (Greenwald and Banaji 2017). In our modern era, explicit prejudice toward most social identities is taboo. This may actually make bringing implicit bias into awareness more challenging.

Most multicultural clinical educators now advocate for *cultural humility,* which involves both intentionally opening oneself to the cultural values, priorities, and experience of another person and making a lifelong commitment to redressing power imbalances (Patallo 2019). This is in contrast to *cultural competence*, which is not possible across all cultural contexts and which can contribute to stereotypes about social groups.

Mindfulness Practices

Kabat-Zinn (2005) describes the practice of mindfulness as "patient attention in a particular way: on purpose, in the present moment, and nonjudgmentally" (p. 4). It is the opposite of acting habitually, multitasking, ruminating about the past or the future, or making snap judgments. Many practices can be done in this way, including breath awareness, walking meditations, and mindful eating. Mindfulness is also applied to thoughts and emotions. Increased skill related to the observation and description of thoughts and emotions is foundational to self-awareness. In addition, there are meditation practices focused specifically on cultivating self-compassion such as the *lovingkindness meditation.*

Personal Psychotherapy

Engaging in personal psychotherapy during training is a time-honored tradition in psychiatry. It is more common in residency training programs where training directors believe in the value of psychotherapy to mitigate personal problems, where there is active encouragement by the training director to seek therapy, and where programmatic support to reduce the cost of therapy is made available (Habl et al. 2010). It is recommended that residents seek out a psychotherapist who does not regularly interact with trainees in a clinical education role. Residency programs may have lists of psychotherapists who have worked with psychiatry residents and who are not a part of the clinical education program. In addition to the potential for increased self-knowledge, another beneficial aspect is increased compassion for the emotional vulnerability inherent in the patient role.

T-Groups

A T-group (sometimes called a process group) is a group that studies its own members' behavior through interactions occurring in the present moment (the here and now) with the goal of understanding and improving individual, interpersonal, and group dynamics (Swiller 2011). When a T-group experience is available within a single residency training program, the group is composed of coresidents. As a result, the stakes can be elevated with regard to interpersonal feedback, and attention to building sufficient *psychological safety* must be a top priority. T-groups are also available in other settings, such as the American Group Psychotherapy

Association and other training organizations. In these cases, the members of the T-group are not usually known to each other ahead of participating in the group.

The T-group offers an environment for interpersonal feedback through examining patterns of behavior with trusted comembers. The Johari window (Figure 23–1), named after its developers Joseph Luft and Harrison Ingham, can be used to illustrate this process with its four quadrants: the *arena* represents behavior that is observable to others and also present in conscious self-awareness; the *blind spot* represents behavior that others have noticed but is outside self-awareness; the *façade* represents that which is known to self but not known to others, such as private unspoken thoughts or personal history; and the *unknown* represents an aspect of self that is not yet known by anyone—an area for personal character growth or acquisition of new cognitive or behavioral skills. In the T-group, members can help each other notice behavior patterns in each others' areas of unawareness, through careful observation and empathic communication (Luft and Ingham 1955).

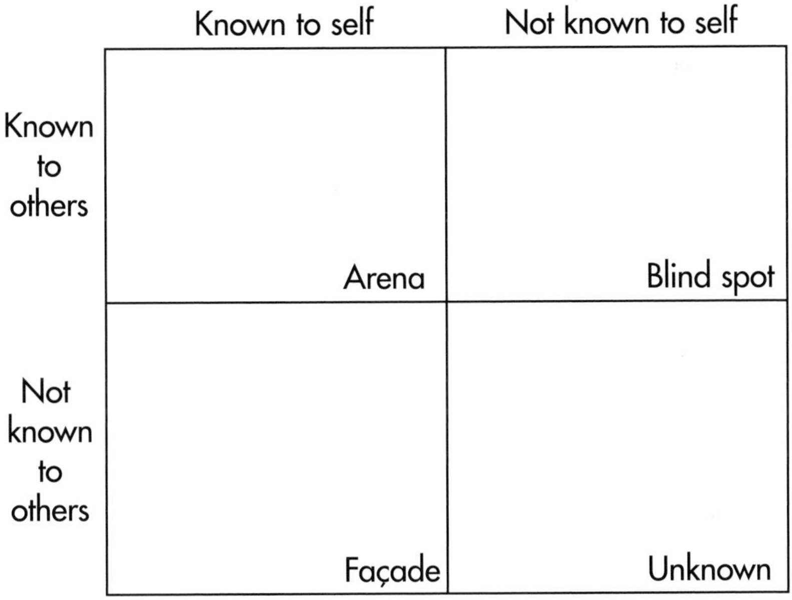

	Known to self	Not known to self
Known to others	Arena	Blind spot
Not known to others	Façade	Unknown

FIGURE 23–1. The Johari window.

This approach also has been used for decades to illustrate the value of an interpersonal focus in group therapy. It has been used more recently in the clinical learning environment to address the culture of feedback (Ramani et al. 2017). In addition, there is a version available online to be completed through email (see "Resources" section).

SPECIFIC CHALLENGES AND STRATEGIES

⌘ **In my second month of residency, I left rounds feeling both ashamed and guilty after getting feedback about missing an important part of the mental status examination.** This is a key time to practice *self-compassion* by speaking with *self-kindness* (remember that this is the second month and that residency is 4 years long for many good reasons), by considering our *common humanity* (check in with trusted co-interns about their inevitable mistakes to recognize that you are all in it together), and by making use of *mindfulness* (the experience of shame and guilt are time limited in this present moment and do not need to be accompanied by sustained self-judgment). By taking on a *growth mindset*, you might view this mistake as both an opportunity for learning about the mental status examination and an opportunity to learn more about yourself.

⌘ **I'm so tired of hearing that my documentation is lacking sufficient detail. I have already tried everything to improve and I keep hearing the same thing.** It is tempting to become defensive when receiving feedback repeatedly, especially when the rigors of residency training inhibit the capacity to hold distressing emotions. However, if you receive the same or similar feedback from multiple people, then it might be worth considering whether you have an area of unawareness perpetuated by *confirmation bias*. It is worth considering "In what way is this feedback accurate?" by seeking out examples of other notes and comparing the level of detail. Try rewriting a note and review it with the attending to make sure you fully understand their comments.

⌘ **I completed a task in a timely and effective way, yet I received harsh feedback during rounds about a minor oversight in protocol.** In settings with low *psychological safety*, it is necessary to identify and cultivate relationships with allies both inside and outside the system. It is less possible to have frank and open conversations if these discussions come at a reputational cost. However, it is still necessary to get support and make sense of what is happening. You can check in with a senior resident and debrief with a trusted colleague. In doing so, it is useful to present both sides and seek what is valid about the feedback and what is not in order to counter *confirmation bias*. However, if a faculty member is known to regularly give harsh feedback, then reaching out to the program director is indicated.

SELF-REFLECTIVE QUESTIONS

1. How did I respond when I most recently had "ink on my face" (shoe untied, shirt untucked, etc.)?
2. When have I noticed myself inhabiting a fixed mindset? A growth mindset? What was happening in the specific situations? What can be learned from this?
3. What helps me feel more psychologically safe in groups and organizations?
4. What experiential practices will I choose to increase my internal self-awareness? What practices will I choose to increase my external self-awareness?

RESOURCES

American Group Psychotherapy Association (AGPA) and local affiliate group psychotherapy societies: www.agpa.org/home/continuing-ed-meetings-events-training

Banaji MR: Blindspot: hidden biases of good people. YouTube video, 6:51, June 4, 2019. Available at: www.youtube.com/watch?v=XK_G-rkXenM. Accessed October 9, 2022.

Brenner AM: The role of personal psychodynamic psychotherapy in becoming a competent psychiatrist. Harv Rev Psychiatry 14(5):268–272, 2006 16990172

Dweck C: Developing a growth mindset. YouTube video, 9:37, October 9, 2014. Available at: www.youtube.com/watch?v=hiiEeMN7vbQ. Accessed October 9, 2022.

Edmonson A: Three ways to create psychological safety in health care. YouTube video, 4:20, August 2, 2017. Available at: www.youtube.com/watch?v=jbLjdFqrUNs. Accessed October 9, 2022.

Hardy K: Tasks of the privileges. YouTube video, 3:05, November 12, 2012. Available at: www.youtube.com/watch?v=MxSsKNHJujs. Accessed October 9, 2022.

Jones C: Allegories on race and racism. YouTube video, 20:31, July 10, 2014. Available at: www.youtube.com/watch?v=GNhcY6fTyBM. Accessed October 9, 2022.

Neff K: The space between self-esteem and self-compassion. YouTube video, 13:07, November 4, 2019. Available at: www.youtube.com/watch?v=pKEtknqHTjo. Accessed October 9, 2022.

Online Johari Window: https://kevan.org/johari—free online website using email to trusted allies to generate the four quadrants (blind spot, arena, façade, unknown)

UCLA Mindful Awareness Research Center: Free guided meditations—online mindfulness practices, including breath awareness, body scan and loving kindness meditation. Available at: www.uclahealth.org/marc/mindful-meditations. Accessed October 9, 2022.

REFERENCES

Calaprice A (Ed): The Ultimate Quotable Einstein, 2nd Edition. Princeton, NJ, Princeton University Press, 2019

Dweck CS: Mindset: The New Psychology of Success. New York, Ballantine, 2016

Edmonson AC: The Fearless Organization: Creating Psychological Safety in the Workplace for Learning, Innovation, and Growth. New York, Wiley, 2018

Edmonson AC, Lei Z: Psychological safety: the history, renaissance, and future of an interpersonal construct. Annual Review of Organizational Psychology and Organizational Behavior 1:23–43, 2014

Eurich T: What self-awareness really is (and how to cultivate it). Harvard Business Review digital articles, January 4, 2018. Accessed June 13, 2022.

Greenwald AG, Banaji MR: The implicit revolution: reconceiving the relation between conscious and unconscious. Am Psychol 72(9):861–871, 2017 29283625

Habl S, Mintz DL, Bailey A: The role of personal therapy in psychiatric residency training: a survey of psychiatry training directors. Acad Psychiatry 34(1):21–26, 2010 20071719

Kabat-Zinn J: Wherever You Go, There You Are, 10th Edition. New York, Hatchette, 2005

Luft J, Ingham H: The Johari window, a graphic model of interpersonal awareness. Proceedings of the Western Training Laboratory in Group Development 246:2014-03, 1955

Morin A: Self-awareness part 1: definition, measures, effects, functions, and antecedents. Soc Personal Psychol Compass 5(10):807–823, 2011

Neff KD: The role of self-compassion in development: a healthier way to relate to oneself. Hum Development 52(4):211–214, 2009 22479080

Patallo BJ: The multicultural guidelines in practice: cultural humility in clinical training and supervision. Train Educ Prof Psychol 13(3):227–232, 2019

Ramani S, Könings K, Mann KV, van der Vleuten C: Uncovering the unknown: a grounded theory study exploring the impact of self-awareness on the culture of feedback in residency education. Med Teach 39(10):1065–1073, 2017 28741446

Swiller HI: Process groups. Int J Group Psychother 61(2):262–273, 2011 21463097

CHAPTER 24

Communication Skills and Managing Conflict

Rebecca Rendleman, M.D.
Oliver M. Stroeh, M.D.

Communication is as fundamental in everyday work in psychiatry as it is in medicine more generally. Effective communication improves patient outcomes, including enhanced patient satisfaction and treatment adherence (Dwamena et al. 2012), and improves our satisfaction with our work as clinicians (Krasner et al. 2009; Saslow et al. 2017). Additionally, effective communication enhances equity in health care (Cordero and Davis 2020) and creates a more inclusive environment for our patients. Increasingly, communication skills training is integrated into medical school curricula, but it is variably integrated into residency education.

How often have you dwelled on a difficult interaction with a patient or family member (or even colleague)? Difficult communications drive down our personal satisfaction and erode our confidence. The good news is that communication skills are teachable and can improve with practice. In this chapter we focus on the fundamentals of communication, provide helpful strategies to use at different points in a physician-patient encounter, and offer examples of how these strategies can be used in our more difficult communications—including those with our colleagues. This framework is based on the relationship-centered communication training that one hospital developed in conjunction with the Academy for Communication in Healthcare.

KEY POINTS

- Communication is a fundamental skill that can be learned and developed through practice.

- Setting an agenda and managing expectations up front maximizes efficiency.

- Empathy and perspective taking deepen the relationship and build trust.

- Delivery of a diagnosis and treatment plan improves when information is delivered in smaller chunks with frequent check-ins and in collaboration with the patient.

COMMUNICATION GOALS FOR THE ENCOUNTER

During your residency, you will have many encounters with patients in a variety of contexts, including in the emergency department, on the medical floors, on psychiatric units, and in ambulatory care settings. In the following sections we focus on effective communication in our daily encounters with patients rather than on methods of communication specific to particular psychotherapies. Although the frame used to demonstrate these skills is the patient-physician encounter, these skills are equally applicable to communications within any relationship, including those with colleagues.

SETTING THE AGENDA

Let's focus on the beginning of the patient-physician encounter. In medical school, you likely learned that the opening of the interview is an opportunity to establish rapport and elicit the patient's chief complaint. However, in practice, patients often have more than one concern. In addition to establishing rapport, the opening of the encounter is an opportunity to elicit *all* of the patient's concerns up front. By doing so, you mitigate the risk of unaddressed concerns and avoid the dreaded doorknob comment or question. Additionally, what is most concerning to the patient may not be what is most concerning to you. Understanding the patient's priorities at the outset allows you to more effectively collaborate on the agenda for the encounter and anticipate potential sticking points later on.

The mnemonic RCA (rapport, concerns, agenda) summarizes the goals for the first patient encounter.

Tool 1: Agenda Setting or RCA

- Establish **R**apport
- Elicit all **C**oncerns
- Collaboratively identify an **A**genda

The importance of establishing rapport is well appreciated by psychiatry residents, but the notion of eliciting all concerns and collaboratively identifying an agenda may not be. Open-ended questions are the best tool for eliciting the full spectrum of concerns. Examples include the following:

- *"What concerns do you have today?"* If you are seeing a patient in a unique context, setting the frame for that context can be helpful.
- *"What concerns brought you to the emergency room today?"* If you are in a consultative setting, you might need to expand on the frame.
- *"Your team (or doctor) has asked for a psychiatry consultation. What do you understand about your team's concerns? What concerns do you have?"* To elicit additional concerns, open-ended questions such as "What else?" or "What other concerns do you have?" are preferable to close-ended questions such as "Any other concerns?," which may signal to the patient that you no longer are interested in hearing additional concerns.

Once the patient has offered all of their concerns, the next step is to work with the patient to collaboratively identify the agenda for the encounter. To do so, it is helpful to repeat the patient's concerns and to inquire which of these concerns is most important to them. This also allows you the opportunity, if your concerns differ from those of the patient, to offer your perspective and propose a path forward that addresses both your and the patient's concerns. The vast majority of patients, if they feel that their concerns are recognized and valued, will be able to collaborate with you on the agenda for the encounter. This entire process sets up a road map for the encounter for both you and the patient and helps you anticipate concerns and manage expectations for the rest of the encounter.

DEEPENING THE RELATIONSHIP

Having established some basic rapport, elicited all of the patient's concerns, and collaboratively constructed an agenda for the encounter, you are ready to transition to the middle of the encounter and learn more about each of the concerns on the agreed-on agenda. This is typically the part of the encounter where you frequently will obtain a lot of information. However, to approach data collection using a battery of unidirectional yes/no questions would be an unfortunate strategy because you likely would end up missing valuable information. Employing techniques to deepen the relationship will facilitate your collection of information, including your understanding of the patient's experience—both at and beneath the surface. This is particularly true in moments of conflict. An understanding of the patient's story and perspective will help you adjust your approach during the encounter, enabling you to treat both the illness *and* the patient. Clinicians who use this approach deliver better care by effectively facilitating the patient's experience of being seen, heard, and understood.

The following two tools facilitate the deepening and building of the patient-physician relationship. One helps you learn about the patient's perspective, and the other helps you explicitly convey empathy to the patient.

Impact, ideas, and expectations (IIE) help you deepen and build the working relationship with a patient through exploration of the patient's perspectives and development of greater understanding of the patient's personal story.

Tool 2: Deepening the Relationship Through Impact, Ideas, and Expectations

- Impact
- Ideas
- Expectations

The tool prompts you to go about this task by asking the patient how their life has been affected by the issue of concern, exploring ideas that the patient may have about a given concern, and/or exploring the patient's expectations of how you might be of assistance to them in addressing the concern. Through exploration of the patient's perspective, you also are likely to reduce any potential reliance on assumptions regarding the patient, including about how their symptoms or illness affect their lives, their understanding of the symptoms or illness, or their expectations regarding what might be accomplished during the visit and, thus, what a "successful" visit would look like. Gaining greater understanding of the patient's perspective decreases the likelihood that you will act on assumptions or biases and, as a result, may mitigate potential sources of health care inequities (Smedley et al. 2003).

PEARLS© is a mnemonic from the Academy of Communication in Healthcare that identifies different types of empathic statements that can be used to deepen the relationship with a patient.

Tool 3: Deepening the Relationship Through Empathic Responses

- **P**artnership
- **E**motion
- **A**cknowledgment and/or apology
- **R**espect
- **L**egitimization
- **S**upport

Have you observed a less experienced medical student or resident speak with a patient and fail to comment in response to the patient's sharing of an emotional, poignant, or meaningful moment? Often, a less experienced learner such as a medical student speeds past the moment, resulting in an empathic failure that introduces greater distance between the learner and the person with whom they are speaking. Although empathy can also be conveyed nonverbally, such a moment highlights the potential importance and utility of making explicit empathic statements ("caring out loud") (Cordero and Davis 2020) and deepening the relationship in support of our goals for the encounter. Indeed, studies have demonstrated that when a patient does share an emotional cue, those physicians who pick up on the cue and make a related empathic statement have greater efficiency in both primary care and surgical outpatient settings (Levinson et al. 2000). The intention is not to make statements that *imply* empathy but rather to make *direct and explicit* statements of empathy, thereby reducing the likelihood of uncertainty or confusion of intention. Table 24–1 outlines different types of potential empathic statements and includes examples of each. Although some types of empathic statements may come more naturally to you than others, practice and use of different types of empathic statements can expand your toolbox such that when faced with a challenging communication encounter, you have a broader array of options from which to draw.

DELIVERING A DIAGNOSIS AND TREATMENT RECOMMENDATION

The end of the physician-patient encounter typically involves the sharing of a diagnosis and/or treatment recommendations. Common reasons for this part of the encounter to go awry include unaddressed concerns, lack of

TABLE 24–1. Examples of PEARLS©

Type of statement	Examples
Partnership	"We'll figure out together what some next steps might be."
Emotion	"You're upset."
Acknowledgment and/or apology	"It's hard to remember to take your medication when so much is going on." "I apologize that I wasn't clear in my communication."
Respect	"I give you a lot of credit for trying to use your new skills."
Legitimization	"Most people I work with would be distressed by that kind of a reaction to the medication."
Support	"I think you're doing a terrific job. I'm here for you."

understanding, or disagreement with the diagnosis and/or treatment plan. During residency, you will develop useful and informative scripts that help you teach patients and families about psychiatric diagnoses and treatment. By the end of training, you likely will be able to pull up these scripts with limited effort. A common pitfall for clinicians is the impulse to recite a script in its entirety with a patient or their family. The information, although useful, is often too much for the patient to absorb. You will be far more effective if you give information in smaller chunks and intermittently check in with the patient to gauge their understanding and to invite questions. We introduce our final mnemonic, ART (also from Academy of Communication in Healthcare), to offer strategies on how you can ARTfully deliver information about diagnoses and treatment recommendations.

At the point in the interview when you plan to deliver your diagnosis and treatment recommendations, it is useful to give a heads-up to the patient and ask permission to share your thoughts. By doing so, you alert the patient that you are going to deliver information.

Tool 4: The ART of Communication

- **A**sk open-ended questions
- **R**espond with a summary or empathic statement
- **T**ell your perspective

For example, you might say, "I have had an opportunity to review all the information that you provided and speak to your family. I have a good idea of what is causing your anxiety and difficulty sleeping. Would you welcome my sharing these thoughts?" You may be wondering what value there is in asking permission. After all, most patients will say yes. In addition to conveying respect, this allows for the possibility that some patients may feel unprepared or afraid to hear a diagnosis or treatment recommendation. Perhaps they would like a friend or family member to join them.

Here is an example of an ART cycle following the delivery of the diagnosis of major depression:

> **Clinician:** What do you know about depression? (*Ask*)
> **Patient:** My mother had really bad depression when I was growing up. I remember that she spent long periods of time in bed and was hospitalized a couple of times. Nothing seemed to work for her. I have always been afraid that would happen to me.
> **Clinician:** I am sorry to hear about your mother and can understand your worries about what depression might mean for you. (*Respond*) Depression, although it can at times be severe, is a highly treatable condition. We have many more treatments available today than were available to your mother. (*Tell*)

By asking an open-ended question, you gain important information about the patient's prior knowledge, can identify potential misconceptions or fears, and can address questions in an ongoing fashion. This allows you to tailor your script to the individual before you. It may be tempting to skip the "R," but this would be a mistake. Our capacity to respond with empathy and to validate concerns deepens the relationship and permits patients to feel safe sharing concerns, especially because so many psychiatric diagnoses and treatments are stigmatized.

Several cycles of ART are often required before you have conveyed the necessary information to conclude the encounter. At this point, it is often helpful, particularly when you have conveyed a lot of information, to make sure that the patient can articulate the plan. This has many elements in common with the teach-back method in patient education. By employing this method, you can correct any errors and reinforce the plan. Here is an example of the conclusion of an encounter:

> **Clinician:** We talked about a lot today, and I want to make sure that I did a good job with my communication. Can you share what you understand about your treatment plan?

SPECIFIC CHALLENGES AND STRATEGIES

⌘ **My patient presents with multiple concerns, and I have only 30 minutes allotted for the visit.** In the section "Setting the Agenda," we emphasized the importance of eliciting the full spectrum of a patient's concern at the outset. Although, on average, patients offer no more than three or four concerns, there are outliers. When this happens, some clinicians respond by cutting off the patient and telling them what they are going to do and what they are not going to do. Other clinicians get lost in the sea of concerns, and a 30-minute visit turns into 60 minutes. Neither response is optimal. In the first scenario, the clinician imposes an agenda and risks the relationship. In the second, the clinician is inefficient and does not help shape priorities. How can you avoid either scenario? As you elicit concerns, summarize the concerns out loud as you go—perhaps visually capturing the number of concerns on your fingers. If you notice that many more concerns are being elicited than can be addressed in the visit, consider responding ARTfully.

> **Clinician:** I am really glad that you are sharing your concerns, and they are important to me. (*Respond*) Given that we only have 30 minutes in this visit, what concerns are most important that we cover today? (*Tell*)

You have alerted the patient to the time constraints. You allow the patient the opportunity to share their priorities as opposed to imposing your priorities on the patient so that you can offer an agenda.

> **Clinician:** That is really helpful for me to know. (*Respond*) Might I suggest that today we focus on these three concerns that you identified? We can set aside time on our next visit to address your other concerns. (*Tell*)

With the patient's participation in decision-making, you can now proceed with the encounter. Sometimes, a patient's concern is outside your area of expertise. Acknowledging this up front and, when possible, offering direction as to how the patient may address these concerns also facilitate agenda setting.

⌘ **I'm on call, and the nurse asks me to see a patient who is angry and wishes to be discharged from the inpatient psychiatric unit.** Assuming that your clinical judgment suggests that the situation is safe for you to engage the patient in communication, you might strategize that it will be important to efficiently build a working relationship with this patient so as to better understand his needs and help him better regulate his emotions. To build this relationship under these stressful circumstances (for both you and the patient), in addition to considering your nonverbal communications (e.g., tone and volume of voice, body stance), you might anticipate using IIE and PEARLS©.

After introducing yourself and asking the patient to share his main concern (such a heated situation is likely not appropriate for an exhaustive elicitation of concerns), you might prompt him to tell you more about his desire to be discharged. You likely should allow him to speak uninterrupted for a minute or two and actively listen to what he shares. You may learn, for example, that he has just finished up a phone call with his wife during which she told him that your coresident had let her know that he likely would be discharged next week. However, the patient had understood from the primary team that he would be discharged before the weekend and in time for his son's first birthday party.

You should consider the PEARLS© tool and make explicit empathic statements when responding to this patient. In particular, statements labeling his emotions and acknowledging and, when appropriate, legitimizing his thoughts and feelings may prove effective at helping this patient feel heard and understood. In turn, this might help him better regulate his emotions and more calmly consider his options. Such empathic statements also will demonstrate that you have heard what he has shared and might facilitate collaboration. You might also try to foster a greater sense of collaboration through the use of partnership statements and, if appropriate, apologize for ways in which you or the team have contributed to the misunderstanding.

You can also bolster the patient's experience of being seen and understood by using the IIE tool to elicit his perspective. To better understand where this patient is coming from, you might ask about impact: "What do you think the impact would be on your child or your family if you missed the party this weekend and completed your treatment here?" Alternatively, or additionally, you could ask about the ideas he might have regarding continued hospitalization: "What are you worried might happen if you stay through the weekend and finish your treatment with us?" You also could consider asking him, "What were you expecting it would be like when you agreed to come into the hospital?" Open-ended questions relating to IIE in combination with ongoing use of the PEARLS© tool will nurture a deepening working relationship between you and this patient. Eliciting his perspective is not the same as agreeing with it. However, an understanding of his story will likely facilitate opportunities for you and him to collaborate, negotiate, and/or compromise.

⌘ **I am newly assigned a patient with major depression who was admitted over the weekend and has been refusing antidepressant medication.** Treatment nonadherence is common. You will encounter it across different settings during your psychiatry training. There are many reasons why patients are nonadherent. Building trust and appreciating the patient's perspective are critical to understanding these reasons. Equally critical is avoiding making assumptions. A good place to start is respectful inquiry. What does your patient know or understand? Your first encounter likely will have several goals, including building rapport, establishing your relationship to the patient's care, reviewing the patient's concerns and history, and discussing diagnosis and treatment.

As you approach the discussion of diagnosis, your respectful inquiry might begin as follows: "What do you understand your diagnosis to be?" or "What did the doctors share with you about your diagnosis on admission?" If the patient does not know, then this is the place to begin. Using the ART skill, share your diagnostic impression and then inquire, "What do you know about depression?" This will allow you to gauge the patient's knowledge and inquire about questions or concerns about this diagnosis before moving on to a discussion of treatment.

Once you have established the patient's understanding of the diagnosis, then you can move to the next ART cycle: "What do you know about the treatment of depression?" or, if the patient's knowledge level is higher, "What do you know about medication to treat depression?" Allowing the patient to share their knowledge and attitudes and validating their concerns may set the stage for inquiring about their nonadherence: "I understand that when the nurses offered you antidepressants over the weekend, you did not take them. What concerns did you have?" You might be surprised by what you learn. Maybe no one explicitly discussed starting the medications. Perhaps medications were discussed, but your patient had unaddressed concerns. Sometimes, no matter what you offer, the patient remains unwilling to take the medications. Assuming that you are not in a situation that might require medication above objection, you may need to slow down and do your best to meet the patient where they are. You may need to spend more time building trust and deepening the relationship to permit you to revisit medication treatment in a subsequent encounter.

⌘ **I just received a call from the internal medicine chief resident, with a consultation request stating, "We have a psych patient here who is not acting right, and my attending wants you to see him."** Relationship-centered communication and its skills have applicability and generalizability to communication in the context of any relationship. Part of the challenge of this request involves a lack of detail and specificity—regarding both the internal medicine team's assessment of the patient "not acting right" and the ways in which the team is hoping that you and the consultation-liaison service can help them and, as a result, the patient. Thus, an appropriate goal of the interaction with the chief resident might be to assist her in communicating her team's needs more clearly. To do so, communication strategies might include 1) using RCA to clarify the concerns of the chief resident and internal medicine team regarding the patient and to establish an agenda for your consultation and 2) using IIE to understand the perspectives of the chief resident and internal medicine team.

To begin, you might consider first establishing basic rapport and a collaborative stance with the consulting chief resident by saying, "Thank you for reaching out. I'd like to help you and your team." To attempt to gather more specific information regarding the team's concerns for the patient, you might then ask, "What concerns do you and your team have regarding the patient?" and/or "What was the patient doing that led you, your attending, and your team to ask for our help?" Using "What else?" and its variants may help you elicit from the chief resident additional information that, prior to calling you, she may not have formulated into specific concerns or questions. Such inquiry may also draw forth information that she and her team, as clinicians with less familiarity with mental health and psychiatry, may not recognize as potentially relevant to the consultation or may not know how to accurately capture or label.

⌘ To help the internal medicine team provide effective care to this patient, it also is essential to understand the perspective of the chief resident and the team regarding this patient and his behaviors. Using IIE, ask, "How are the patient's behaviors *impacting* your team's abilities to provide medical care to him?" This might help you prioritize targets of psychiatric assessment and treatment and provide practical guidance to the internal medicine team. Asking, "What is your idea of what might be going on and leading this patient to act the way he is?" might serve as an invitation for the chief resident to share her and/or her team's current clinical impressions and associated notions regarding the patient's behaviors. The chief resident's answers may reveal issues such as inaccurate or incomplete understanding of mental illness; inadvertent stigmatization of patients with mental illness; or underrecognized thoughts, feelings, or judgments (i.e., countertransference) that may be impeding the team's abilities to provide better and more effective care. Thus, as a consultant, you may discover opportunities to intervene—ultimately contributing to more effective care for the patient. Finally, asking the chief resident about her and the team's *expectations* of you and your team (e.g., "How are you hoping that we can be of greatest use to you and your team?") increases the likelihood that she and her team will be content with the assistance you and your team provide. Maybe they are hoping that you can provide concrete suggestions to nursing staff about how best to interact with a patient with particularly challenging behaviors. Alternatively, maybe they are hoping that you can provide guidance about how best to manage the patient's restlessness so that he can tolerate an indicated and essential MRI scan. Their expectations of you may not be self-evident and are worth making explicit.

SELF-REFLECTIVE QUESTIONS

1. What type of interaction presents a communication challenge to me?
2. Which skills might I employ during challenging interactions to enhance communication?
3. What barriers do I anticipate in trying to improve my communication and conflict management?

RESOURCES

Academy of Communication Healthcare: https://achonline.org. This professional organization is dedicated to research and teaching of relationship-centered communication.

Chou C, Cooley L: Communication Rx: Transforming Healthcare Through Relationship-Centered Communication. New York, McGraw Hill, 2018. This book, published in conjunction with the Academy of Communication in Healthcare, expands on relationship-centered communication and its application beyond the clinical encounter.

VitalTalk: www.vitaltalk.org. VitalTalk offers evidence-based trainings to enhance communication about serious illness, including goals of care at the end of life. This is particularly useful to psychiatrists interested in palliative care.

REFERENCES

Cordero DM, Davis DL: Communication for equity in the service of patient experience: health justice and the COVID-19 pandemic. J Patient Exp 7(3):279–281, 2020 32821779

Dwamena F, Holmes-Rovner M, Gaulden CM, et al: Interventions for providers to promote a patient-centred approach in clinical consultations. Cochrane Database Syst Rev 12:CD003267, 2012 23235595

Krasner MS, Epstein RM, Beckman H, et al: Association of an educational program in mindful communication with burnout, empathy, and attitudes among primary care physicians. JAMA 302(12):1284–1293, 2009 19773563

Levinson W, Gorawara-Bhat R, Lamb J: A study of patient clues and physician responses in primary care and surgical settings. JAMA 284(8):1021–1027, 2000 10944650

Saslow M, Sirota D, Jones D, et al: Effects of a hospital-wide physician communication training workshop on self-efficacy, attitudes, and behavior. Patient Exp J 4(3):48–54, 2017

Smedley BD, Stith AY, Nelson AR (eds): Unequal Treatment: Confronting Racial and Ethnic Disparities in Healthcare. Institute of Medicine (US) Committee on Understanding and Eliminating Racial and Ethnic Disparities in Health Care. Washington, DC, National Academies Press, 2003

CHAPTER 25

Embracing Uncertainty

A Prescription Toward Clinical Expertise

Vinod H. Srihari, M.D.
Robert Rohrbaugh, M.D.

> The great pleasure of ignorance is the pleasure of asking questions. The [person] who has lost this pleasure or exchanged it for the pleasure of dogma, which is the pleasure of answering, is already beginning to stiffen.
>
> *Robert Lynd (1921, p. 18)*

Residency training is a time of rapid professional growth. You learned much in medical school, but you have now entered the practice of psychiatry. A vast repertoire of knowledge, skills, attitudes, and values must be retrieved, acquired, and tested in the service of your patients. As you gain independence from your supervisors, you will also discover your dependence on interprofessional teams within health care organizations that are in turn embedded within complex regional networks of stakeholders. You must learn how to leverage medical and also social determinants to advance the health of your patients. It is natural to feel unmoored in the face of all these demands. In this chapter we focus on uncertainty, specifically that common, pervasive situation wherein answers are not readily available, yet decisions need to be made. Our hope is to provide you with tools to practice learning from such uncertainty in a supportive community of peers and supervisors.

KEY POINTS

- Uncertainty is pervasive in clinical practice and is a catalyst for learning. Case formulations can help convert inchoate mysteries into tractable problems.

- If you deliberately take plural perspectives on a challenging scenario (problem framing), this can organize your priorities for resolution (problem solving).

- Evidence-based medicine is a set of tools (not rules) to help you build and respond to those questions that require responses from systematic studies of populations.

- It is important to develop an active and reflective approach to your own learning.

NAVIGATING UNCERTAINTY: USE OF A TASK-BASED MAP

Uncertainty is common in our work as clinicians, researchers, administrators, and educators, and your response to uncertainty will influence whatever career path you choose after residency training. A taxonomy of three tasks—empathic, interpretive, and scientific—in the clinical encounter will help you navigate uncertainty (Srihari 2008).

Empathic Task

The empathic task helps you understand what it is like in your patient's mind. It can be enabled by your own experiences (e.g., of low mood or severe anxiety) and by valuable depictions in novels, movies, or other media that can powerfully extend your capacity to imagine what your patient is thinking and feeling and, thus, to communicate more effectively with them in the midst of their suffering. Additionally, when challenged to comprehend mental states that are likely to be qualitatively more alien to common human experience (e.g., hallucinations), you will need to read accounts from descriptive psychopathology. These accounts from a vast accumulated literature are necessary not just to help your own appreciation of these states of mind but to help your patients put words to and, thus, gain some agency over an otherwise confusing internal landscape. This can have immediate therapeutic value in reducing your patient's sense of isolation while also retrieving essential data for personalized care.

Interpretive Task

The interpretive task asks, how can *this* presentation be understood within *that* model of disease or personality or behavior or narrative (McHugh and Slavney 2012)? It is best begun via case formulation. This topic is detailed in the "Resources" at the end of the chapter and elsewhere in this book (see Chapter 7, "Learning to Develop a Case Formulation"); in this subsection we emphasize the value of a pluralistic approach to each case (Ghaemi 2007). The predicaments we face in our clinical work should not be reduced exclusively to an impersonal disease process (What does this patient have?); maladaptive choices (What did this patient do?); personality or cognitive vulnerabilities (Who is this person?); or larger cultural, historical, social, or economic forces to which the patient has been subjected (How did the environment shape this person?) (McHugh and Slavney 2012). In practice, however, you might find yourself or your peers gravitating toward one or another of these perspectives. The common temptation to take either a purely biological or purely psychodynamic approach to all cases can offer the comfort of a routine or a familiar template to apply in the face of what can feel like a chaotic avalanche of information, but this can come at the price of ignoring significant information that can compromise your care of patients.

Good formulation practice thus might need to include the discipline of deliberately taking several perspectives on each case. Different views will highlight and drive consideration of different problems to be targeted within a comprehensive treatment plan, as in the following vignette.

Case Vignette

Mr. S has been admitted recurrently with alcohol withdrawal. A rigorously behavioral perspective can provide a coherent, theoretically satisfying account of the genesis and sustenance of his addiction and will organize specific treatment approaches (e.g., naltrexone combined with peer groups to address the biological mechanism and situational triggers for craving). However, a separate effort to honor and thereby fully elicit Mr. S's own narrative understanding may reveal a strong conviction that his disordered use was precipitated by the painful loss of his wife. The only treatment he wants for staying sober is therapy targeting this unresolved grief, despite acknowledging years of severe addiction. Knowing this allows the clinical team to better understand Mr. S's lack of enthusiasm for their proposed treatment plan, which has frustrated his outpatient clinicians and family and threatens to derail the discharge planning process. It becomes clear that his narrative of why he chose to drink needs to be reconciled with the clinical team's learning theory–based model.

Such explanatory conflicts are indeed commonplace, if often only implicit, and they can also occur within clinical teams. It is thus important to find ways to share your developing formulations. Disagreements about what to do can often be traced to the different perspectives being taken on the predicament, and, when explicitly articulated, can be addressed (e.g., it is possible to allow for Mr. S's narrative while also enriching it with a behavioral and neurobiological account of the onset and persistence of his addiction to alcohol). When disagreement occurs among clinicians, it is similarly important to clarify whether this is because different perspectives are being used to formulate different aspects of a case (Are you framing different problems and talking past one another?) or because different evidence or appraisals of the same evidence are being applied within a singular perspective (Are you disagreeing about how to solve the same problem?). In both cases, unearthing these disjunctions can stimulate useful debate and enrich the treatment plan. Sharing your formulations with your supervisors and peers and processing their feedback will help you develop expertise in this important task.

Scientific Task

Formulations can clarify which are the most relevant issues and what perspectives might best apply (problem framing), and they also will raise specific questions about diagnosis (e.g., What is the best way to distinguish alcoholic hallucinosis from a primary psychotic disorder?), prognosis (e.g., How likely is a completed suicide after a first attempt by hanging?), risk (e.g., How likely is a fetal abnormality with lithium use in pregnancy?), or treatment (What is the relative effectiveness of drug A vs. drug B?). These questions cannot be resolved solely with information from a single case or even a vast series of cases encountered by an experienced clinician, but they require knowledge from systematic studies of populations. The scientific task involves integrating evidence from clinical research into treatment for the patient(s) under your care and is an essential element of expert clinical practice.

The heuristic of evidence-based medicine was first articulated to guide clinicians through this challenging third task. The "Resources" at the end of this chapter provide case-based examples to help your practice in each of the following steps:

- *Ask:* Convert specific uncertainties into questions structured to facilitate answers from clinical research using the PICOT method, referencing a patient or population (P), an intervention or exposure (I), a comparison (C), relevant outcomes (O), and a clinically relevant time period (T).
- *Access:* Efficiently retrieve the most rigorous and relevant scientific evidence, such as by first reviewing syntheses (systematic reviews, practice guidelines) before reading individual studies.
- *Appraise:* Critique this evidence for quality, size, and precision of effect and applicability.
- *Apply:* Use this evidence to inform decision-making by your patients in a manner that respects and integrates their values and preferences.
- *Audit:* Assess the actual impact of this evidence-informed practice on the outcomes of patients in your practice setting.

Evidence from the scientific literature will rarely provide a definite answer or resolution of uncertainty. More commonly, you will find provisional answers that can inform imminent decisions, and your appraisal of this evidence will also prepare you to update this answer as future studies are completed. Applying population-based data to the individual under your care (who may differ from those included in the best available studies) requires judgment and a commitment to elicit the values and preferences of your patient.

REFLECTIVE PRACTICE: DEVELOPING A LEARNING HABIT FOR YOUR CAREER

The task-based approach outlined in the previous section can provide a map for organizing your initial responses to uncertainty, one that you will no doubt modify as you gain more experience with the territory of clinical psychiatry. You should expect to arrive at these tasks with a variable degree of fluency and comfort, and you may find that your skill varies across different patients and in different clinical settings. Recognize and embrace the tasks as an opportunity to practice and curate your own trajectory of improvement across the widening variety of situations you are likely to encounter over your career. These tasks do not exhaust all the domains of work you may be engaged in as a psychiatrist, but they provide a good starting place to make operational an approach to lifelong, practice-based learning.

A growing literature on reflective practice offers some useful ideas on how to develop and sustain such an approach. One definition describes this as "practice conducted with personal and professional self-awareness and reflection; with awareness of competencies; with appropriate self-care" (Fouad et al. 2009, p. S10). However, a critical review of the varied uses and implementations of this broad concept reveals that it is far from clear how to do this in a manner that best serves your patients and your own professional development (Lilienfeld and Basterfield 2020). The following subsections provide some provisional suggestions, cautions, and questions to guide your own critical approach to learning.

Engage in Self-Directed Feedback

Self-reflection or introspection on your strengths and weaknesses is an unreliable path to improvement (Eva and Regehr 2008). A rich literature on universal cognitive biases strongly supports seeking feedback from others to avoid areas of unawareness in our thinking and learning. There are no easy answers on how to construct workplaces that make such feedback safe and routine, but residency training is an excellent time to experiment with different approaches to seeking feedback and engaging in self-directed learning.

Seek Direct Observation

Look for opportunities to have others observe your work and to present your thinking to patients (across all three tasks) in verbal and written form. Resist the urge for mere approval but instead invite criticism from peers and supervisors. Consider also inviting feedback from allied professions (e.g., nursing, social work) in your workplace.

Build and Nurture Your Approach to Uncertainty

Keep track of questions as they arise, reach out to medical librarians or mentors who can help you efficiently track down empirical evidence when necessary, and set aside time to follow up on questions that are recurrent, important for clinical care, or just interesting.

Be Kind to Yourself and Never Worry Alone

Use supervision to process both your clinical experiences (as sources of tacit learning) and the scientific evidence (as sources of effortful learning that can correct or extend your clinical experience).

Avoid Relying on One Expert

Consider Eraut's (2005) critique of the myth of clinical expertise residing in the head of one clinician. Your work with most patients will be as a member of a multidisciplinary team, which, in turn, is embedded in a health care organization. Consider how your pluralistic formulation can help you liaise within and outside your health care organization to obtain additional input and to advocate for your patient.

Audit Outcomes

Consider regularly auditing the outcomes of patients under your care. Sometimes, the barrier to high-quality care is not your personal uncertainty about what to do but inadequate implementation. Seeing to what extent the best available evidence is or is not applied in a particular setting can reveal opportunities for learning and quality improvement at the personal and the system levels.

Be Critical About the Pedagogical Impact of Clinical Settings

Clinical settings can be "wicked learning environments" (Hertwig et al. 2018; Hogarth et al. 2015) that limit opportunities for repetitive, deliberative practice with feedback and can thus inhibit the development of expertise. For example, your brief interactions with patients in emergency departments or inpatient units may negatively bias your assessment of your own effectiveness: you may interact most with those patients who were least responsive to your interventions at a prior visit. Relatedly, such settings can also make you excessively gloomy about the prognosis of the illnesses you treat because you are exposed to the most treatment-refractory cases. Think of how you can guard against this "clinician's illusion" (Cohen and Cohen 1984). You might balance initial overexposure to acute, tertiary settings by choosing elective rotations in community clinics where you are more likely to see a broad range of illness severity. Continuity clinics early in your training, where you get to follow as outpatients those patients who do not frequently need rehospitalization, can also ameliorate this source of prognostic bias.

Hopefully, this framework will help you embrace and use the uncertainties that are common and indeed constitutive of clinical work and will help you foster your own development toward clinical expertise. Using an explicit approach to uncertainty can also help you in your role as an educator and leader of clinical teams. It can empower those who look to you for guidance to realize that you are comfortable with not having all the answers, can model a response to uncertainty (evidence-based medicine), and can demonstrate your willingness to learn from peers and from the measured outcomes of the patients under your care.

SPECIFIC CHALLENGES AND STRATEGIES

⌘ **I'm afraid to ask for feedback.** It is important to actively seek critical feedback from supervisors and team members, but this is possible only in learning environments where you feel respected and safe to acknowledge ignorance or confusion. If you do not feel this safety in your training program, reach out to trusted faculty or your program director. Incidentally, the practice of psychotherapy provides an excellent example of how to create a safe environment for your patient to learn within, and you should expect the same for yourself during residency training.

⌘ **What if my supervisors disagree?** You may present the same patient to more than one supervisor and receive conflicting recommendations. Consider whether they are disagreeing about how to respond to the same problem or are actually highlighting distinct problems from different perspectives. In either case, their counsel can help you develop your skills in pluralistic case formulation and treatment. A more challenging situation is when a supervisor cites evidence for a recommendation that rests solely on personal experience and is thus difficult to appraise. Even in that situation, you might attempt to understand the theoretical framework from which this recommendation ensues and weigh it against the quality of competing evidence. A corollary is a supervisor who confuses an evidence-based approach with a rigid adherence to published guidelines. Even the most rigorous evidence from a relevant clinical study is never enough and must be integrated with the unique circumstances and preferences of the patient. This inevitably requires judgment. The key here is that you should feel supported in querying, thereby appreciating both the evidentiary basis and the related arguments for multiple or competing courses of action, even as you implement the recommendations of the supervisor who is designated as legally responsible for the care of the patient by the institution. If, however, you feel this approach compromises patient care, you should ask for a confidential consultation with your training director.

⌘ **What if there is little to no published evidence to guide my decision?** This is a situation where you may find the empathic and interpretive aspects of the task-based map useful. In the empathic task, consider what it would be like to be in the patient's mind and try to help your patient articulate their experience. This can increase rapport and focus your therapeutic efforts. In the interpretive task, consider a pluralistic approach to case formulation to guide your comprehensive treatment plan. You will likely need to rely more on the advice of experienced clinicians and, as in all cases, the values and preferences of your patients. In the absence of strong evidence on how to engender the best outcome, you should be even more diligent in regularly assessing your patient's progress and changing course as necessary.

SELF-REFLECTIVE QUESTIONS

1. Have I invited and received useful feedback from my supervisors, allied health professional staff, peers, and patients? What are the barriers to gathering such feedback?
2. Do I have peers and supervisors with whom I feel safe to acknowledge uncertainty? If not, how can I remedy this?
3. How can I audit my impact on patient outcomes?

RESOURCES

Empathic Task

Oyebode F: Sims' Symptoms in the Mind: An Introduction to Descriptive Psychopathology, 6th Edition. New York, Elsevier, 2018. Supplement this resource with textbooks, journals, and accounts in literature, film, and the wider humanities as you encounter specific presentations of illness.

Interpretive Task

The following two manuals provide a practical approach to developing pluralistic formulations of your cases. Use one of these templates, present your cases, get feedback and refine them as you care for patients.

Campbell WH, Rohrbaugh RM: The Biopsychosocial Formulation Manual. New York, Routledge, 2006
Chisolm MS, Lyketsos CG: Systematic Psychiatric Evaluation: A Step-by-Step Guide to Applying the Perspectives of Psychiatry. Baltimore, MD, Johns Hopkins University Press, 2012

Scientific Task

Journal of the American Medical Association: JAMA users' guide to the medical literature. Chicago, IL, American Medical Association, 2022. Available at: https://jamanetwork.com/collections/44069/users-guide-to-the-medical-literature. Accessed September 1, 2021.
Oxford University Center for Evidence-Based Medicine: www.cebm.net
Yale Psychiatry Residency Program: Evidence-based mental health (designed for psychiatrists in training), https://guides.library.yale.edu/EBMH

REFERENCES

Cohen P, Cohen J: The clinician's illusion. Arch Gen Psychiatry 41(12):1178–1182, 1984 6334503

Eraut M: Expert and expertise: meanings and perspectives. Learn Health Soc Care 4(4):173–179, 2005

Eva KW, Regehr G: "I'll never play professional football" and other fallacies of self-assessment. J Contin Educ Health Prof 28(1):14–19, 2008 18366120

Fouad NA, Grus CL, Hatcher RL, et al: Competency benchmarks: a model for understanding and measuring competence in professional psychology across training levels. Train Educ Prof Psychol 3:S5–S26, 2009

Ghaemi SN: The Concepts of Psychiatry: A Pluralistic Approach to the Mind and Mental Illness. Baltimore, MD, Johns Hopkins University Press, 2007

Hertwig R, Hogarth RM, Lejarraga T: Experience and description: exploring two paths to knowledge. Curr Dir Psychol Sci 27(2):123–128, 2018

Hogarth RM, Lejarraga T, Soyer E: The two settings of kind and wicked learning environments. Curr Dir Psychol Sci 24(5):379–385, 2015

Lilienfeld SO, Basterfield C: Reflective practice in clinical psychology: reflections from basic psychological science. Clinical Psychology: Science and Practice 27(4):e12352, 2020

Lynd R: The Pleasures of Ignorance. New York, Scribner's Sons, 1921

McHugh PR, Slavney PR: Mental illness: comprehensive evaluation or checklist? N Engl J Med 366(20):1853–1855, 2012 22591291

Srihari V: Evidence-based medicine in the education of psychiatrists. Acad Psychiatry 32(6):463–469, 2008 19190290

CHAPTER 26

The Resident as Teacher

Erick Hung, M.D.

One of the wonderful traditions in medicine is the emphasis on teaching the next generation of physicians. Teaching and the identity of being an educator are central to our daily work. And teaching, like all professional skills, is a skill that can be refined and improved throughout your career.

As a resident, you play a key teaching role in the clinical learning environment. Residents teach medical students. Senior residents teach less experienced residents. Residents teach across specialties, such as on a consultation-liaison psychiatry service. What makes residency unique is that you are often socially and cognitively more congruent with early learners compared with your senior faculty (Lockspeiser et al. 2008). For example, you may better appreciate the academic demands of a medical student preparing for a shelf examination. Or, in a sea of information, you may be able to identify the appropriate amount of information to teach to a nurse practitioner student learning how to categorize antidepressant medications for the first time.

So what makes for a great resident teacher? Think back to a time when you were most influenced by a teacher. Perhaps you will remember a teacher who was able to make complex concepts simple. Or perhaps a teacher was able to clearly communicate goals and expectations. Or perhaps a teacher was able to make everyone in the room feel included in the conversation, even when the conversation was difficult. Or perhaps a teacher was able to motivate you when you felt like giving up. Regardless of the role model that comes to mind, the takeaway from this chapter is to embody that great teacher. In this chapter we describe two elements that constitute great teaching: 1) creating a positive learning climate and 2) giving effective feedback.

KEY POINTS

- The foundation to all great teaching and learning is creating a positive learning climate. You can create a positive learning climate through stimulation, expectation setting, involvement and inclusion, and a growth mindset.

- Feedback comes in many forms. For residents, one way to give effective feedback is through coaching. The coaching conversation should be anchored to expectations, specific and reinforcing as well as corrective, limited to a few points, and focused on behaviors rather than presumed motivation.

- Use the ADAPT model (ask, discuss, ask, plan together) for giving effective feedback.

CREATING A POSITIVE LEARNING CLIMATE

A positive learning climate is the foundation for effective teaching and learning. Without a positive learning climate, learners don't want to learn, teachers don't want to teach, and opportunities for growth are lost. Although fostering a positive learning climate is a concept everyone can agree on, actually creating a positive learning climate is not easy. So what is a learning climate? The learning climate is the tone or atmosphere of the clinical teaching setting, including whether it is stimulating and whether learners can comfortably identify and address their limitations. A simple way of measuring whether the learning climate is positive (promotes learning) or negative (inhibits learning) is asking and answering the following questions: Does the learner want to be there? Is the learner excited to be with you in clinic or on rounds?

We have all been in situations when we have not been challenged. Things have been too safe. And we have also been in situations when we have felt criticized or attacked. Things have been too stressful. The optimal learning climate is somewhere in between safe and stressful. We will call this the stretch zone. In the stretch zone, learners are neither apathetic nor afraid to speak up. Figure 26–1 provides a helpful diagram in thinking about this zone of optimal learning (Yerkes and Dodson 1908).

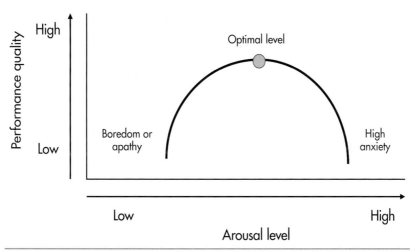

FIGURE 26–1. Yerkes-Dodson law.

Learning and performance are highest when the arousal level is in this stretch zone, this middle ground. Too little arousal fosters boredom, apathy, and minimal learning and performance. Similarly, too much arousal fosters high anxiety and minimal learning and performance. Therefore, it is critical to reflect on how your behaviors can help learners stay in this stretch zone.

The following four strategies can foster a positive learning climate and keep us in the stretch zone: stimulation, setting expectations, involvement and inclusion, and growth mindset. Be aware of the behaviors that promote or distract from these strategies.

Stimulation

You can stimulate learners by showing enthusiasm, being aware of your body language, and providing a conducive physical environment. If you are not enthusiastic, then your learners will not be enthusiastic. Enthusiasm is more than what you say; it is also in your body language. Make eye contact with students. Be mindful of your arm placement and whether it invites asking questions or not asking questions. Open up the space in the room so that everyone can see each other and be part of the conversation.

Setting Expectations

Setting expectations is both an art and a science. Let's first talk about the science. From what cognitive load theory tells us about how people process information, we have to focus our learners on essential information and de-emphasize extraneous information. Extraneous information is a distraction. It is the nonessential elements of a learning setting that misdirect attention and effort. Therefore, setting expectations helps to bring focus. Think about a medical student prerounding to give a presentation on a patient with a complex mental health history for the first time. Having clear expectations about what information the student should look for reduces the extraneous load in the task. Setting expectations helps learners focus on what really matters at their stage of learning.

Now let's talk about the art. What are the expectations you think are important to make clear to your learners? Some categories you might consider are how to approach patient care, communication within the team, the structure of rounds, how to present, reviewing clerkship objectives, feedback, well-being, allyship and upstanding, and evaluation criteria. Once you have considered what expectations to set, then think of how you will set them. Will this be done in person? Will it be delivered by email? Will you have a document for learners to refer to? Do you have different sets of expectations for different sets of learners? Remember, setting expectations is a dynamic process. You should change and revise them over time. Find time to meet with each learner to go over specific expectations of them and also of you. When we are rushed on busy clinical services, it is often tempting to skip expectations. Don't skip them. Setting expectations and carving out sufficient time to review and discuss them are essential to a positive learning climate.

Involvement and Inclusion

You can involve learners by building rapport and being inclusive. *Rapport* is about building positive relationships. Rapport is not just making learners feel warm and fuzzy. It is getting to know each other as people that helps us to work together and communicate. Ways to do this include looking at your learners, encouraging participation, and asking questions. Team icebreakers can be an introductory approach to put this into action. For example, when leading a team, you might ask each learner to share their preferred name (including what that person prefers *not* to be called), pronouns, where one calls home, schooling, career interests, goals, and hobbies. *Inclusion* is making everyone feel valued. The most important word in everyone's vocabulary is their own name. Use names and pronounce them correctly. Elicit learner goals and actually focus on them. Make sure everyone contributes to the conversation.

Growth Mindset

You can foster growth on your team by avoiding ridicule, intimidation, or interruption; acknowledging the learner's situation; and role-modeling your own errors and limitations. The basic gist of a growth mindset is that we are all works in progress. Improving proficiency in almost any skill is possible with deliberate practice, receptivity to feedback, and hard work. If we acknowledge this and focus on consistent improvement as opposed to results, good things will come. Adopting a growth mindset does a few things to help create a positive learning climate. It allows for mistakes. No one is expected to be perfect because we are all a work in progress. This opens people up to feedback because if someone knows it is OK to make mistakes, then that person will be more willing to accept feedback as coaching, as opposed to an indictment of that person's performance. It makes people more willing to disclose mistakes because they know that they will not be judged. This allows for better learning and better patient care.

FEEDBACK

Providing feedback is one of the most valuable activities we do as teachers. Remember, practice does not make perfect. Practice makes permanent. But it is practice *with feedback* that allows us to grow and get better. If feedback is so critical, then why do learners feel that it is done poorly, and why do teachers not like to give it? Well, feedback conversations are tough. As a feedback deliverer, we are sometimes afraid of hurting the learner's feelings. Or we may be afraid of learner retaliation if they are not satisfied with what has been said. Both these aspects potentially get in the way of having authentic feedback conversations. Effective teachers acknowledge these feedback challenges and find a way to have the conversation, often using a relationship-centered, coaching mentality (Sargeant et al. 2015). And speaking of coaching, feedback comes in different types. Feedback can be *appreciation* (e.g., "I see you and value your dedication and effort"). Feedback can be coaching (e.g., "Here are the things you should do to meet your goals"). Feedback can be *evaluation* (e.g., "Here is how you measure up against a particular standard"). All three types of feedback are important (Heen and Stone 2012), but especially for you as a resident; you can be a great coach because you often directly observe students and may be best poised to give specific, change-oriented feedback.

These ten tips can improve your effectiveness in providing meaningful feedback to students (Ende 1983):

1. Make educational goals explicit up front.
2. Maintain a safe and respectful learning environment.
3. Provide feedback before the details are forgotten.
4. Label feedback as feedback at the beginning.

5. Provide feedback that is specific and both reinforcing and corrective.
6. Limit feedback to two to three objectives at a time.
7. Provide feedback on behaviors rather than presumed motivation.
8. Limit feedback to behaviors that are changeable.
9. Include student self-appraisal.
10. End with a mutual action.

How do you put these 10 feedback tips into action? There are several frameworks for engaging in a feedback conversation. A framework *not* to use is the feedback sandwich (positive-negative-positive). We all roll our eyes when we hear feedback shared in this particular format—which, for the cynics in the room, is often heard as inauthentic ego boosting followed by "Tell me what you really want to say." This feedback has been shown to *not* improve performance (Parkes et al. 2013).

An effective feedback model for improving performance is ADAPT (ask, discuss, ask, plan together) (Fainstad et al. 2018). ADAPT is an approach to asking for, receiving, and providing feedback in the clinical learning environment. ADAPT is a theory-informed conversational approach to feedback based on the "ask-tell-ask" discourse pattern that providers often follow with patients. Here is how it works: Prepare for the observed clinical task. Tell your student that this is a two-way conversation rather than a one-way dump of information. Ask your student to reflect on learning goals and communicate those goals to you. Similarly, you can reflect on program and student goals and orient them to your expectations. After observing a clinical task, engage your student in a conversation following the steps described in the following subsections.

Ask

Have the student reflect on the observation. Hopefully, the student will ask for specific feedback. Reflect on the student's readiness for feedback. Ask for the student's thoughts about the observation, with questions such as the following:

- "Are you open to some feedback?"
- "How do you think that went?
- "What went well that you want to keep doing? What didn't go so well that you would like to stop doing or change?"

Discuss

Engage the student in a conversation about the observation. Coach the student on observed, modifiable, specific behaviors related to the task(s). In this discussion, you can put several of the 10 feedback tips into action.

Ask

If the student does not ask for clarification on what was discussed, ask them to clarify points as necessary. You might ask,

- "Does this feedback make sense? Does it resonate?"
- "Do you agree with this feedback? Do you disagree with it?"
- "Have you heard this feedback before? Or is it a surprise to you?"

Plan Together

Plan next steps with the student. As you engage in feedback conversations, remember that we all observe different tasks. What an attending physician observes with a medical student (e.g., presenting on rounds) may be very different from what you observe (e.g., the process in which a medical student gathers information to prepare for rounds). All of these observable tasks are moments for coaching. And it is all right if different parties give feedback on different tasks or even disagree because their points of observation are different. If a medical student is really struggling, it is also helpful to know that no single person on a team should feel the sole responsibility to resolve the issue. Involve your coresidents, attendings, and site directors to help a struggling learner.

In summary, you play a huge role in the clinical learning environment. Creating a positive learning climate and engaging in effective feedback conversations are two important teaching skills to develop in residency. Remember, make teaching fun. Check out the list of teaching resources at the end of this chapter to further develop your skills as an educator. We can all improve our teaching skills so that we can act as role models for and best inspire and coach the next generation of learners.

SPECIFIC CHALLENGES AND STRATEGIES

⌘ **Our team is focused more on the tasks of being in the hospital (or clinic) rather than on the people doing those tasks.** Build team rapport early through team icebreakers. For example, ask team members to share about food that reminds them of home, a current favorite restaurant, the most recent thing they remember cooking, a book or movie they enjoyed recently, a trip they really loved or a trip they are dying to take, or what they would you do with their life if they couldn't be in medicine. Find out about your learners' lives *outside* work. For example, "How was your day off? How did you spend it?" "How are you adjusting to a new city?" "What rotation are you finishing? How was it?" You can also hold space for current events and acknowledge the context of the world we live in. Acknowledging life outside the hospital is important for grounding the team and providing perspective.

⌘ **Some students on the team are not speaking up.** We all want to create inclusive teams and learning environments, yet this is easier said than done. Power and privilege (based on gender, race, ethnicity, sexual orientation, socioeconomic status, ability, and other factors) can influence who on the team speaks first or who on the team speaks at all. As a teacher, listen for such problems and address issues openly when they arise.

⌘ **My students are very performance-driven and focus on the final evaluation and grade.** The performance mindset is difficult to let go of (after all, this mentality likely served us well getting into medical school). You will need to demonstrate a growth mindset in order for others to buy into the concept. Discuss the importance of trying things out and making mistakes. For example, you might ask your learners, "What are you working on?" Tie evaluation to growth rather than performance. Share where you are growing. Provide an example of feedback that changed your practice.

⌘ **I thought I gave specific, constructive feedback, but the student seems to have shut down.** Feedback conversations can be tough at times. But that does not mean that we should shy away from them, especially if they are an opportunity for growth and improvement. Even when delivered well, feedback sometimes (or, dare we say, often) flops because it comes as a surprise to a student (and that takes effort to fully appreciate) or may be perceived as an identity attack and sets off a series of insecurities or doubts. It is for this reason that the second ask in the ADAPT model is so important. It allows for (hopefully) a conversation about the feedback conversation. And it may take multiple conversations. Just remember, all of this is in the spirit of growth, which can be uncomfortable.

SELF-REFLECTIVE QUESTIONS

1. What would be my top three strategies to build rapport with my student or my team?
2. Reflecting on my privilege and power, how do they influence how I foster an inclusive learning environment?
3. Thinking of a time when someone gave me feedback and I rejected it, how can that inform my engagement in a challenging feedback conversation in the future?

RESOURCES

Harvard Macy Institute Program for Educators in Health Professions (interactive virtual course): www.harvardmacy.org/index.php/hmi-courses/educators

Heen S, Stone D: Thanks for the Feedback: The Science and Art of Receiving Feedback Well. New York, Penguin, 2012.

Ramani S, Leinster S: AMEE Guide no. 34: teaching in the clinical environment. Med Teach 30(4):347–364, 2008 18569655

Resident as Teacher Curriculum on MedEdPORTAL: www.mededportal.org/doi/10.15766/mep_2374-8265.10001

Snell L: The resident-as-teacher: it's more than just about student learning. J Grad Med Educ 3(3):440–441, 2011 22942984

REFERENCES

Ende J: Feedback in clinical medical education. JAMA 250(6):777–781, 1983 6876333

Fainstad T, McClintock AA, Van der Ridder MJ, et al: Feedback can be less stressful: medical trainee perceptions of using the prepare to ADAPT (ask-discuss-ask-plan together) framework. Cureus 10(12):e3718, 2018 30906679

Heen S, Stone D: Thanks for the Feedback: The Science and Art of Receiving Feedback Well. New York, Penguin, 2012

Lockspeiser TM, O'Sullivan P, Teherani A, et al: Understanding the experience of being taught by peers: the value of social and cognitive congruence. Adv Health Sci Educ Theory Pract 13(3):361–372, 2008 17124627

Parkes J, Abercrombie S, McCarty T: Feedback sandwiches affect perceptions but not performance. Adv Health Sci Educ Theory Pract 18(3):397–407, 2013 22581568

Sargeant J, Lockyer J, Mann K, et al: Facilitated reflective performance feedback: developing an evidence- and theory-based model that builds relationship, explores reactions and content, and coaches for performance change (R2C2). Acad Med 90(12):1698–1706, 2015 26200584

Yerkes RM, Dodson JD: The relation of strength of stimulus to rapidity of habit-formation. J Comp Neurol Psychol 18(5):459–482, 1908

CHAPTER 27

Navigating Technology in Residency

Patrick McGuire, D.O.

E. Ann Cunningham, D.O.

Technology and its advancements are an integral part of medicine in the twenty-first century. Proper utilization of technology can greatly enhance the residency experience in a multitude of ways, but it is equally important to recognize potential pitfalls to ensure proper, professional, and effective usage.

KEY POINTS

- Technology can make resident life easier with improved workflows, improved organization, and decreased time spent on extraneous tasks.

- Personal learning and didactic experiences can be bolstered using technology.

- Technology tools can be harnessed to improve quality of patient care as well as to enhance communication with the treatment team.

- Use of technology can have drawbacks and pitfalls.

ORGANIZING

The change in responsibility from student to physician is significant, and establishing a foundation of strong organization when starting in residency is critically important. Residency requires adaptation to a smaller, more individualized learning environment compared with medical school. This brings both new opportunities and challenges. Using technology to maximize organization can greatly reduce what otherwise might feel like an overwhelming number of new responsibilities, assignments, meetings, and deadlines.

An online calendar can serve as a lifeline throughout residency. Your calendar should be used to help you and others keep track of your daily schedule and complete customized reminders that suit your needs. Your residency program and/or hospital systems will likely use a single, combined email and calendar application for all employees, such as Google Mail (Google, Mountain View, California) or Microsoft Outlook (Microsoft Corporation, Redmond, Washington). Adopting this application as your primary calendar and email is highly recommended and likely will be a requirement. Others in your organization and residency can use this application to send meeting invitations, deadlines, and other events straight to your calendar, which is a huge convenience. Most major email-calendar applications have the ability to be synchronized, which can be very helpful if you used a different electronic calendar prior to residency. Residents would benefit from adding as much as possible to their calendar prior to the start of each academic year, including rotation schedule, didactics, paid time off, on-call schedule, and other residency events such as grand rounds, journal club, and adviser meetings. Consider adding 1-month reminders for any upcoming presentations and 1-week reminders for smaller to-do items to improve preparation.

Another benefit of the most popular email and calendar applications is the ability to upload files to the cloud so they link to an account instead of being accessible on only one device. Examples of well-known cloud storage programs include Microsoft OneDrive, Google Drive, and Apple iCloud Drive (Apple, Cupertino, California). Applications such as Calendly (Calendly, Atlanta, Georgia) make scheduling meetings more efficient and eliminate users having to email each other repeatedly trying to find a time that works for everyone's schedule. Other applications independent of email, such as Dropbox (Dropbox, San Francisco, California), can be of similar use if preferred. Ultimately, online storage applications can serve as a handy repository of resources such as electronic books, forms, residency manuals, and lectures.

Cloud storage can serve as a file-sharing service as well. You should consider having a cloud storage folder location for yourself, your class, and any other group that may benefit from having a designated space. A file storage service can make materials easy to locate for future use, and residents can pass these materials down to other residents. Some hospitals may have general security restrictions with cloud storage, so you should ask the information technology team for more information on what is permissible with the institution.

Online survey software such as SurveyMonkey (SVMK, San Mateo, California), Qualtrics (Qualtrics, Provo, Utah), and Google Forms are other options for improving both personal and professional organization. For example, Google Forms may be used as an event invitation with RSVP. This platform can be used when planning a residency social event or a personal event using an editable template, or you can create your own invite. Additionally, platforms such as SurveyMonkey can be used to assess residents' interest in various well-being activities or resident retreat activities.

LEARNING AND TEACHING

The primary purpose of a psychiatry residency is to become a competent psychiatrist, and technology can aid you in achieving this goal. Technology can help you quickly find clinical information among countless available academic resources. Each residency and hospital organization will generally provide residents with various information resources. It would benefit you to discover what options are available to you and to access them early in your training. A good starting place would be to contact the hospital librarian and/or navigate the employee services website to identify which journals, books, and other resources are available. Upper-level residents and faculty can often point less experienced residents in the right direction as well. Additionally, librarians who can assist with accessing materials and conducting literature searches are available in some health care settings. The National Neuroscience Curriculum Initiative (www.nncionline.org) and YouTube, which features channels such as Khan Academy (www.youtube.com/user/khanacademy), are great resources for learning but can also be used for your teaching of others. MedEdPORTAL and the American Psychiatric Association (APA) Learning Center have other great teaching and learning resource collections that are contributed to by health care professionals across specialties. Consider Twitter, Slack, and Microsoft OneNote for digital note-taking in didactics.

Technology has changed how education can be delivered. It can improve the quality of teaching as well as increase engagement and participation of an audience (Brooks 2020). You can use technology for teaching points during a team huddle, delivering formal lectures to medical students, speaking at grand rounds, or presenting a patient safety and quality improvement project. Virtual meetings are becoming more reliable, and video platforms such as Cisco Webex (Cisco Systems, San Jose, California), Zoom (Zoom Video Communications, San Jose), and Google Meet combined with increased familiarity among medical providers has led to virtual lectures and meetings becoming a viable alternative to in-person attendance. Residents can join or host meetings or lectures they might not otherwise have been able to attend because of schedule constraints or the need to travel to different sites, all due to the advent of virtual video. Moving forward, the standard likely will become some combination of in-person and virtual attendance (Torous et al. 2018). Virtual meetings can improve the delivery of lectures by allowing screen-sharing options for rapid shifts in content as needed. Additionally, you should consider enhancing presentations by making use of applications that increase engagement. Poll Everywhere (Poll Everywhere, San Francisco) is an easy-to-use audience response system used online or even embedded within a Microsoft PowerPoint lecture for instant audience polling and results. As an example, a resident group studying for the Psychiatric Resident-In-Training Examination (PRITE) used an audience response system that led to improvement in the group studying experience as well as improved scores (Hettinger et al. 2014). Also, many virtual video platforms have a feature allowing users to create small group discussion via breakout rooms as well as other features to increase engagement such as chat features and whiteboard drawing options controlled by presenters.

Technology has also allowed most residency programs to use an electronic evaluation system for rotation evaluations, faculty reviews, program evaluation, didactic feedback, and more. It will be important for you to fill out evaluations and surveys as requested for the program to provide constructive feedback for others and to implement changes within the program. If you would like to receive evaluations for your own teaching, your residency administrator may be a great resource to walk you through how to navigate the particular system used in your program. Many of the systems have the ability to aggregate evaluation forms and comments, so you can track your performance over time.

Another option to your program's evaluation system may be using one of the many different survey software options provided free with basic functionality that is sufficient for most users. Paid versions allow for upgraded customizability if desired. Survey software can be a huge quality-of-life improvement when it comes to giving and asking for feedback by eliminating the distribution and collection of paper forms. Survey software, as noted in the section "Organizing," can also be used to quickly poll residents or faculty on various topics, such as ways to improve residency-led didactics. These services allow the option of anonymous responses in certain cases, which can alleviate potential hesitation about providing honest feedback (Mahoney et al. 2018).

FACILITATING CLINICAL WORK

Technological advancements are readily apparent in patient care, with the broad adoption and continual improvements of electronic medical records (EMRs), telemedicine, and more.

EMRs serve as a location for the entire treatment team to access shared documentation that is updated continuously. EMRs that offer options that help with efficiency during documentation are becoming more common. They are increasingly allowing implementation of customizable forms that can be prefilled or auto-populated. For example, having a prefilled mental status examination form that can be altered and individualized can prevent you from having to free-type and format for every patient encounter. Learning the details and options of an EMR is a worthwhile investment of energy that can lead to greater efficiency in clinical documentation. Residents can spend more time with patients if they are spending less time on documentation, which can lead to improved rapport with patients and overall patient care (Siegler et al. 2015). You would benefit from taking time early on in your residency to learn what options are available to you within the EMR to enhance documentation efficiency. It is important to recognize that the efficiency provided by EMRs can also lead to oversights and errors. For example, a physical examination documented from a previous day may be copied forward efficiently to a new day, but if you did not conduct or update the physical examination on the new day, then you may be documenting care that was not provided, and the examination may no longer be accurate.

Virtual video appointments have been on the rise and will continue to play a large role in health care to improve patient access moving forward. Zoom Medical, Doximity (Doximity, San Francisco), and Cisco Webex are just several examples of Health Insurance Portability and Accountability Act (HIPAA)–compliant virtual appointment applications that have become mainstream. You can use them for quick and easy access to faculty supervision through such features as three-person video and audio calling to bring faculty into patient encounters. Ultimately, patients' options for virtual appointments will vary. Possible methods are audio-only phone calls, a computer with video, and smartphones. You should discuss with your supervising attending physician the options and preferences for patient encounters (see Chapter 18, "Telehealth Services").

Many providers like to suggest apps to patients to help with a variety of symptoms they are experiencing. It is important to recognize that most of the clinical apps available that target patients have not been studied and, therefore, do not demonstrate clear evidence for efficacy. The APA offers guidelines on how to evaluate apps for clinical practice (see "Resources" section).

SPECIFIC CHALLENGES AND STRATEGIES

⌘ **When teaching my medical students online, it is hard to keep them engaged.** It can be challenging to hold the attention of an audience virtually because of such factors as physical distance and nonverbal communication and environmental distractions among individual members of the audience. A general diffusion of responsibility can occur in a large virtual group setting, where it is easier for lack of engagement to go unnoticed. You can set yourself up for success by having a prepared agenda; discussing goals at the start of a presentation; encouraging audience participation; requesting that cameras be turned on; and using tools such as audience polling, breakout rooms, chat, and/or the whiteboard for more active participation.

⌘ **My patient expected a response to their email immediately, but I've been in clinic all day.** The convenience of telemedicine is a major benefit for both residents and patients, but it can also create new gaps and challenges. What may once have been a message left with the front office with the expectation of a call at the end of the day now may be a patient wanting or expecting to connect with a physician more directly through email, an EMR, or other means. It can be helpful to have conversations with patients surrounding healthy professional boundaries and to set clear expectations on when and how both parties will communicate based on the technology that is available to them. In addition, patients often benefit from knowing how to reach someone urgently, if necessary, when you are not immediately available.

⌘ **I am overwhelmed navigating the abundant and ever-changing technology options.** Ultimately, no set of tools and services is unanimously agreed on to be the best. Keeping up to date with technology requires maintaining a pulse on digital advancements, which can be done in a variety of ways, such as online web reviews, social media, and peer listservs. Consider asking mentors, advisers, faculty, and coresidents of all years for their experiences and input. You should also strongly consider using the same tools as colleagues to improve teamwork and collaboration. Tools that are familiar within a program may end up being the most effective, simply because most electronic applications have a learning curve and getting all users up to speed can be a difficult undertaking. It is not uncommon for people to get lost in the details or features of a tool and feel bogged down rather than sped up. Adopting new technology can be challenging, so it is always worth continually evaluating whether a tool is helpful enough to warrant investing the time to learn to use it. It is also important to consider whether the tool is the right fit for the task at hand. For example, although SurveyMonkey has a number of impressive and detailed features such as integration with other applications, advanced result analysis, map data visualizations, and custom logo and color options, it may not be the right tool or approach for quickly polling residents to see what team-building activities they want to do for their retreat. Always make sure the technology is doing what you need it to—sometimes, more is not necessarily better.

SELF-REFLECTIVE QUESTIONS

1. In what aspects of my workflow could I use technology to improve quality or efficiency?
2. Am I using my calendar to maximal capacity to aid in preparedness for residency-related activities?
3. Am I informed of rules, regulations, and policies related to telehealth visits in my state and within my program?

RESOURCES

General Technology Resources

American Medical Association: Digital health implementation playbook series. Chicago, IL, American Medical Association, 2022. Available at: www.ama-assn.org/amaone/ama-digital-health-implementation-playbook. Accessed January 14, 2021.

American Psychiatric Association: App Advisor: www.psychiatry.org/psychiatrists/practice/mental-health-apps. This tool can help you evaluate any app you might be considering. By using this methodology, you will be able to make an educated decision about a particular app and its suitability in the care of your patient.

Shore JH, Yellowlees P, Caudill R, et al: Best practices in videoconferencing-based telemental health April 2018. Telemed J E Health 24(11)827–832, 2018 30358514

Technology Review Sites

American Psychiatric Association: Telepsychiatry blog, www.psychiatry.org/psychiatrists/practice/telepsychiatry/blog
American Psychiatric Association: Telepsychiatry toolkit, www.psychiatry.org/psychiatrists/practice/telepsychiatry/toolkit
CNET: www.cnet.com
TechCrunch: https://techcrunch.com
Torous J, Chan S, Luo J, et al: Clinical Informatics in psychiatric training: preparing today's trainees for the already present future. Acad Psychiatry 42(5):694–697, 2017 29047074
The Verge: www.theverge.com

REFERENCES

Brooks V: COVID-19's effects on emergency psychiatry. Curr Psychiatr 19(7):33–29, 2020
Hettinger A, Spurgeon J, El-Mallakh R, Fitzgerald B: Using Audience Response System technology and PRITE questions to improve psychiatric residents' medical knowledge. Acad Psychiatry 38(2):205–208, 2014 24563242
Mahoney N, Walaszek A, Caudill R: Incorporating technology into the psychiatric residency curriculum. Acad Psychiatry 42(6):847–851, 2018 30203152
Siegler JE, Patel NN, Dine CJ: Prioritizing paperwork over patient care: why can't we do both? J Grad Med Educ 7(1):16–18, 2015 26217415
Torous J, Chan S, Luo J, et al: Clinical informatics in psychiatric training: preparing today's trainees for the already present future. Acad Psychiatry 42(5):694–697, 2018 29047074

CHAPTER 28

Navigating Use of Social Media

Daniel E. Gih, M.D.

Jeana Benton, M.D.

Laura Flores, Ph.D.

Social media is ubiquitous, and its use continues to expand in medicine. Academic health centers, provider organizations, medical journals, research centers, and physicians are increasingly deploying it in numerous ways (Liu et al. 2019). Each rising generation has increased its consumption of social media, with 88% of Americans ages 18–29 years using social media, as compared with 78% of Americans ages 30–49 and 64% of Americans ages 50–64 (Smith and Anderson 2018).

Many residents have social media accounts for personal reasons and may not have considered professional uses. Anecdotal reports suggest that programs and departments with a well-curated online presence receive positive impressions from residency applicants and patients, pointing to the growing impact of social media. The COVID-19 pandemic likely increased the usage of social media in response to the expanded need for virtual connectedness to others. Psychiatry residents can benefit from these platforms professionally. Strategic use of social media can include developing a professional identity, networking, communicating science to the public, augmenting residency education, and assisting with residency recruitment. Advocacy is another major use of social media (see Chapter 32, "Advocacy"). Although social media has many benefits, residents may be hesitant to expand their social media presence because of professionalism concerns and antipsychiatry views.

KEY POINTS

- Each social media platform has a different audience and emphasis in content.

- Thoughtful social media use can benefit the public and residents professionally.

- A strong social media presence can build a professional brand.

- Content may generate negative reactions or attract trolls; however, this can offer an opportunity for reflection and dialogue.

- Residents can address misinformation and normalize conversations around mental health through social media.

PLATFORMS

One of the rewarding aspects of social media is the immediate engagement with other users without hierarchical barriers. All users on a given platform essentially have the same access and controls. Therein lies a democratization of ideas and exchanges. Several social media platforms are commonly used and vary by audience, content, and format, as demonstrated in Table 28–1.

EDUCATION USES

The current generation of residents has become more adept at collating and crowdsourcing educational materials online. Because most residents carry smartphones and other internet-connected devices on their person, closing gaps in clinical knowledge is no longer bound to having to carry printed materials, with their issues of portability and accessibility. High-quality and updated content can be obtained from "tweetorials" on Twitter, podcasts, and YouTube videos (Sterling et al. 2017). Real-time exchanges through social media can broadcast questions globally and highlight the immediacy of inquiries, producing answers within minutes. A framework for social media and networking in psychiatry has

TABLE 28–1. Comparison of popular social media platforms and utility for psychiatrists

Platform	Description	U.S. adults using the platform	Advantages for psychiatry professional use	Disadvantages for psychiatry professional use	Noteworthy statistics
YouTube	• Video-based platform • Allows for subscription to users and channels	73%	• Unlimited video length allows for clear messaging • High user base	• Video content only • Sponsored ads	Many medical societies have a YouTube channel
Facebook	• Free platform supporting text, photos, and video sharing • Can be used by individuals, interest groups, or organizations	69%	• Variability in content • High user base • Ability to designate private groups	• Professionalism boundaries can be harder to maintain because many use the platform for personal life • Algorithmic selection of newsfeed limits control of what users see and can inadvertently increase misinformation	Facebook has the most users globally of any social media platform
LinkedIn	• Free platform supporting text, photos, and video sharing • Can be used for professional and job-sharing information	28%	• Limited to professional interactions • Can be used for job search to connect with employers	• Conversations tend to be slower and more formal	51% of U.S. adults with college degrees use LinkedIn

TABLE 28–1. Comparison of popular social media platforms and utility for psychiatrists (continued)

Platform	Description	U.S. adults using the platform	Advantages for psychiatry professional use	Disadvantages for psychiatry professional use	Noteworthy statistics
Snapchat	• Free image- and video-based platform	25%	• High user base, particularly with millennials and Generation Z • May be used for recruitment purposes and to reach younger populations	• Images and videos expire within 24 hours of posting • Considered an informal platform	65% of Snapchat users are between 18 and 29 years old
Twitter	• Free individual user platform • Allows members to share messages shorter than 280 characters	23%	• Ease of use • Hashtags can be used to index information • Many psychiatric organizations and physicians use the platform to share news and live events	• Fewer Generation Z and millennials on the platform	500 million tweets are sent per day
TikTok	• Free video-based platform • 15-second videos with captioning ability	21%	• Increasingly used in younger populations • Many providers make short informational videos about specific psychiatric illnesses	• Questions of security risks for users • Dangers of diagnosing mental illness using short clips	48% of users are between 18 and 29 years old

Source. Center 2021.

been proposed for training programs that provides suggested competencies for residents (Zalpuri et al. 2018). Furthermore, the sociopolitical movement of Black Lives Matter and other issues related to diversity, equity, and inclusion have added a rich dialogue and perspectives to larger issues in medicine not covered in the traditional medical curriculum. Supplementing clinical training with social media can be an opportunity for growth; however, it is important to note that social media can also be a rich source of misinformation, so careful consideration of use is important.

NETWORKING AND PROFESSIONAL DEVELOPMENT

Social media is a tool for rapidly connecting with others across multiple backgrounds, disciplines, and settings. By using social media, you can find peer support, mentors, and sponsors outside your institution and can encourage collaboration in a less formal venue. Social media also provides visibility to inform others about professional accomplishments alongside personal interests, offering a window into a person's larger professional identity. This is of particular importance for residents from historically marginalized groups because it allows for additional networking opportunities and subsequent professional advancement that may not be accessible within their own institutions or communities. Cultivating a strong social media presence in training can be an asset when transitioning to independent practice because residents will have an early opportunity to demonstrate a professional identity or brand before hitting the job market. Although building a recognizable online presence may offer career building opportunities, it is important to consider potential impacts on the patient-provider relationship. For example, a patient may disagree with certain postings or become uncomfortable with personal knowledge about their provider, leading to a disruption in their care. This is important in psychotherapy relationship building and establishing boundaries, particularly with resident self-disclosure. Professional judgment is important as residents cultivate their online presence.

SCIENCE COMMUNICATION

With access to the internet, patients are becoming more empowered in researching their conditions and treatments. However, they are also finding advice from unreliable or even dangerous sources in addition to stigmatizing views. Therein lies an opportunity for residents to assist with science communication and raise awareness about conditions and effective treatments. Residents likely have more education and training in psychiatry than a layperson and most individuals in medicine. Explaining the science behind the disease and treatment processes may be a reinforcing step in helping patients to retain information and an opportunity to practice clear communication. Likewise, providing a summary or commentary on a research article or current event may be valued by the public. Establishing a regular line of content generalized from daily clinical care duties can potentially dispel myths about psychiatry and decrease stigma.

RESIDENT RECRUITMENT USES

The recent COVID-19 pandemic has been a motivator for programs to expand their presence online as students were denied the opportunity to visit or do rotations at programs outside their home institution. In the decade before the pandemic, there was a rapid opening of new training programs accredited by the Accreditation Council for Graduate Medical Education. Currently, there are more than 280 psychiatry training programs, and each program is likely seeking an opportunity to differentiate and showcase itself to applicants.

Newer programs are likely at a competitive disadvantage over more established ones. The latter group may have a developed word-of-mouth reputation built over several decades. Social media may help to level the playing field, and residents can play a major role in attracting excellent applicants and future colleagues. Moreover, social media is typically a budget-neutral marketing option that can help connect potential trainees.

Students want nuanced information to help determine where to apply and whether a potential program will be a good fit. Characteristics such as resident cohesion, the availability of mentoring, community outreach, and social interaction among residents and faculty can be difficult to ascertain. Social media provides an accessible forum to advertise the unique aspects of a program and is likely more impactful than a static or institutional website. It is also an opportunity to describe the "personality" of a program. Depending on how social media is managed for the training program, a resident can submit content to the department or training account about their rotations, teaching pearls, quality of life, and recreational opportunities in the area. There may also be opportunities to contribute to a broader institutional account, which can expand the program's reach online. As a resident, sharing lived experience can shape the perceptions of the program and provide direct and specific information for prospective residents. These are often curated with the help of the program director, so complementary information provided by current residents in other ways remains useful.

PITFALLS

At least a decade ago, most employers were already using Facebook, Instagram, or Twitter to supplement information on job candidates (Bosslet 2011). Demonstration of a long-standing interest or expertise in a particular area could be an asset. Overly casual use of social media by physicians is common and potentially problematic (Lefebvre et al. 2016). Often, there is a blurring of professional and personal content and subsequent exchanges by the creator and the reader. Content can be a liability. Embarrassing, insensitive, or derogatory material or pictures may cause applicants in competitive positions to be eliminated from consideration or to have their employment be terminated. Therefore, residents should monitor their use of and interactions on social media. No matter the disclaimers posted on account biographies, viewers may associate your content with the training program and institution you belong to, which could damage your professional reputation and violate your employer's social media policies. As such, posts should be constructed to avoid negative consequences. Finally, misinterpretation or misappropriation of content happens, and as the creator, you may receive a volley of undesirable responses, including online trolling and leadership concerns about you as a resident. You should be prepared for these consequences. These types of online interactions can be overwhelming, and management of negative consequences might involve your training program's leadership, legal and risk management departments, and the Graduate Medical Education office in potential responses and solutions.

Permanency is best summed up as "a misstep online has the potential to spread globally and to be preserved indefinitely" (Daviss et al. 2015, p. 170). All content online can be archived, and past postings can be easily disseminated long after they are deleted by the original poster. Tools such as the Internet Archive website and screenshots can be potent reminders of missteps. Trainees can protect themselves by revisiting the THINK acronym before they post: is the post true, helpful, inspiring, necessary, and/or kind? (see "Specific Challenges and Strategies" at the end of the chapter).

Protecting information and privacy is an additional consideration. It is never appropriate to post direct or ancillary information that could violate patient privacy laws. Posting of clinical content or cases can inadvertently provide identifiers (e.g., date, clinical setting) that could be traced back to specific patient encounters, and care should be taken to avoid such details. Likewise, anonymity, particularly for physicians, is not guaranteed. Most physicians can be found online with public details about their professional credentials and clinical work affiliations. Although personal information and disclosures can provide moments of vulnerability and authenticity to highlight points, privacy may not be regained once lost. Having separate social media accounts for personal and professional use and corresponding content is advisable. Many trainees use accounts without using their real names ("anon") as an additional layer of separation and privacy, but this is not entirely foolproof.

Residents should also be familiar with the "Goldwater Rule," which is found in section 7 of the American Psychiatric Association's Principles of Medical Ethics (American Psychiatric Association 2010; Kroll and Pouncey 2016). The rule declares it unethical for psychiatrists to give a professional diagnosis about a public figure whom they have not personally examined. A professional opinion given publicly without consent from the individual violates confidentiality. Similarly, the temptation to provide any direct medical advice to individuals seeking care outside a formal medical treatment setting should be avoided.

Any questions about professionalism standards and how to best represent oneself and the medical profession may be rich opportunities to engage in dialogue with training leadership and colleagues.

SPECIFIC CHALLENGES AND STRATEGIES

⌘ **Should I be concerned about having a large number of followers?** Follower count is a rough proxy for influence. Having a larger audience can increase opportunities for collaboration and expand the reach of content beyond traditional colleagues and into the public. The higher-level aim should be connection opportunity. This process starts with creating an inviting profile. Create your account using a clear username and a professional picture and follow interest-matching accounts and users. Replying with thoughtful content to others' posts, reposting or amplifying helpful posts, and creating regular individual content will grow your audience.

⌘ **I'm worried about what content to include in my social media posts for fear of negative feedback.** Prior to posting, recall the THINK acronym in considering the wide ways content may be interpreted. T—is it true? H—is it helpful? I—is it inspiring? N—is it necessary? K—is it kind? Staying in the position of positivity, using the evidence base, and being patient centered will probably never be disadvantageous. Conversely, weaponizing shame and guilt are unlikely to win people over.

⌘ **A user is making antagonizing remarks toward me about a posting and I'm not sure how to respond.** Take the high road. The best course is to ignore and to not engage in online discussions that are unlikely to produce a respectful resolution. Many platforms offer such options as blocking and muting. Blocking will prevent you from seeing the user's content and vice versa. Note that Twitter will notify the other account that it has been blocked, which might further fuel that person's actions toward you. Muting will cause the platform to not notify you of any content and responses the user makes but does allow you to manually search for their postings. For the public, much of the information about psychiatry is stigmatizing and misinformed, and residents have an opportunity to use social media to help decrease stigma and normalize dialogue around mental illness.

SELF-REFLECTIVE QUESTIONS

1. What are three main goals for the social media account I am using?
2. Who would I like to be connected to and what audience do I seek?
3. What boundaries will I set for my social media account (e.g., posting non-work-related personal facts?)

RESOURCES

Farnan JM, Snyder Sulmasy L, Worster BK, et al: Online medical professionalism: patient and public relationships: policy statement from the American College of Physicians and the Federation of State Medical Boards. Ann Intern Med 158(8):620–627, 2013 23579867
Stukus DR, Patrick MD, Nuss KE: Social Media for Medical Professionals: Strategies for Successfully Engaging in an Online World. Cham, Switzerland, Springer, 2019

REFERENCES

American Psychiatric Association: The Principles of Medical Ethics: With Annotations Especially Applicable to Psychiatry. Washington, DC, American Psychiatric Association, 2010. Available at: www.psychiatry.org/File%20Library/Psychiatrists/Practice/Ethics/principles-medical-ethics.pdf. Accessed October 13, 2022.
Bosslet GT: Commentary: the good, the bad, and the ugly of social media. Acad Emerg Med 18(11):1221–1222, 2011 22092907
Daviss S, Hanson A, Miller D: My three shrinks: personal stories of social media exploration. Int Rev Psychiatry 27(2):167–173, 2015 25906990

Kroll J, Pouncey C: The ethics of APA's Goldwater Rule. J Am Acad Psychiatry Law 44(2):226–235, 2016 27236179

Lefebvre C, Mesner J, Stopyra J, et al: Social media in professional medicine: new resident perceptions and practices. J Med Internet Res 18(6):e119, 2016 27283846

Liu HY, Beresin EV, Chisolm MS: Social media skills for professional development in psychiatry and medicine. Psychiatr Clin North Am 42(3):483–492, 2019 31358127

Pew Research Center: Social Media Fact Sheet. Washington, DC, Pew Research Center, 2021. Available at: www.pewresearch.org/internet/fact-sheet/social-media. Accessed October 4, 2022.

Smith A, Anderson M: Social media use in 2018: demographics and statistics. Washington, DC, Pew Research Center, March 2018. Available at: www.pewresearch.org/internet/2018/03/01/social-media-use-in-2018. Accessed August 31, 2021.

Sterling M, Leung P, Wright D, et al: The use of social media in graduate medical education: a systematic review. Acad Med 92(7):1043–1056, 2017 28225466

Zalpuri I, Liu HY, Stubbe D, et al: Social media and networking competencies for psychiatric education: skills, teaching methods, and implications. Acad Psychiatry 42(6):808–817, 2018 30284148

CHAPTER 29

Leadership

Michael DeGroot, M.D.
Katharine J. Nelson, M.D.

You are committed to making things better for people. You live this value every day in your work to care for your patients. If you are motivated to expand the impact of your caring through taking part in strategies and initiatives that benefit others beyond the patient sitting in front of you, you are probably a leader (whether you identify with this label or not). In this chapter you will learn how the benefits of leadership in psychiatry extend far beyond you, the leader, having an impact on the systems in which you practice and even on the outcomes of your patients. You will learn how to recognize skills that you have already acquired, on which you currently rely in your day-to-day work as a psychiatrist, to become an effective leader. And you will be provided a road map to cultivate these skills and aptitudes to pursue meaningful and specific leadership roles within your residency program and beyond.

As the adage goes, great leaders are made, not born. It is developmentally appropriate if you do not yet have full confidence in your leadership bona fides at this point in your career. Leadership skills, like all skills in medicine, can be learned and polished. The process of becoming an effective physician leader will span the duration of your residency and continue long into your professional career.

KEY POINTS

- The pursuit of leadership can add meaning to your career, promote agency and autonomy, optimize the efficiency and effectiveness of the setting in which you practice, and improve the quality of care your patients receive.

- Important traits and skills of successful leaders (e.g., emotional intelligence, empathy, the capacity to validate others) also happen to be vital for effective psychiatrists.

- When pursuing a leadership position as a psychiatry resident, consider your leadership niche and the scope of your goals.

- Effective leaders set good boundaries, rely on the advice and guidance of mentors, and know when and from whom to seek help.

WHY LEADERSHIP?

Whether or not you plan to pursue a formal leadership position as a psychiatry resident or in your work as an attending physician, leadership aptitude is a requisite skill for effective psychiatrists because of the multidisciplinary nature of the specialty. There will be times in residency and beyond when peers, nurses, social workers, trainees, or other members of a treatment team depend on you to make a difficult clinical decision. This is leadership. But beyond functioning effectively in your role as a physician leader on a multidisciplinary team, the pursuit of a formal leadership position can improve the personal satisfaction of your work in a myriad of ways. From reducing burnout to improving patient outcomes, physician leaders have the agency to improve the quality of their lives while having meaningful impacts on those of the patients for whom they care.

Physician leadership and the opportunity to influence or make decisions in your professional environment counteract feelings of loss of control and autonomy that have been documented to contribute significantly to physician burnout (West et al. 2018). Undoubtedly, there have been times in your training when you have recognized a systems failure in the hospital where you were practicing. Or perhaps you identified an opportunity to improve the educational experience for yourself and your peers in your residency training program. It is equally likely that you may have felt insufficiently empowered to speak up in these instances. This is a recipe for frustration and burnout. Now imagine being given the platform to share your ideas in a formal setting such as a residency curriculum committee or on a quality improvement project team. Leadership roles afford you the opportunity to find your voice and to effect change, enhancing your autonomy and professional satisfaction.

In addition, one study found that hospitals with physician leadership had higher *U.S. News and World Report* patient quality ratings across all specialties than did hospitals with nonphysician leaders (Tasi et al. 2019). Too often in medicine, the priorities of physicians misalign with those of hospital administration. This research suggests that the recruitment of physician leaders should be a shared goal of both medical practitioners and hospital administrators, making you as the resident-leader a more attractive professional candidate.

PSYCHIATRISTS ARE PRIMED FOR LEADERSHIP

The wonderful (and perhaps reassuring) thing about endeavoring to become a leader in psychiatry is that there is no standard leadership archetype. The diversity of psychiatric leaders is as broad as the specialty itself. You already may have the qualities necessary for strong leadership.

Emotional Intelligence

There does appear to be a foundational characteristic shared by many successful leaders (and effective psychiatrists): emotional intelligence. One study of nearly 200 large global companies found that 90% of the differences between outstanding employees and average ones could be attributed to emotional intelligence (Goleman 1998). Therefore, whether you tend toward introversion or extroversion, whether you love public speaking or your palms grow sweaty with the thought, you can lean on the emotional intelligence you already possess (and use daily to connect with your patients) to build your foundation as a psychiatric leader.

Validation

The practice of identifying the legitimate perspectives of another individual and accurately demonstrating an understanding of this experience is a technique called validation. Validation in psychiatry refers to the often-difficult process of setting aside one's initial reaction to a challenging interpersonal situation while affirming the valid aspects of another person's perspective (Linehan 1993). Psychiatrists are often in the position of fielding the concerns, hopes, needs, and wants of others. Such requests might come from the patients you treat or a colleague requesting a consultation. It can be tempting to offer solutions or perspectives to resolve these requests outright. Psychiatrists are, in fact, frequently rewarded and conditioned to offer solutions and advice in such matters. However, dilemmas will arise that are not easily solved with a prescription, research article, protocol, or procedure. In these cases, the most effective intervention is often the validation of the experiences of others. Similarly, in a leadership role, this attunement to the unique perspectives of other team members will demonstrate empathic leadership and enhance cohesion and collaboration.

A ROAD MAP TO LEADERSHIP IN RESIDENCY AND BEYOND

You may now have a better understanding of how the pursuit of leadership opportunities can enhance your residency experience. You may even recognize a few personal attributes that could make you an effective resident leader. But if the concept of leadership still feels a bit nebulous, take the following key steps in order to set more concrete leadership goals: identify your leadership niche, find a mentor, identify leadership development opportunities, and identify leadership opportunities.

Identify Your Leadership Niche

Perhaps you are passionate about psychiatric research or clinical education. Maybe your interests lie more at the systems level of psychiatric care, or you are committed to social justice, equity, and diversity in psychiatry. In order to embark on your leadership journey, you must first identify a niche that motivates you to lead.

Find a Mentor

Once you have identified an area you can champion, find a mentor within your niche capable of guiding you in your pursuits (see Chapter 33, "Mentorship and Sponsorship"). Your mentor can then help you identify the scope of your leadership goals. For example, do you wish to be a leader within your residency, within the hospital system where you practice, among the psychiatric specialty, or in the field of medicine in general? Your residency training director; clinical supervisor; resident colleagues; and/or local, state, or national psychiatry organizations might be able to connect you with a mentor. If your leadership aspirations lie more in the research domain, seek out a mentor who is also a primary investigator in a research study or in studies at your institution.

Identify Leadership Development Opportunities

Once you have found your leadership niche and a mentor to guide you, you might consider seeking out leadership training opportunities within your residency and beyond if you are not comfortable jumping directly into a leadership position. Leadership development opportunities can help you acquire valuable skills, fine-tune your personal leadership style, and set leadership goals for your residency tenure and eventual career. Training is not necessarily required at this stage because experience is invaluable. Some leadership development opportunities include the following:

- Resident leadership didactics and/or tracks within a psychiatry residency program
- Resident leadership programs within local graduate medical education committees
- Resident leadership programs within hospitals or schools of medicine
- Resident leadership programs at the national level (see "Resources" section at the end of the chapter)

Identify Leadership Opportunities

Many leadership opportunities will be available to you within your residency training program or the hospital system where you practice. Some universal opportunities that exist across training programs include chairing a quality improvement project or assisting in the development of the resident or medical student didactic curriculum. You might also consider volunteering for a committee position within your training program or department or at an institutional level. Many residency training programs actively encourage resident participation in such committees. For a less formal leadership opportunity in research, consider inviting a clinical mentor to collaborate on a case report or brief report for publication in a peer-reviewed journal (see Chapter 31, "Publishing"). One prototypical leadership role is the chief resident position. If becoming chief resident is a potential leadership goal for you, talk to your current chief resident(s) to inquire about their path to the position.

Opportunities to participate in leadership or to be paired with a leadership mentor at the national level are also available. The American Psychiatric Association (APA) offers several opportunities:

- Local APA district branch or state association:
  - Become a resident representative in the local chapter (if available)
  - Attend local or state meetings
  - Become involved in a committee or task force
- National APA level:
  - Apply to become an APA resident-fellow member trustee (available to all psychiatry residents who are APA members; trustees

serve a 2-year term on the APA Board of Trustees, the governing body of the APA)

- Join the Assembly Committee of Area Resident-Fellow Members (confers APA Assembly representation to psychiatry residents in order to include the resident perspective on APA actions or proposed actions with the potential to affect resident-fellow members; residents are chosen for participation by their APA district branches or state associations)
- Apply for an APA fellowship or award

In addition, national fellowships and awards are yet another way for residents to pursue leadership, mentorship, and networking opportunities. Many organizations offer fellowships and awards to trainees to foster their growth as psychiatric leaders (Table 29–1). These programs are typically tailored toward a specific subpopulation of physician leaders such as underrepresented minorities, women in psychiatry, psychiatric researchers, or emerging leaders in psychiatric education. Check to see if any of the fellowships or awards align with your leadership aspirations before you consider applying. These programs often provide mentorship, the opportunity to serve on a national committee, and an invitation to attend an annual meeting at reduced or no cost to the fellow. Participation in national fellowships also affords you the opportunity to network with a diverse group of co-fellow peers from outside your home residency program who are also likely to be emerging leaders in your field. If you are interested in applying for one of the fellowships or awards, reach out to your program director or mentor and request that they nominate you. Also, consider contacting residents who are current or former fellows or award recipients for more information.

SPECIFIC CHALLENGES AND STRATEGIES

⌘ **It's up to me as a leader to fix all of these problems *immediately*.** Frequently, leaders fall into the trap of the "Don't just sit there, do something!" mantra. Leadership is a process. And being a leader does not imply that you could or should have all of the answers right off the bat. Take time to put sufficient thought into a leadership challenge and incorporate the insight of mentors and peers before taking action. You may find yourself better served by the alternative mantra "Don't just do something, sit there!"

⌘ **I don't look like a lot of the leaders in psychiatry at my training site.** As undergraduate and graduate medical training programs contin-

TABLE 29–1. Fellowships and awards from national psychiatry organizations

Topic	Name	Organization	Link
Addiction	MERF scholarship	Medical Education and Research Foundation for the Treatment of Addiction	www.merfweb.org
	Ruth Fox Endowment Memorial Scholarship	American Society of Addiction Medicine	www.asam.org/membership/asam-award-programs/ruth-fox-endowment-fund
	Sheldon Miller Early Career Award	American Academy of Addiction Psychiatry	www.aaap.org/training-events/annual-meeting/2020-annual-meeting/schedule-of-events/awards/conference-awardees
Child and adolescent psychiatry	AACAP Educational Outreach Program for Child and Adolescent Residents	American Academy of Child and Adolescent Psychiatry	www.aacap.org/aacap/Awards/Resident_and_ECP_Awards/AACAP_Educational_Outreach_Program_for_CAP_Residents.aspx
	Child and Adolescent Psychiatry Fellowship	American Psychiatric Association (APA)	www.psychiatry.org/residents-medical-students/residents/fellowships/available-apa-apaf-fellowships/child-and-adolescent-psychiatry-fellowship
	Peter Henderson M.D. Memorial Award	American Association of Directors of Psychiatric Residency Training	www.aadprt.org/annual-meeting/awards-fellowships/award-detail?awardsid=72
Education	Gold Foundation Humanism and Excellence in Teaching Award	Association of American Medical Colleges	www.gold-foundation.org/programs/humanism-and-excellence-in-teaching-award

TABLE 29–1. Fellowships and awards from national psychiatry organizations (continued)

Topic	Name	Organization	Link
	George Ginsberg Fellowship	American Association of Directors of Psychiatric Residency Training	www.aadprt.org/annual-meeting/awards-fellowships/award-detail?awardsid=79
	NNCI Scholar	National Neuroscience Curriculum Initiative	https://nncionline.org/nnci-ambassadors
	PRITE Fellowship	American College of Psychiatrists	www.acpsych.org/resident-fellowships/the-prite-fellowship-program
	Resident Psychiatric Educator Award	Association for Academic Psychiatry	www.academicpsychiatry.org/resident-psychiatric-educator-award
Forensic psychiatry	Edwin Valdiserri Correctional Public Psychiatry Fellowship	APA	www.psychiatry.org/residents-medical-students/residents/fellowships/available-apa-apaf-fellowships/edwin-valdiserri-correctional-psychiatry-fellowship
	Douglas Mossman Research Award	Midwest Chapter of American Academy of Psychiatry and the Law	https://midwestaapl.org/the-douglas-mossman-research-award
	Rappeport Fellowship	American Academy of Psychiatry and the Law	www.aapl.org/rappeport-fellowship
Geriatrics	AAGP Scholars Program	American Association for Geriatric Psychiatry	www.aagponline.org/index.php?src=gendocs&ref=AAGPScholarProgram
International health	Ellen Violett International Fellowship	Association of Women Psychiatrists	https://associationofwomenpsychiatrists.com/awards

TABLE 29–I. Fellowships and awards from national psychiatry organizations *(continued)*

Topic	Name	Organization	Link
Leadership	World Psychiatric Association Fellowship	World Psychiatric Association	https://wcp-congress.com/fellowships
	Jeanne Spurlock, M.D. Minority Fellowship Achievement Award	APA	www.psychiatry.org/psychiatrists/awards-leadership-opportunities/awards/spurlock-minority-fellowship-achievement-award
	AWP Fellowship	Association of Women Psychiatrists	https://associationofwomenpsychiatrists.com/awards
	Commonwealth Fund Fellowship in Minority Health Policy at Harvard University	Harvard University	https://cff.hms.harvard.edu
	Diversity Leadership Fellowship	APA	www.psychiatry.org/residents-medical-students/residents/fellowships/available-apa-apaf-fellowships/diversity-leadership-fellowship
	GAP Fellowship	Group for the Advancement of Psychiatry	www.ourgap.org/gap-fellowship
	Organization of Resident Representatives at the Association of American Medical Colleges	American Association of American Medical Colleges	www.aamc.org/professional-development/affinity-groups/orr

TABLE 29–1. Fellowships and awards from national psychiatry organizations (continued)

Topic	Name	Organization	Link
	Resident Recognition Award	APA	www.psychiatry.org/psychiatrists/awards-leadership-opportunities/awards/resident-recognition-award
Philosophy	Karl Jaspers Award	Association for the Advancement of Philosophy and Psychiatry	https://aapp.press.jhu.edu/jaspers
Psychotherapy	APsaA Fellowship	American Psychoanalytic Association	https://apsa.org/fellowship
	Austen Riggs Award for Excellence in Psychotherapy	Austen Riggs Center	www.austenriggs.org/education-research/training
	The Group Foundation Scholarship Program (including the Barbara and Albert Dazzo Scholarship and Robert E. White, M.D., and Sara Jane White, Ph.D., Scholarship Fund)	American Group Psychotherapy Association	https://agpa.org/foundation/scholarships
	Scott Schwartz Award	American Academy of Psychodynamic Psychiatry and Psychoanalysis	www.aapdp.org/education/scott-schwartz-award
	Southwestern Group Psychotherapy Scholarship	American Group Psychotherapy Association	https://agpa.org/Foundation/scholarships/scholarship-list

TABLE 29–1. Fellowships and awards from national psychiatry organizations (*continued*)

Topic	Name	Organization	Link
Public psychiatry	Public Psychiatry Fellowship	APA	www.psychiatry.org/residents-medical-students/residents/fellowships/available-apa-apaf-fellowships/public-psychiatry-fellowship
	SAMHSA Minority Fellowship	APA and Substance Abuse and Mental Health Services Administration	www.psychiatry.org/residents-medical-students/residents/fellowships/available-apa-apaf-fellowships/samhsa-minority-fellowship
Recognition for overall excellence	AWP Fellowship	Association of Women Psychiatrists	https://associationofwomenpsychiatrists.com/awards
	Indo-American Psychiatric Association Outstanding Resident Award	Indo-American Psychiatric Association	myiapa.org/announcements/awards/
	Laughlin Fellowship	American College of Psychiatrists	www.acpsych.org/resident-fellowships/the-laughlin-fellowship-program
	Nyapati Rao and Francis Lu International Medical Graduate (IMG) Fellowship	American Association of Directors of Psychiatric Residency Training	www.aadprt.org/annual-meeting/awards-fellowships/award-detail?awardsid=78
Research	APA Research Colloquium for Junior Psychiatrists	APA	www.psychiatry.org/psychiatrists/practice/research/research-colloquium/u-s-and-canada-application

TABLE 29–1. Fellowships and awards from national psychiatry organizations *(continued)*

Topic	Name	Organization	Link
	Clinical Trials in Psychopharmacology	American Society of Clinical Psychopharmacology	https://ascpp.org
	Klingenstein Third Generation Fellowship	Kathleen Pomerantz at Klingenstein Foundation	klingenstein.org/klingenstein-third-generation-foundation/fellowship-program/applying
	NIMH Outstanding Resident Award Program	National Institute of Mental Health	www.nimh.nih.gov/research/research-conducted-at-nimh/scientific-director/office-of-fellowship-and-training/outstanding-resident-award-program
	Nina Schooler Early Career Research Award	American Society of Clinical Psychopharmacology	https://ascpp.org/resources/httpswww-ascpp-orgresourcesnina-schooler-early-career-research-awardpreviewtruepreview_id2345preview_noncef09c5c12e5
	Outstanding Resident Award Program	National Institute of Mental Health	www.nimh.nih.gov/research/research-conducted-at-nimh/scientific-director/office-of-fellowship-and-training/outstanding-resident-award-program
	Psychiatric Research Fellowship	APA and APA Foundation	www.psychiatry.org/residents-medical-students/residents/fellowships/available-apa-apaf-fellowships/psychiatric-research-fellowship
	Science and SciLifeLab Prize for Young Scientists	SciLifeLab	https://scienceprize.scilifelab.se

TABLE 29–1. Fellowships and awards from national psychiatry organizations *(continued)*

Topic	Name	Organization	Link
	Travel Fellowship Award—Early Career Investigator—Domestic	Society of Biological Psychiatry	https://sobp.org/travel-fellowship-award-early-career-investigator-domestic
Women's health	Alexandra and Martin Symonds Foundation Fellowship	Association of Women Psychiatrists	https://associationofwomenpsychiatrists.com/awards

ue to recognize and address the importance of diversity, cultural sensitivity, and inclusion among their population of medical trainees, there is growing awareness that comparable diversity among physician leadership is lagging. Do not let this discourage you. The medical students and residents of today, emerging from increasingly diverse socioeconomic, cultural, and racial backgrounds, will be the psychiatric leaders of tomorrow. Work with your training program or medical school to find a diversity champion who can serve as a mentor or ally.

⌘ **I am too exhausted to take on anything else in addition to my primary duties as a resident.** The rigorous academic and clinical demands of residency can make the idea of taking on additional roles or responsibilities seem overwhelming. Take inventory of your schedule and preexisting commitments before taking on new leadership tasks. Don't be afraid to talk to your residency program director or others in your training program about support or protected time that may be required to pursue leadership opportunities. Frequently, residency training programs are happy to accommodate such endeavors.

⌘ **I'm not really leadership material.** Feelings of self-doubt and imposter syndrome hinder the pursuit of leadership and are more common early in your career and during transitional phases such as residency training. Be aware that imposter syndrome disproportionately affects marginalized and minoritized trainees. Take inventory of all the accomplishments that you have made to this point in your career. Don't let perfectionism lead to paralysis. Try to separate feelings from facts. And if all else fails, rely on your mentor. Remember that although you are new to the specialty of psychiatry and the field of medicine in general, all individuals currently in medical leadership one day stood where you stand now.

SELF-REFLECTIVE QUESTIONS

1. How might the pursuit of leadership opportunities enhance my personal residency experience and improve the setting in which I work?
2. Thinking of a time when I used my emotional intelligence to help a patient or colleague through validation, can I envision using this strategy in a leadership role?
3. When thinking about my leadership niche and the scope of my goals, can I identify three potential mentors who could support me in my journey?

RESOURCES

Academic Medicine Leadership

KD Coach blog: https://kemidoll.com/blog. Dr. Kemi Doll is a physician who writes a blog for women of color in academic medicine.

Leadership Training

Karpinski J, Samson L, Moreau K: Residents as leaders: a comprehensive guide to establishing a leadership development program for postgraduate trainees. MedEdPORTAL, August 19, 2015. Available at: www.mededportal.org/doi/10.15766/mep_2374-8265.10168. Accessed September 27, 2021.

Rotenstein LS, Sadun R, Jena AB: Why doctors need leadership training. Harvard Business Review, October 17, 2018. Available at: hbr.org/2018/10/why-doctors-need-leadership-training. Accessed September 27, 2021.

National Resident Leadership Programs and Resources

CHIEF RESIDENTS

Chief resident program sessions at the Annual Meeting, American Psychiatric Association: www.psychiatry.org/psychiatrists/meetings/annual-meeting

Accreditation Council on Graduate Medical Education Leadership Skills Training Program for Chief Residents: www.acgme.org/Meetings-and-Educational-Activities/Other-Educational-Activities/Courses-and-Workshops/Leadership-Skills-Training-Program-for-Chief-Residents

Annual Chief Residents Leadership Conference (formerly known as the Tarrytown Meeting): www.einsteinmed.edu/departments/psychiatry-behavioral-sciences/psychiatry.aspx?id=32653

Chief resident leadership curriculum: https://libraryinfo.bhs.org/CRleadership_curriculum. Website with learning objectives and resources developed by the Baystate Medical Center.

LEADERSHIP IN ACADEMIC RESEARCH

Career Development Institute for Psychiatry (CDI): www.cdi.pitt.edu. A multifaceted longitudinal training experience for young psychiatrists and Ph.D. researchers interested in successful research careers in academic psychiatry. Participants work with senior faculty and mentors from the Departments of Psychiatry of the University of Pittsburgh and Stanford University, representatives from the National Institute of Mental Health, and past CDI participants.

REFERENCES

Goleman D: What makes a leader? Harv Bus Rev 76(6):93–102, 1998 10187249

Linehan MM: Cognitive-Behavioral Treatment of Borderline Personality Disorder. New York, Guilford, 1993

Tasi MC, Keswani A, Bozic KJ: Does physician leadership affect hospital quality, operational efficiency, and financial performance? Health Care Manage Rev 44(3):256–262, 2019 28700509

West CP, Dyrbye LN, Shanafelt TD: Physician burnout: contributors, consequences and solutions. J Intern Med 283(6):516–529, 2018 29505159

CHAPTER 30

Scholarship

Melissa R. Arbuckle, M.D., Ph.D.
James I. Rim, J.D., M.D.
Deborah L. Cabaniss, M.D.

According to the Accreditation Council for Graduate Medical Education (2020), all residents and faculty must participate in scholarship. Although this might sound intimidating if you have limited research experience, engaging in scholarship is both easier to implement than you might think and of significant benefit to you as a trainee. There are numerous types of scholarship and many ways that you can get involved. Engaging in scholarship is also an important way for you to feel energized and connected to a larger network of colleagues. It can enhance the residency training experience by providing a deep dive into a particular area of interest, connecting you to meaning in your work (an important strategy for preventing burnout) (Wei et al. 2020) and creating an opportunity to develop an area of expertise. In this chapter we describe various types of scholarship, with specific examples, and provide practical tips for engaging in scholarship and strategies for tackling some of the challenges you might face along the way.

KEY POINTS

- Scholarship is the acquisition and sharing of knowledge through research, synthesis, practice, and teaching.

- Many kinds of scholarship that can easily connect to your interests are available, and engaging in scholarship during residency is more feasible than you might think.

- Engaging in scholarship enhances the experience of residency training in psychiatry by providing a deep dive into a particular area of interest and a model for engaging with the psychiatric community.

- Working with a mentor and a team can help you to overcome many perceived challenges to pursuing scholarship.

WHAT IS SCHOLARSHIP?

Scholarship is the acquisition and sharing of knowledge through research, synthesis, practice, and teaching (Boyer 1990). Traditional views of scholarship generally refer to the *scholarship of discovery*, or the acquisition of knowledge through basic research. However, there has been increasing recognition of a broader range of scholarship (Figure 30–1).

- The *scholarship of integration* involves making connections across disciplines. This type of scholarship includes literature reviews and meta-analyses (or comparing results across studies). Pursuing scholarship almost always starts with integration. Understanding the landscape of previous work is critical to setting the stage for any scholarly effort.
- The *scholarship of discovery* is the acquisition of knowledge through basic research.
- The *scholarship of application* is applying basic research and integrated knowledge to real-world problems. Case reports, quality improvement, and implementation science are examples of this type of scholarship.
- The *scholarship of teaching* is educating future scholars. This includes developing and assessing new curricula, innovative teaching approaches, and methods for evaluation.

Many departments recognize scholarship across these various domains, with distinct academic tracks focused on research, clinical practice, and education. Thinking across this spectrum highlights the

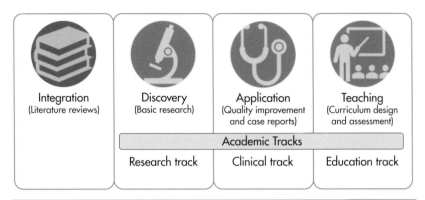

FIGURE 30–1. The four major types of scholarship and their relationship to academic tracks in medical settings.

different ways in which you can engage in scholarship beyond working in a traditional laboratory setting. Residents can take a scholarly approach to any area of interest sparked by their clinical work or medical training. For example, residents are frequently involved in case conferences and quality improvement efforts—activities that can easily be transformed into scholarship. In addition, residents are often involved in teaching medical students and other learners—another area particularly ripe for scholarship.

GETTING STARTED IN SCHOLARSHIP: NUTS AND BOLTS

Your best approach to scholarship depends on your own long-term goals. Before you get started, it is important to ask, *How much time do I imagine devoting to research after I graduate?* If you imagine doing research for the majority of your time, you likely will pursue scholarship in a different way than if you intend to have a career focused predominantly on clinical work or education.

If you envision pursuing research for the majority of your time, you are planning a *research-focused career.* The traditional path for a research-focused career usually starts with finding a mentor who is pursuing research that is of interest to you and getting involved in their work. Scholarship is well defined within a traditional research career, and many psychiatry residency and fellowship training programs have formal research tracks that allow residents to have protected time for a mentored research experience (Blacker and Morgan 2018). The National

Institutes of Health provide funding for institutional training grants (T32 programs) and individual awards for mentored career development (K-awards) that provide postresidency opportunities for ongoing mentorship and support for developing research expertise and scholarship.

If you do not envision pursuing research for the majority of your time but are still interested in an academic career, you are likely planning a *clinical- and/or education-focused career*. Although protected time and funding for research may be more limited in this career path, you can engage in scholarship by focusing on a few key strategies.

- *Focus on what you know.* Residents often have a unique perspective and vantage point that can easily be translated into scholarship by engaging in a project and disseminating the results (through either presentations or publications). For example, residents may have important ideas about improving residency training, and resident-led projects focused on program administration might include evaluating and improving a residency advisory or mentorship program (Berry et al. 2017), exploring factors that influence resident morale (Caravella et al. 2016), and developing a system to improve resident feedback (Havel et al. 2017). Additional areas for scholarship may focus specifically on improving clinical training, such as by examining psychiatric training in primary care (Jones-Bourne and Arbuckle 2019) or in psychotherapy (Blumenshine et al. 2017). The resident role as a teacher is also an area of resident expertise (Latov et al. 2018), as is resident moonlighting (Robinson et al. 2019).
- *Focus on what gets you excited.* Pursuing scholarship in an area about which you are passionate is most likely to be productive. For example, if you are interested in pursuing fellowship training (such as consultation-liaison or child psychiatry), you might consider pursuing scholarship in this area, such as case report or a quality improvement project. This not only allows you to capitalize on specific interests but helps to build an area of expertise that can enhance your future fellowship application. It can also provide you with an opportunity to network with faculty and fellows with expertise in your area of interest.
- *Join an ongoing project.* Speaking with faculty and other trainees about existing and recent scholarly projects can also help to generate ideas about particular topics that may pique your interest. Joining a project under way can also be a great way to get involved and to learn some of the basic approaches to scholarship.
- *Find a mentor.* Mentorship is also critical for any scholarly effort. Mentors may offer additional expertise in the *content area* you are interested in or in the *process* of conducting scholarship, whether it is

how to conduct a literature review or how to implement a local survey. You can find a mentor in many ways. Potential mentors might include your residency supervisors, members of a project in your program that interests you, scholars in your program who are doing work in your area of interest, and scholars outside your program who are researching your area of interest. Seeking guidance from your residency training director or other leaders in your department can be helpful (see Chapter 33, "Mentorship and Sponsorship").

- *Connect to a larger network.* Although it is often ideal to identify local opportunities for collaboration and mentorship, you may need or want to join with individuals outside your home institution. Connecting to a larger community of experts by attending the annual meetings of various organizations, such as the American Psychiatric Association (APA) or the Association for Academic Psychiatry, can be another way of identifying potential mentors and projects. The APA and other organizations, such as the American Association of Directors of Psychiatric Residency Training and the National Neuroscience Curriculum Initiative, also provide fellowship opportunities that connect residents to mentors and an opportunity to get more involved in a particular area of interest. Some of these fellowships (such as the APA Substance Abuse and Mental Health Services Administration Minority Fellowship) also provide funding for innovative projects. The recent expansion in videoconferencing has opened up opportunities for connecting to a national network of potential mentors and collaborators. Although outside faculty may not be available for an ongoing mentorship relationship, they are often very open to speaking with trainees and providing general guidance and advice on scholarly pursuits in line with their expertise (see Chapter 29, "Leadership").

START WITH THE END IN MIND: DISSEMINATING SCHOLARLY EFFORTS

Sharing knowledge, or dissemination of your work, is a critical part of scholarship. Before starting a scholarship project, thinking ahead to what your final product will be allows you to organize your efforts and enhances the chances of sharing your knowledge effectively. Several options are available:

- *Presentations* (which include workshops, talks, and posters) vary depending on the type of scholarship as well as the intended audience. *Posters* usually require some data but are often well suited for small studies that focus on a single site or studies with preliminary outcome data. *Workshops* are less data-driven and more focused on skill-building. For example, novel approaches to medical education are often shared through workshops. *Seminars, grand rounds,* or *lectures* are usually more in-depth presentations focused on a particular area of expertise.

- *Publications* include journal articles, book chapters, websites, or pieces for the popular press. Traditionally, within academic circles, *peer-reviewed manuscripts* of original work published in a scientific journal have been the gold standard for measuring scholarly activities relevant for academic promotion. *Original research articles* generally report on work that is data-driven and is often evaluated on its innovation and sample size (with a larger sample size suggesting more generalizable findings). However, there are other types of peer-reviewed publications. *Brief reports* are often shorter research pieces focused on smaller data sets that highlight preliminary data. *Review articles* synthesize the most up-to-date information on a topic of interest. *Viewpoints* are short pieces framed around a particular opinion, with supporting data. *Letters to the editor* are brief pieces that respond to recently published articles or highlight a topical issue. *Case reports* often highlight relatively unique clinical situations (see Chapter 31, "Publishing").

HOW WILL YOU DEMONSTRATE THAT YOUR SCHOLARLY EFFORTS HAVE VALUE?

Once you have identified a project of interest and considered how you hope to share the results, it is time to demonstrate the value of your work. For example, if describing a new resident-led course for medical students, you would need to provide some evidence that your course is successful in meeting the intended learning objectives. In medical education, we generally measure outcomes across the domains of knowledge, skills, and attitudes. Comparing trainee performance across these domains before and after an educational intervention is one way of demonstrating the potential value of your efforts.

Most published scholarship requires data of some sort. When pursuing a scholarly project, think up front about what types of data you will collect. The type of data may depend on the type of scholarship you are conducting, whether it is basic science, clinical research, quality improvement, or program development in medical education. Data generally fall into two categories:

- *Quantitative data*, which consist of specifically measurable information such as the percentage of responses on a survey
- *Qualitative data*, which are generally more descriptive, such as data obtained from focus groups or responses to open-ended survey questions

Quality improvement studies often include both quantitative data (e.g., looking at uptake of new evidence-based practices over time) and qualitative data (e.g., barriers and facilitators to change).

Before you collect data, you will need to determine whether your study qualifies as *human subjects research* and therefore requires approval by your institutional review board (IRB). *Don't be afraid of this step*—it is typically very straightforward and will generally help you to consolidate your project. Quality improvement and program development projects are generally considered by IRBs to be exempt from review. However, any project you may want to present or publish in the future should be submitted in advance to your department's IRB to determine if it requires IRB review and, if so, verifying that it meets appropriate standards in protecting the rights and welfare of participants.

Once you have collected your data, you are ready to share your work in the format you identified at the start of your scholarly project. This process often will include submission of your scholarly work for review and acceptance into the format of dissemination, whether it is a publication in a journal, a workshop or poster at a conference, or grand rounds at your institution. If your work is accepted right away, congratulations—you have contributed to the growth of our field and have started a scholarly dialogue with your community of fellow psychiatrists. If your work is not accepted immediately, don't despair—you may receive feedback or suggestions from journal editors or faculty mentors that enable you to enhance your work and resubmit. Engaging in this work of revision and resubmission is a core part of scholarly effort and is often a deep learning experience for you as a trainee. Remember, scholarship not only satisfies training requirements outlined by the Accreditation Council for Graduate Medical Education, it also gives you an opportunity for learning and engagement with colleagues and, ultimately, further enhances the care of your patients.

SPECIFIC CHALLENGES AND STRATEGIES

⌘ **I don't have the skills to be successful in scholarship.** Even if you don't feel confident in your ability to do a thorough literature search, analyze statistical data, or write up results, don't be intimidated. Individuals in full-time research careers know you must have a team. Everyone has areas of strengths and areas of need, and a team approach allows you to leverage one another's skills. Because everyone in academia is expected to engage in scholarship, try partnering with a colleague. Scholarship is more fun when done with a peer. It is also important to get mentorship early and seek advice. A mentor can assist in team formation and can help you network outside your program. Your local medical librarian, if you have one, can also be a resource for getting started with literature reviews.

⌘ **I don't have the time for scholarship.** With so many demands on your time, it can be difficult to figure out how to add a scholarly project. It is useful to think about capitalizing on the work you are already doing. Rather than thinking of scholarship as something extra that you do on the side, integrate it into the work you are already doing. Some examples include writing up case reports, assessing your residency experience, conducting quality improvement projects in clinical rotations, and assisting in the education of early learners. Additional strategies for addressing time limitations include working with a team, building in regular meetings for accountability, and focusing on something that really motivates and excites you. Investing in what you love pays major dividends in terms of job satisfaction and well-being.

⌘ **Now that I have elective time for scholarship, how do I make the most of it?** Many residency programs provide some elective time for residents to pursue research or scholarship during residency. This might be a block rotation (e.g., 2 months of full-time scholarship) or a certain percentage of time longitudinally over a longer time frame (e.g., 20% of time over the entire year). If you have a percentage of time available to you, you should try to block out that time each week on your calendar so that it is truly protected. Because it is tempting to catch up on clinical work (e.g., writing notes, following up on prescription orders) during open, unstructured scholarly project time, it is often helpful to set goals for each week and meet regularly with your mentor and team for accountability. In addition, it is generally better to consolidate your time for scholarship as much as possible. Frequent task shifting can quickly degrade the quality of the time you have available to focus on scholarship. Having an entire day each week dedicated to scholarship is likely to be more effective than having small bits of time throughout the week.

⌘ The scope of your project should match the amount of time you have available. Try to set specific SMART (specific, measurable, achievable, relevant, time-bound) goals for yourself. In addition, it is critical to anticipate steps that might delay digging into a project and to do as much as possible in advance of your protected elective time. Getting IRB approval (if necessary) can sometimes take months. You may want to use elective time to prepare and submit an IRB proposal. Or you may want to do this in advance in order to maximize your protected time for the project itself.

SELF-REFLECTIVE QUESTIONS

1. What topics make me most excited when I think about scholarship?
2. How might a scholarly project simply extend the work I am already doing?
3. Who might be a good mentor for a scholarly project?

RESOURCES

Browne JE: Getting started with research "Beginning: defining a research question and preparing a research plan." Ultrasound 21(2):102–104, 2013

Browne JE: Getting started with research "Writing-up the results of your research." Ultrasound 22(1):70–72, 2014

Papanas N, Georgiadis GS, Demetriou M, et al: Creating a successful poster: "beauty is truth, truth beauty." Int J Low Extrem Wounds 18(1):6–9, 2019 31064287

Pautasso M: Ten simple rules for writing a literature review. PLoS Comput Biol 9(7):e1003149, 2013 23874189

Sastry A, Tagle A: The right mentor can change your career: here's how to find one. NPR, September 9, 2020. Available at: www.npr.org/2019/10/25/773158390/how-to-find-a-mentor-and-make-it-work. Accessed July 10, 2021.

Shah BB: "Just write it up"—the art of writing a case report in gastroenterology. Gastrointest Endosc 70(5):977–979, 2009 19879404

UC San Diego Department of Psychology: Writing research papers. San Diego, University of California, Available at: https://psychology.ucsd.edu/undergraduate-program/undergraduate-resources/academic-writing-resources/writing-research-papers/writing-research-papers-videos.html. Accessed July 10, 2021.

Vandenbroucke JP, Pearce N: From ideas to studies: how to get ideas and sharpen them into research questions. Clin Epidemiol 10:253–264, 2018 29563838

REFERENCES

Accreditation Council for Graduate Medical Education: Common program requirements (residency). Chicago, IL, Accreditation Council for Graduate Medical Education, 2020. Available at: www.acgme.org/Portals/0/PFAssets/ProgramRequirements/CPRResidency2020.pdf. Accessed April 2, 2021.

Berry OO, Sciutto M, Cabaniss D, et al: Evaluating an advisor program for psychiatry residents. Acad Psychiatry 41(4):486–490, 2017 28197983

Blacker CJ, Morgan RJ: Research tracks during psychiatry residency training. Acad Psychiatry 42(5):698–704, 2018 29520584

Blumenshine P, Lenet AE, Havel LK, et al: Thinking outside of outpatient: underutilized settings for psychotherapy education. Acad Psychiatry 41(1):16–19, 2017 27283018

Boyer EL: Scholarship Reconsidered Priorities of the Professoriate. New York, Carnegie Foundation for the Advancement of Teaching, 1990

Caravella RA, Robinson LA, Wilets I, et al: A qualitative study of factors affecting morale in psychiatry residency training. Acad Psychiatry 40(5):776–782, 2016 27251705

Havel LK, Powell SD, Cabaniss DL, et al: Smartphones, smart feedback: using mobile devices to collect in-the-moment feedback. Acad Psychiatry 41(1):76–80, 2017 27160895

Jones-Bourne C, Arbuckle MR: Psychiatry residents' perspectives of primary care in the psychiatric setting. Acad Psychiatry 43(2):196–199, 2019 30560349

Latov DR, Levine M, Cutler JL, et al: Developing an observed structured teaching exercise for psychiatry residents. Acad Psychiatry 42(6):867–868, 2018 30066244

Robinson LA, Osborne LM, Hsu AJ, et al: Moonlighting by psychiatry residents: a survey of residents and training directors. Acad Psychiatry 43(1):46–50, 2019 30456706

Wei H, Kifner H, Dawes ME, et al: Self-care strategies to combat burnout among pediatric critical care nurses and physicians. Crit Care Nurse 40(2):44–53, 2020 32236429

CHAPTER 31

Publishing

Matthew G. Yung, M.D.
Adam Brenner, M.D.

Publishing your work can initially feel like a daunting task, but by the end of this chapter you will have a general framework for approaching your first manuscript. Before we discuss the specific steps to publishing, it is important to examine the purpose of writing. One of the primary purposes of writing is to make scholarly contributions and promote the advancement of knowledge, both of which are essential to the medical profession. However, other purposes for writing are equally valid. Effective writing can influence clinical practice, provide educational opportunities, illuminate gaps in knowledge and challenges in the field, advocate for the underserved, and influence policy and promote change (Roberts and Coverdale 2020).

Writing is also an important tool for professional and personal growth. Successful writing requires you to refine, test, and sharpen your ideas in order to bring something of value to the community with rigor. Writing can shape career interests and path, develop self-reflection and empathy, and deepen a commitment to lifelong learning. Publishing can also enhance your reputation and lead to the expansion of professional opportunities. Finally, collaborative writing can be an enriching experience for fostering collegial relationships, mutual learning, and mentorship.

CHOOSING A TOPIC AND FORMAT

One of the first tasks in publishing is determining the topic and format of your work. When considering a topic, reflect on your clinical, research, and advocacy interests as well as long-term career directions and goals. It can also be helpful to review your prior writings or presentations that have brought a sense of personal gratification. Experience with classroom essays, conference papers, posters, or thesis work can all be fertile ground for eventual publication. Sometimes the topic is already determined because you will be reporting the new data and findings of your research. But it is important to remember that many valuable types of publications do not consist of presentation of data (e.g., commentaries, case reports). All professions and sciences advance through a communal conversation that takes place in the pages of its journals; it can be helpful to think about which current discussions you would like to add your voice to.

CHOOSING A JOURNAL

Before starting the writing process, it is often helpful to select a target journal in which to publish your work. Each journal has a specific audience, aims and scope, reputation, and author guidelines for manuscripts. Therefore, it is important to consider all of these factors when selecting where to submit your work. One helpful strategy to determine which journal is most suitable is to review your cited references and see where they were published. Another approach is to review a year's worth of manuscripts in a target journal, with a primary focus on the titles and types of manuscripts, to determine if your work fits the scope of the journal. Other factors to consider include a journal's review process, publishing outlet, metrics (e.g., impact factor, productivity, longevity, rejection rate, time to publication), and publication fees (Belcher 2019). It can be very helpful to ask for recommendations from faculty and colleagues for appropriate journals for your work. Selecting a target journal before writing will allow you to use its instructions to authors to shape your initial draft to the publication's expectations and to use similar articles published in that journal as models to emulate.

APPROACHING THE WRITING PROCESS

Authorship

Collaborative writing can be an enriching learning experience for trainees; however, challenging ethical issues regarding authorship may arise. International guidelines help to clarify the criteria for authorship. The International Committee of Medical Journal Editors (ICMJE) has four criteria for authorship. All authors must 1) make "substantial contributions to the conception or design of the work" or "the acquisition, analysis, or interpretation of data for the work," 2) be involved in writing the work or "revising it critically for important intellectual content," 3) approve the ultimate version of the publication, and 4) consent to be "accountable for all aspects of the work," including its integrity and accuracy (www.icmje.org/recommendations/browse/roles-and-responsibilities/defining-the-role-of-authors-and-contributors.html). Team members who do not meet all four criteria but have significantly contributed to the project should not be authors but should be recognized in a formal acknowledgment (Roberts 2017).

Another important issue to address is the order of authors. In general, the first author will lead the writing, revision, and submission of the manuscript; respond to comments from peer review; and function as the corresponding author. The senior author, generally listed last, usually helps to establish the framework of the manuscript and provides feedback and iterative revisions. The middle authors should have specific roles that maximize their unique skills and strengths. It is generally advised to address authorship order early and to collaboratively define each member's expected contributions and avoid ambiguity. However, in some situations, work burden and professional responsibility shift during the writing process. For instance, a collaborator may not fulfill their expected role, and another team member may take on these responsibilities. Addressing these situations through direct conversation can be difficult but is a crucial skill to practice. In these situations, it is recommended to reapply the ICMJE criteria post hoc after a manuscript draft is developed to reevaluate whether each member has contributed enough work to be considered an author and whether authorship order should be rearranged (Roberts 2017).

Writing

Clear and effective writing forms a bridge to an audience and allows the writer to communicate ideas and results and generate discussion, change, and action. However, a number of barriers to effective writing may be encountered by even the most seasoned of writers (Viglianti et al. 2019). One of the most common problems is not having enough time. Experienced and successful writers prioritize writing by scheduling designated times each day for writing without distraction. Writing sprints, in which one writes as much as possible in a short period of time without editing, is another way to jump-start the writing process. Other strategies to support the writing process include joining a writing group and writing the easiest section first.

Another particularly insidious barrier is the expectation that your first draft will be coherent and readable. Often it is neither, but the goal should be simply to put all your ideas and thoughts on paper. Ultimately, the goal is to have a draft that can be revised and improved with successive iterations. It can help to set the draft aside for several days and then reread it, asking yourself what the important ideas are and what you most want to say to the reader. The rewriting cycle, although arduous at times, is essential for clarifying and deepening your thinking and ideas.

COMMON TYPES OF MANUSCRIPTS

Original Reports

Original reports are the most common type of manuscript. These pieces are ideal for full and completed research studies. In general, these reports have few restrictions on the number of authors, references, and tables and figures. The general structure consists of an abstract, introduction, methods, results, and discussion.

Brief Reports

Brief reports are ideal for small-scale projects or research in early development. Usually, the design is relatively simple, and sample size may be modest. Brief reports typically contain one or two significant findings, and the overall structure mirrors that of original full reports.

Systematic and Literature Reviews

Systematic reviews aim to retrieve, synthesize, and critically appraise existing knowledge on a particular subject. This particular type of review is unique in that it has a well-defined research question formulated using the PICO framework (population/problem, intervention, comparison, outcome), including explicitly defined inclusion and exclusion criteria (Coverdale et al. 2017; Møller and Myles 2016). In addition, a written protocol of how the review was conducted should be registered with the International Prospective Register of Systematic Reviews (PROSPERO) database (www.crd.york.ac.uk/prospero), and the methodology should be replicable and transparent. The Preferred Reporting Items for Systematic Reviews and Meta-Analyses (PRISMA) guidelines (www.prisma-statement.org) should be used when reporting findings. Undertaking a systematic review generally requires at least three team members with various levels of expertise related to the review question and a system for blinded review of retrieved sources and usually takes 10–18 months to complete.

A literature review, often referred to as a narrative review, seeks to describe and review the existing literature without the rigidity of defined parameters of a systematic review. These reviews have a wide scope and a nonstandardized methodology.

Case Reports

A case report is a detailed description of symptoms, signs, diagnosis, and treatment of an individual patient. Case reports represent one of the most traditional forms of medical communication, and, although they are considered the lowest on the hierarchy of evidence in medical literature, they have served as a platform for identifying rare and emerging diseases and treatment complications. One of the first and most challenging decisions to make is whether your clinical case is appropriate for publication. It can be helpful to discuss the case with mentors and colleagues to identify the interesting aspects and learning points and determine if the case is unique enough for presentation. Although a rare condition almost always meets criteria for a case report, few of us have the opportunity to report on an entirely new condition. Thus, another reason to report a case is to teach a lesson. Consider whether your case increases awareness of a particular condition, suggests a proper diagnostic strategy or cost-effective approach to management, or describes unusual presentation or complications of relatively common conditions (American College of Physicians 2021).

In terms of structure, case reports generally include the following components: abstract, introduction, case description, and discussion. The introduction should briefly describe the context of the case and its relevance and importance, citing relevant literature when appropriate. The case description should describe in sequential order the patient, history, physical examination, laboratory studies or imaging, treatment plan, progress, and ultimate outcome. The key is to include all essential components of the case and exclude any extraneous information. The discussion is the most important part of the report and should explain why decisions were made and convey the lesson from the case.

Commentaries

Commentaries generally include opinion pieces or narratives. Commentaries do not follow the traditional format and structure of a research article. Instead, they are meant to be thoughtful and tightly reasoned pieces on an important issue in the field. The breadth of topics is wide, with possibilities including issues related to narrative medicine, clinical practice, and social injustice.

A summary of the types of manuscripts is provided in Table 31–1.

OTHER PUBLICATIONS

Posters

Posters are widely used in the academic community, particularly at conferences. The purpose of a poster is to summarize research clearly in a visually appealing way and thus generate discussion. Ideal posters contain a mixture of short text and tables, figures, or diagrams. Before constructing a poster, it is important to review the conference's poster guidelines on sizing. In general, key information should be readable from 6–10 feet away. Keep text brief and concise and use bullet points, numbering, and headings. Posters are usually organized into sections and include an introduction, objective or goals, methods, results, conclusion, acknowledgments, and references. In terms of design, aim for a visually appealing, clean, and consistent layout and design. Consider including a QR code, URL, or printed handout of your poster that audience members can reference after the conference (NYU Libraries 2022). Various design software programs are available to help you create your poster, including PowerPoint, Keynote, and Adobe Illustrator or Photoshop, to name a few.

Medical Writing for the Public

Effectively communicating with the general public is an important skill that is unfortunately not routinely taught in medical training. Yet writing for the public is essential if trainees seek to correct misperceptions of science and mental health, have an impact on policy making, and bridge the gap between research and implementation. For instance, trainees may write about the stigma facing people with psychiatric illness or the structural forces contributing to mental illness. When you are writing for the public, there are key differences in writing style and approach to be considered. It is important to recognize that in order to adapt your writing to target a broader audience, you must sharpen and refine the story. In general, the thesis should focus on addressing the questions *How does this affect me?* and *What can we do with this knowledge?* More spe-

TABLE 31–1. Overview of different manuscript types

Manuscript type	Purpose	Word count	Number of tables and/or figures	Number of references
Original reports	Communicate results from original research structured with an introduction, methods, results, and discussion	2,400–4,000	≤5	40–50
Brief reports	Similar in structure to original reports but for smaller-scale projects with one or two significant findings	1,250–1,500	≤2	≤20
Systematic and literature reviews	Systematic reviews: clearly defined research question formulated with the PICO framework with clearly delineated inclusion and exclusion criteria Literature reviews: summary and synthesis of existing knowledge on a specific topic with less rigidly defined parameters	3,000–5,000	≤5	50–60
Case reports	Unique clinical case with the goal of presenting a key teaching point regarding diagnosis, management, or potential complications; obtain informed consent from the patient prior to writing and maintain patient anonymity throughout the report	1,250–2,250	2–3	≤20
Commentaries	Focused pieces on recent events, opinion, or narratives	1,000–3,000	1–2	10–30

Note. Data compiled in this chart are based on various journals in the field of psychiatry.
PICO=population/problem, intervention, comparison, outcome.

cifically, keep the story relatively simple in order to have a clearly defined thesis with a focus on the implications your story has for the public or society at large. A front-loaded structure (lead, development, and resolution), which is commonly used in journalism, will quickly engage your reader (Schimel 2012). With this approach, the lead (the core of the story) is presented early in the piece, and the rest of the piece develops the story. Remember to simplify your language and avoid jargon.

PEER REVIEW PROCESS AND RESPONDING TO REVIEWS

Defining Peer Review

Peer review is a unique and vital part of the scientific and medical community. It ensures that scholarly works meet scientific and ethical standards and evaluates their relevance and rigor. Reviewers are typically experts in their field and are expected to review only manuscripts that fall within their scope of expertise or practice. Although some beginning writers may view reviewers as adversaries, it is better to think of them as colleagues and consultants whose primary purpose is to improve a piece. Although peer review is subjective and vulnerable to bias, it is the standard by which academic works are judged and can improve the quality of scholarly work. Learning from and responding to reviewers' comments can be a formative experience that not only improves a manuscript but also deepens your understanding, thinking, and communication.

Responding to Initial Outcomes

In general, a manuscript may be returned with the following outcomes: rejection, major revisions, minor revisions, or acceptance. It is exceedingly rare that a piece is accepted without any revisions; therefore, an invitation to revise and resubmit is generally a positive result.

RESPONDING TO MINOR REVISION

A request for minor revisions is quite rare and is cause for celebration. Sometimes, the journal will explicitly say that your submission will be acceptable for publication if you successfully make the requested changes. Other times, this is not stated explicitly, but signs of this decision can be detected in the decision letter urging you to resubmit by a certain date to be included in a particular issue or describing relatively minor revisions to only certain sections of the manuscript (e.g., defining specific terminology, expanding on methodology, adding references). It is in your best interest to revise promptly and resubmit without delay.

RESPONDING TO MAJOR REVISION

A request for major revisions should also generally be regarded as a positive sign. This means that the editors see substantial, sometimes structural, concerns raised by the reviewers, but they believe these issues are potentially correctable. If they did not see a path forward, the decision would have been to reject the piece at this stage. It is best to respond positively, nondefensively, and in detail. As you read the decision letter and comments from reviewers, ensure that you understand the feedback and suggestions and ask for clarification from the editor if needed. In approaching your revisions, you may feel that entire sections need to be rewritten or overhauled. Instead, it is often best to take a targeted and measured approach to revisions, even to major objections or recommendations from reviewers.

In a revision cover letter, demonstrate clearly point by point what changes were made. The tone of the letter should be respectful and demonstrate a commitment to improving the quality of your work on the basis of the received feedback. Frame the letter in a series of bullet points organized individually or by category, with corresponding revisions addressing the problem. If you choose to not make all the suggested changes, list the reasons for not addressing those recommendations at the end of the letter and ensure that your rationale is objective, well-reasoned, and academic. If different reviewers gave conflicting recommendations, it is appropriate to ask the editor for further guidance. It can also be helpful to share your work with a mentor or writing group for feedback. Aim to resubmit your revised work within 1–2 months unless the journal requests an earlier return, and keep in mind that two or three iterations of revisions may be required before your manuscript is accepted (Belcher 2019).

HANDLING REJECTION

Receiving a rejection letter is understandably a disappointing result. Read the reviewers' comments and editor's letter carefully to understand why your manuscript was rejected; it will help to ultimately improve your piece. Unfortunately, you will not always receive this feedback. It is good to remember that sometimes your paper is simply not a good fit for the scope and focus of the journal. Other times, the journal may have recently published similar or overlapping material. Deciding how to proceed after a rejection is highly variable. In general, most authors revise their article on the basis of the feedback and send it to another journal. The decision on whether to submit to a higher- or lower-ranked journal (on the basis of impact factor or acceptance rate) depends on whether you think the revisions have substantially improved the quality of your work; however, the majority of authors submit to a less prestigious journal (Belcher 2019). When submitting to a target journal, it can be helpful to review other factors using the Belcher Journal Evaluation Form (available online at https://wendybelcher.com/writing-advice/workbook-forms).

SPECIFIC CHALLENGES AND STRATEGIES

⌘ **Although I initially agreed to a middle author position, I ended up writing most of the manuscript.** At times during the development of the manuscript, you might assume responsibility for more sections than initially agreed on. It is recommended that authors reapply the ICMJE criteria for authorship after a manuscript is developed to evaluate whether each member has contributed enough work and taken sufficient responsibility to be considered an author and whether authorship order needs to be rearranged accordingly. Although these conversations can be difficult, they are crucial. It may help to rehearse with a peer or mentor before any difficult conversations. In this case, it is good to be straightforward: "I have been thinking about the order of authorship of the paper. Do you have some time to talk about this? We agreed that I would be a middle author when the plan was that I would contribute X. But as the work progressed, I was also asked to do Y and Z. My sense is that I may now be the author who has contributed the most to this paper. What is your perspective?"

⌘ **After receiving a rejection letter, I'm not sure I have it in me to resubmit my manuscript to another journal.** Receiving a rejection letter is understandably disappointing; however, carefully and objectively review the reviewers' comments because they can be invaluable in your subsequent revisions. The decision on whether to submit to a higher- or lower-tier journal is a personal one. Most authors submit to a lower-tier journal after an initial rejection, but these decisions will be guided by the interval improvement of your manuscript after revisions.

⌘ **I'm writing my first manuscript and have writer's block.** Even if you are working on a manuscript about a topic you are passionate about, you may struggle to make progress in writing and find yourself with writer's block. Consider setting a consistent time to read and write, engaging in "writing sprints" in which you write as much as you can in a short period of time without editing, or joining a writing group.

SELF-REFLECTION QUESTIONS

1. What are my specific interests within the field of psychiatry?
2. What prior pieces of writing am I working on or have I completed that received positive feedback, generated a sense of gratification, or instilled a sense of curiosity and passion that might result in a publishable article with further revision?
3. Which mentors or faculty members could help guide me in my writing and provide feedback?
4. What are perceived fears or obstacles I envision regarding the writing process? How might I address these obstacles?

RESOURCE

The OpEd Project: www.theopedproject.org

REFERENCES

American College of Physicians: Writing a clinical vignette (case report) abstract. Philadelphia, PA, American College of Physicians, 2021. Available at: www.acponline.org/membership/residents/competitions-awards/acp-national-abstract-competitions/guide-to-preparing-for-the-abstract-competition/writing-a-clinical-vignette-case-report-abstract. Accessed June 16, 2022.

Belcher WL: Writing Your Journal Article in Twelve Weeks: A Guide to Academic Publishing Success. Chicago, IL, University of Chicago Press, 2019

Coverdale J, Roberts LW, Beresin EV, et al: Some potential "pitfalls" in the construction of educational systematic reviews. Acad Psychiatry 41(2):246–250, 2017 28188504

Møller A, Myles P: What makes a good systematic review and meta-analysis? Br J Anaesth 117(4):428–430, 2016 28077528

NYU Libraries: How to create a research poster. New York, NYU Libraries, April 1, 2022. Available at: https://guides.nyu.edu/posters. Accessed June 16, 2022.

Roberts LW: Addressing authorship issues prospectively: a heuristic approach. Acad Med 92(2):143–146, 2017 27355782

Roberts LW, Coverdale J: Why write? Acad Med 95(2):169–171, 2020 31990715

Schimel J: Writing Science: How to Write Papers That Get Cited and Proposals That Get Funded. New York, Oxford University Press, 2012

Viglianti EM, Admon AJ, Carlton EF, et al: Publishing a clinical research manuscript: guidance for early career researchers with a focus on pulmonary and critical care medicine. Chest 156(6):1054–1061, 2019 31265833

CHAPTER 32

Advocacy

Ann Crawford-Roberts, M.D., M.P.H.

Nichole Goodsmith, M.D., Ph.D.

Jennifer E. Manegold, M.D., M.S.

Isabella Morton, M.D., M.P.H.

Enrico G. Castillo, M.D., M.S.H.P.M.

> When you see something that is not right, not fair, not just, you must have the courage to stand up, to speak up, and find a way to get in the way.

—*John Lewis (2016), civil rights leader and Congressional representative*

> When physicians believe a law violates ethical values or is unjust they should work to change the law.

—*American Medical Association (2016)*

Although advocacy may conjure up lofty visions of speaking at the nation's capital, this is just one of many ways physicians can advocate. Broadly speaking, advocacy encompasses any action taken in support of a specific cause. As you will see, there are numerous ways to take that action, at levels ranging from your individual patients to national legislation and everything in between. In this chapter we focus on advocacy in support of health equity; similar tools can be used to advocate for other goals.

No formal training is required to become an advocate. As a physician, you possess medical expertise, an intimate understanding of patients' lived experiences, and public respect. These assets give you the power to make a difference. As you begin to view advocacy as a state of mind, you will find yourself identifying countless opportunities "to promote those social, economic, educational, and political changes that ameliorate the suffering and threats to human health and well-being" (Earnest et al. 2010, p. 63).

KEY POINTS

- Advocacy can occur at multiple levels: individual, clinical, community, institutional, and governmental.

- Advocacy interrupts the pathway to burnout and is an important form of clinical practice and leadership.

- Advocacy skills can be learned and are essential to being an effective physician advocate.

- Advocacy has challenges, but information and experiences can help you overcome them.

ROLE OF ADVOCACY IN THE RESIDENT EXPERIENCE

As you progress through training, you will bear witness to the ways health and health care are inequitable. You will see that at this moment in America, so much of our patients' health is influenced by their race, the zip code in which they live, how much money they have, their citizenship status, and the language they speak. You will grow in structural competency—an appreciation of the ways that laws, institutional policies, and social forces such as stigma influence the social determinants of health and perpetuate health inequities.

At the same time, you will become an expert in the systems in which you work: your residency program, clinic, emergency department, and hospital system. That expertise, known as systems-based practice, will improve your care for your patients but will also raise your awareness of the limitations of those systems. This awareness can lead to burnout—not only from overwork but also from feelings of disempowerment or moral injury, which occurs when one's experiences and actions go against one's own ideals.

Advocacy transforms experiences that could lead to burnout, such as working within flawed institutions or witnessing patients' suffering due to an unjust society, into opportunities to act (Eisenstein 2018). The advocacy described in this chapter encourages us to re-envision our roles as physicians to heal not only individual patients but also systems, policies, and institutions. In this way, advocacy is truly an advanced form of practice and leadership.

Advocacy may take us out of our comfort zone as we confront difficult truths, initiate challenging conversations, and recognize actions or policies that do not live up to our values. Complicit silence, however, ensures that unjust laws and institutions are left unchecked to harm our patients. As with clinical skills, increased comfort with advocacy will come with practice; residency is the perfect time to begin to build and hone advocacy skills that will serve you throughout your career.

We believe that advocacy is anchored not in any particular political party or professional organization but, rather, in the basic principles of social accountability and equity. Society imbues physicians with trust, and we must use that trust to dismantle the injustices we see and work to achieve equity for our most vulnerable patients. Advocacy combined with structural competency ensures that this work is done with and for the benefit of communities to address the fundamental causes of health inequities.

MULTIPLE LEVELS OF ADVOCACY

As you will see in this section, there are numerous ways to take action and several levels of advocacy, from the individual to the legislative. You may realize that you have been engaging in advocacy without realizing it. See Figure 32–1 for examples of psychiatry residents advocating at each level.

At the *individual* level, you can educate yourself on issues impacting your patients, such as local housing or law enforcement policies. You can take simple actions, such as wearing a badge buddy with your gender pronouns or wearing a pin promoting voter registration.

At the level of *clinical care*, you can advocate for a patient by connecting them with needed housing or legal services or completing disability paperwork. You can work in a multidisciplinary team and integrate so-

Government
Policy at the local, state, or national level
UCLA psychiatry residents testify in front of the Los Angeles Board of Supervisors to advocate against jail expansion in favor of a *care first* approach.

Community
Social mobilization
Alongside New Haven community organizers, Yale psychiatry residents help found the Semilla Collective, a grassroots collective fighting for immigration and labor justice.

Organization
Policy within a clinic, hospital, health system, or professional organization
UCSF psychiatry residents advocate against use of excessive force by security in the hospital.

Clinical Care
Advocacy in the clinical encounter
A Columbia psychiatry resident completes disability paperwork and thereby advocates for an individual patient.

Individual
Addressing personal attitudes and beliefs
A UNC psychiatry resident wears a badge buddy with preferred pronouns to promote inclusivity at an individual level.

FIGURE 32–1.   Levels of advocacy.

Note.   UCLA=University of California, Los Angeles; UCSF=University of California, San Francisco; UNC=University of North Carolina.

cial interventions into your treatment plan. You can stand up against racism, sexism, homophobia, transphobia, and other forms of bias that you witness a patient encountering within the health care system.

At the *organizational* level, you can promote policies to improve health equity within your hospital, clinic, department, or professional organization. As frontline workers, residents are particularly well positioned to advocate for policy change to combat health care inequities within their own health systems.

At the *community* level, you can connect with like-minded individuals around you—within your program, department, neighborhood, community-based organizations, and city—to educate each other, identify areas of needed change, and organize for action.

Finally, at the *government* level, you can use your voice to make a significant impact on local, state, or national policy. Local policies often have the deepest impact on our daily lives and the lives of our patients and present real opportunities to make a difference. You can call, write to, or meet with your local representatives. You can attend and speak at public hearings or legislative meetings. And if you are a citizen, you can vote in your local, state, and national elections.

BUILDING SPECIFIC ADVOCACY SKILLS

You might be hesitant to engage in advocacy work because you feel that you simply do not have the skills. The good news is if you can learn to prescribe clozapine and do psychotherapy, you can learn to do this. The best way to build a skill is to learn the basics, practice the skill, and, one day, teach it.

Patient Advocacy

Helping your patients navigate systems and connect to resources to help them better address their health and social needs is an essential form of physician advocacy. Often, such tasks are delegated to social workers and case managers, but advanced clinicians are themselves knowledgeable about available resources for their patients and work closely with a multidisciplinary team to incorporate social interventions into a comprehensive treatment plan. You can start by systematically screening for the social determinants of health using evidence-supported screening tools (see the "Resources" section at the end of the chapter). You can also learn how to connect your patients to financial benefits, legal aid, housing, food, peer support services, and other community resources. These skills include writing letters of advocacy for your patients, which can help them receive financial benefits such as Supplemental Security Income, fight off eviction, or inform judicial discretion in criminal court cases, to name a few examples (see "Resources"). Community partnerships (as detailed in the following subsection) are also important for patient advocacy because developing strong relationships with community-based organizations and local agencies can help you better address the needs of your patients. You can advocate that your training program include educational sessions on the activities listed in this chapter. You can improve your clinic's and hospital's policies so that screening patients for the social determinants of health and connecting patients to resources are incorporated into routine clinical care pathways. You can advocate for patients who are historically oppressed in medicine (see Chapter 8,

"Working With Historically Oppressed Patient Populations"), attending to their particular socioeconomic needs and speaking up against racism, sexism, homophobia, transphobia, and other forms of bias. Finally, you can advocate for patients in your role as a psychiatric consultant (e.g., in the emergency department or consultation-liaison service), knowing you may understand their medical and social circumstances more thoroughly than their primary team does. You can communicate your patients' needs directly and clearly to consulting teams, advocating for longer stays, effective treatment, or more appropriate disposition plans.

Finding Partners

Finding peers, faculty, administrators, and community members with common interests can help you build a small community of co-organizers to support and encourage each other in advocacy work. Seek out residents with shared interests and learn from senior residents about their experiences. Residents in other specialties, particularly pediatrics and family medicine, may already be involved in advocacy. Residency-wide and graduate medical education–wide social events can be important venues for meeting residents outside your program and clinical teams. Search faculty's online profiles, and ask faculty you already know to recommend others with shared interests. Residents can also discuss their advocacy interests with program directors, who may help connect residents to others already doing advocacy. Identify residents or faculty at other institutions through professional organizations or conferences. Community members and organizations can be found through social media, local news, and existing partnerships with faculty. Following social media accounts can help you learn about which individuals and groups are already doing advocacy work, and they can help connect you to local resources, events, and actions. Don't be afraid to send a direct message to social media accounts—this can be an easy way to connect. Last, email listservs are important tools to find advocacy-related events and individuals with similar interests; they can be particularly useful for learning about events involving community members and organizations.

Power Mapping

A crucial skill in advocacy is identifying your target audience, whether that be institutional leadership, elected representatives, coresidents, your specialty organization leaders, or members of your broader geographic community. Power mapping is a process that identifies key players, their relative power, and their level of support of or opposition to your goals (Figure 32–2). It helps you identify the key decision-makers who can change policies, the individuals and organizations that influence them, and the connections you and your group hold to those primary and secondary targets. Start with power mapping, then select an appropriate medium for influencing the key players, such as social media, the local newspaper, or an academic journal. You will want to select a medium that your key targets or their supporters read. For example, your city council member may be influenced by an op-ed in the local newspaper that their constituents read; a specialty organization leader may be affected by a letter to the editor in the specialty's top journal. The "Resources" section provides helpful examples.

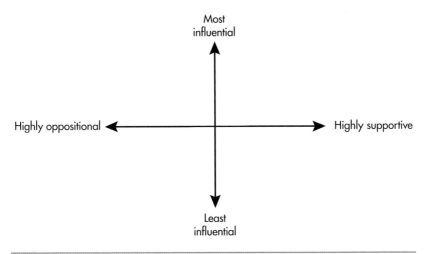

FIGURE 32–2.   Blank power mapping template.

Op-Eds and Letters to the Editor

Opinion pieces, editorials, and letters to the editor are important tools and serve to empower individuals to express their ideas. Effective letters to the editor and op-eds are timely, personal, and designed to influence the intended audience. See "Resources" for an excellent training on writing op-eds and letters to the editor.

Social Media

Social media creates a platform for individuals to share their opinions and experiences with a wider community. Identify one to three issues in which you want to develop a public expertise on social media, and use your voice to provide education and to signal boost relevant advocacy campaigns. See "Resources" to find a webinar on social media best practices for psychiatrists.

Legislative Advocacy

A survey of congressional staffers identified that private citizens can most influence Congress members by 1) providing consistently reliable information and 2) presenting a concise argument (Rehr 2012). As physicians who deliver important medical information to patients and families, we know how to do both, and these same activities can have a greater influence on elected representatives. When congressional staffers were asked how valuable different sources are for them when learning about policy issues, the second most valuable source was academic or issue experts (Rehr 2012). When it comes to our patients and their health needs, physicians are certainly seen as experts, and when it comes to medicine, we are academics. When speaking to policymakers, it is important to come prepared with specific stories you will share, a clear and concise message you will deliver, and written resources you will leave with staff (see "Resources").

How Find and Contact Your Representatives

First, a brief background on your government representatives: You have executives and legislators representing you at local, state, and national levels. There are four main types of local government: counties, municipalities (cities, towns, boroughs, and villages), special districts, and school districts. Counties are the largest units of local government and are usually led by a board of supervisors. Cities are often led by a mayor and a city council. Local government structure varies by region and population size. You also have state assembly members, state senators, and a governor who represent you in your state government. Finally, you have two senators, one U.S. House representative, and one president whom you elect on the national level. Engage with your elected officials:

1. Enter your address on a website such as https://ballotpedia.org/ Who_represents_me and find out who represents you.
2. Store your elected officials' contact information in your phone for easy access ("My Representative A").
3. Call their offices, meet with them, attend a board of supervisors or city council meeting to give public testimony, and/or write them letters. These elected officials represent you, and it is their responsibility to listen to you and take your concerns seriously.

SPECIFIC CHALLENGES AND STRATEGIES

⌘ **I'm so busy, I can't imagine having time for advocacy work during residency.** Start small. As a doctor, you have a powerful voice, and people want to hear from you. Build connections with other residents or faculty. Volunteer for a small and manageable role in an advocacy project that is already under way. Build confidence by getting your feet wet. Advocating for your patients, within your own institution or at a local level, can feel more accessible and be more immediately impactful on your patients' lives than national or statewide advocacy work. You also may find ways to create dedicated time within your schedule for nonclinical work. Advocate for protected time for residents, such as through advocacy-related didactics or scholarly projects. Set up a meeting with your program director if this is not yet an option—and show them this chapter. You would be surprised how much change is possible if you ask for it.

Here are some suggestions of how to advocate with little time:

- *Engage in passive advocacy.* Wear a badge buddy to encourage voting or a lapel pin to show solidarity with a particular group.
- *Advocate for your patients.* Ask about and acknowledge your patient's social needs. Fill out paperwork to help them achieve housing, paid time off work, or disability benefits, as appropriate.
- *Educate yourself.* Reflect on the impacts of national, local, and institutional systems and policies on your patients. Discuss these issues with your colleagues and supervisors.
- *Follow the lead of an organization you trust.* Sign up for mailing lists for local advocacy groups working on issues you care about. They will offer straightforward actions, such as emailing or calling your representative using a template that you can quickly modify.
- *Find opportunities.* Advocacy can begin with simply mentioning an issue to a peer or your program director. If others share your concerns, continue the dialogue and see where it goes. Look for opportunities for change not only at the legislative level but also in residency, clinic, or hospital policies. Find your voice and make an impact.

⌘ **I'm the only one who cares about this, and I'm worried my supervisors will find my ideas controversial.** Building a community of like-minded colleagues and community members can be a powerful antidote. Advocacy work is best carried out by a group of individuals with a diversity of skill sets, roles, perspectives, and life experiences. Mentorship in advocacy, support from program leadership, and individual advocacy champions are important elements for supporting the development of advocacy programs within residencies (Vance and Kennedy 2020). Refer to the subsection "Finding Partners" to see how to identify others with shared advocacy interests.

⌘ **I'm not sure what my role is in a partnership with a community organization.** Community organizations are often made up of and led by individuals who experience the challenges that they and you are advocating to change. Their work may be informed by their own life experiences. As physicians, we are habituated to being leaders on the clinical team. However, physician advocates can be allies, and we do not necessarily need to lead advocacy work ourselves. Many community organizations work full-time on advocacy issues, with a deeper understanding of the historical background, the relevant actors, and the opportunities for change. It is important that physicians approach community organizations with a posture of humility and an awareness of both the privileges and the power that a physician carries.

⌘ **I'm uncertain if I can identify my hospital or academic institution affiliation when I'm advocating publicly.** It is important to know your rights. First, know that the right to free speech applies to you as an individual, meaning that you are free to advocate as you wish under your own name, leveraging your credentials as a physician. At the same time, you should do so while making clear that your views are your own, and not those of affiliated institutions. Second, take the time to learn about relevant institutional policies, particularly when engaging in advocacy activities that may be perceived as representing your institution. For example, you and your coresidents may wish to write a letter to your local, state, or national elected officials explaining the mental health impacts of a particular policy. Although you can choose to sign the letter simply as "concerned physicians," it may be more powerful to name your training program *if this is allowed by your institution*. You can find your institution's policies around physician advocacy on its media relations or communications website. When in doubt, contact your program director or Graduate Medical Education, Human Resources, or Media department to get clarification on the relevant policies. One piece of advice is to not take anyone's word for it but to find the specific written policy relating to free speech and political expression at your program or institution.

SELF-REFLECTIVE QUESTIONS

1. What structural determinants (e.g., laws, institutional policies, social forces such as racism) impact my patients' mental health? Their access to resources? Their access to medical care?
2. In what ways have I engaged in advocacy in the past? How can I build off my prior experiences to apply them to a different level of advocacy or a different advocacy topic?

3. Who in my professional community do I share interests with? How can I build those relationships and support my peers in advocacy work?

4. What barriers have I faced when doing advocacy in the past? How can I use the tools in this chapter to overcome those challenges?

RESOURCES

Advocacy skills workshops hosted by the American Psychiatric Association (APA), American Medical Association, Doctors for America, and other medical and community organizations

Anti-Racism Daily: www.antiracismdaily.com—an email newsletter that includes daily education and easy ways to engage in antiracism advocacy

Federal Legislative Advocacy Manual: www.psychiatry.org/psychiatrists/advocacy/congressional-advocacy-network/resources—a guide from the APA's Congressional Advocacy Network, which includes tips on communicating with members of Congress and conducting facility tours, with an overview of the federal legislative process and key psychiatry federal committees

Letters of support for benefits applications: Ask colleagues and attendings for templates for letters of support for Supplemental Security Income (SSI), Social Security Disability Insurance (SSDI), and other benefits applications. When writing a letter of support for your patient, do not simply copy and paste your note; instead, organize your letter such that the information you include directly addresses the benefit program's eligibility criteria (e.g., see descriptions Paragraphs B and C criteria for SSI/SSDI mental health disability evaluations: www.ssa.gov/disability/professionals/bluebook/12.00-MentalDisorders-Adult.htm).

The OpEd Project: www.theopedproject.org—an organization that provides trainings on writing opinion pieces and offers ongoing editorial support; even if you cannot attend a training, their website is a helpful resource that includes tips on writing an op-ed and pitching it to newspapers

Power mapping tools: a short video from Resistance School on power mapping (www.resistanceschool.com/lesson/lesson-8-power-mapping-and-identifying-targets-for-organizing) and a handout with visual exercises from the Union of Concerned Scientists (www.ucsusa.org/sites/default/files/attach/2018/07/SN_Toolkit_Power_Mapping_Your_Way_to_Success.pdf)

Social Media Best Practices for Psychiatrists: www.psychiatry.org/
psychiatrists/practice/social-media—a training by the APA's Council
on Communications on how to use social media professionally,
including advocacy work

Resistance School: www.resistanceschool.com—a collection of online
videos on theory and skills of community organizing, including
team building, sustaining action, and effective communication

Social determinants of health screening tools: Protocol for Responding to
and Assessing Patients' Assets, Risks, and Experiences (PRAPARE;
www.prapare.org) and the Institute of Medicine Measures of Social
and Behavioral Determinants of Health (www.ncbi.nlm.nih.gov/
pmc/articles/PMC5253326)

REFERENCES

American Medical Association: Code of Medical Ethics Preface and Preamble.
Chicago, IL, American Medical Association, 2016. Available at: www.ama-
assn.org/delivering-care/ethics/code-medical-ethics-preface-preamble.
Accessed November 16, 2022.

Earnest MA, Wong SL, Federico SG: Perspective: physician advocacy: what is it
and how do we do it? Acad Med 85(1):63–67, 2010 20042825

Eisenstein L: To fight burnout, organize. N Engl J Med 379(6):509–511, 2018
29924700

Lewis J: John Lewis' 2016 commencement address at Washington University in St.
Louis. St. Louis, MO, Washington University in St. Louis, May 20, 2016. Available at: https://source.wustl.edu/2016/05/john-lewis-2016-commencement-
address-washington-university-st-louis. Accessed November 16, 2022.

Rehr D: The Congressional Communications Report, 3rd Edition. Arlington,
VA, Columbia Books, 2012

Vance MC, Kennedy KG: Developing an advocacy curriculum: lessons learned
from a national survey of psychiatric residency programs. Acad Psychiatry
44(3):283–288, 2020 31950369

PART 5

Developing a Career

CHAPTER 33

Mentorship and Sponsorship

Lia Thomas, M.D.

Mohona Sadhu, M.D.

As you embark on psychiatry residency training, you may wonder how to manage clinical work, administrative duties, educational goals, and research demands, as well as how to find the "perfect" balance between work and personal life. You are not alone. During your training, you are surrounded by coresidents, fellows, and attending physicians at various stages of this journey. Although it is important to learn DSM-5 criteria for psychiatric diagnoses (American Psychiatric Association 2022), it can be just as important to seek guidance and input from your colleagues in the form of mentorship as you shape your career.

KEY POINTS

- Selecting a mentor who fits your career needs and is able to provide guidance is fundamental to your professional development.

- Addressing challenges in mentoring relationships will facilitate deeper and more helpful professional connections.

- Continuing to reflect on your goals as you progress in your career will allow you to make adjustments on the basis of your values.

WHAT IS A MENTOR?

Although mentorship can be defined in multiple ways, mentorship in medicine often takes the form of an experienced senior physician (i.e., *mentor*) who is responsible for nurturing the development of an early career physician (i.e., *mentee*). Traditionally, this is a dyadic model between the mentor and mentee in which the mentor's intent is to support the career and professional development of the mentee through a series of meetings, reflections, and academic collaborations (Sambunjak et al. 2006). The concept of a mentor can be traced back to Homer's *Odyssey*, in which the young Telemachus, son of Odysseus, was given an adviser named Mentor who was responsible for his upbringing when Odysseus left for the Trojan War. On Odysseus's return 20 years later, he found Telemachus to be brave, respectable, and honorable, which was attributed to Mentor's influence and guidance. Since then, the definition of mentor as an experienced and trusted adviser has been adopted and has evolved in various career fields. The role of mentorship in medicine has become one of the most important factors in reducing burnout and increasing job satisfaction and is also linked to productivity, academic success, higher rates of promotion, and resiliency (Straus et al. 2006). Additionally, the role of the mentor transcends the role of an educator or role model, with the mentor serving as a guardian or promoter of the mentee's personal and professional development. Mentorship also involves more than coaching, which often is used to impart specific knowledge or a skill for a defined goal. Surviving residency is no easy feat, and finding a mentor who can assist in identifying career goals, promote healthy self-reflection, create a safe place for discussing challenges, offer exposure for growth and opportunity, and provide encouragement along the way can help ensure a rich, rewarding, and successful career.

"IDEAL" MENTOR AND MENTEE

As with any successful partnership, both the mentor and the mentee have an equal role to play in making the relationship effective. When looking for a mentor, be on the lookout for qualities that can be helpful in promoting your growth and development. A systematic review evaluated qualitative characteristics for both mentors and mentees in academia (Sambunjak et al. 2010). An "ideal" mentor is described in terms of three dimensions, including personal, relational, and professional. On the personal front, an ideal mentor is someone who is altruistic, honest, open, trustworthy, an active listener, and nonjudgmental. Regarding relational characteristics, the mentor is accessible, approachable, and sincere in wanting to develop the mentee's strengths and goals. Last, on a professional level, the ideal mentor is well respected, knowledgeable, and a senior in their field.

However, *your* ideal mentor may be different from your coresident's ideal mentor. As you continue your journey through training, you will also find other aspects that may be important to you when looking for your mentor, including gender, race, ethnicity, or cultural background. Some of these shared qualities also may play a large role in finding the right fit for you (see Chapter 4, "The Underrepresented in Medicine Experience").

Sambunjak et al. (2010) also found that qualities that make for an ideal mentee include honesty, reliability, eagerness to learn, flexibility, punctuality, passion to succeed in their career, appreciation for the time the mentor provides and the effects of mentorship, taking initiative, being proactive, being understanding, and demonstrating seriousness in the relationship.

HOW TO FIND A MENTOR

As you begin to conceptualize your career goals and the qualities you are looking for in a mentor, finding a mentor can also be a challenge. Some tips for finding a mentor include discussing with other residents, fellows, faculty, and/or program director your specific areas of interest in order to identify other senior physicians with similar interests and career goals. You may want to send emails to faculty introducing yourself, informing them that you are interested in career guidance and mentoring and asking for 30–60 minutes of their time to meet and discuss your goals. You may use this time as an opportunity to assess goodness of fit for the mentor-mentee relationship. Additionally, getting involved in projects that align with your career goals is another way to be introduced to faculty with similar interests and a chance to assess their compatibility as a mentor for you.

Asking a senior physician to be your mentor can cause some anxiety, and it is also important to understand that mentoring can occur both formally and informally. Formal mentoring involves asking a senior faculty to be your mentor, with specific expectations and objectives targeting your career goals. It often involves structured, regular meetings. A formal mentor may provide more guidance on specific tasks along with a more thorough understanding of your career goals. Informal mentoring often involves less structure, with fewer set expectations over a shorter period of time. Informal mentoring may be instrumental in your exposure to clinical practice and different psychiatry roles. Some examples of an informal mentor may include one-time guidance on a project, talking with a presenter at a conference, or discussing a specific aspect of a project with a supervisor during a clinical rotation.

Given the increasing importance of mentorship in medicine, some psychiatry residency programs may have structured mentorship programs. They may provide a list of faculty interested in serving as mentors and/or assign mentors early in residency to ensure that residents have guidance and support. Although having an assigned mentor can have benefits, mentees who are able to identify their own mentors may have a more comfortable and effective relationship in the long term. Having assigned mentors can lead to less effective relationships due to mismatches in the process, incompatibility in career directions, and lack of open communication (Straus et al. 2009). Another potentially successful model may be a hybrid system in which residents are assigned a mentor to provide support in their early career, but as the mentee's career goals change over time, they are able to organically find other mentors more suited to their goals.

Although it can be helpful to share common aspects of your personal identity with your mentor, it may also be a rich experience to have mentors from different backgrounds. In cross-cultural mentoring, you and your mentor acknowledge the personal attributes that you both bring to the relationship, such as socioeconomic status, race, ethnicity, language, nationality, sex, gender identity, sexual orientation, religion, geography, disability, and age, and make them part of the mentoring experience through learning each other's perspectives based on those differences and how those differences can impact clinical care (Geraci and Thigpen 2017). This acknowledgment comes from a place of humility and understanding and a desire to grow and change. It is about celebrating diversity of experiences.

MENTORING MODELS

As you begin searching for your mentor, it is important to remember that a single mentoring relationship may not guide you in every aspect of your professional life, but rather may guide you in just those aspects in which the mentor has expertise. Furthermore, it is also important to determine which mentoring model would be the most helpful depending on the stage of your career: dyadic mentoring, multiple mentoring, peer mentoring, functional mentoring, or a hybrid of all four. See Table 33–1.

WHAT TO EXPECT FROM A MENTOR

Regardless of the mentorship model you choose, the initial step of a mentoring relationship is setting goals and expectations (for sample goals, see Table 33–2). Ask yourself, *For which goals or aspects of my career am I specifically asking for guidance? Does this mentor have expertise in that area? What are some benchmarks to indicate I am progressing in this aspect?* Furthermore, it is important to have a conversation with your mentor about your expectations. Consider how your mentor can be helpful, how often you would you like to meet, and how you prefer to receive feedback. You will also want to discuss your mentor's expectations. Do they expect you to join their projects? How often are they able to meet? Who sets the agenda? Although initial chemistry can be assessed prior to discussing specific expectations, more formal discussions about goals and expectations allow you to further evaluate and foster a relationship based on trust, openness, bilateral communication, and listening.

As with any working relationship, each participant has their roles and responsibilities in order to make the mentorship successful. Nevertheless, even with both the mentor and the mentee's best intentions, challenges may still arise. The key is to understand the forces behind these challenges and to develop some strategies to address them. Additionally, be cautious about certain pitfalls. One of the most common pitfalls is choosing a mentor primarily on the basis of their prominence in your department rather than other qualities that might lead to a good fit with your career goals and personality. Another common pitfall is rushing to solidify a mentoring relationship after just a few meetings. The process of assessing whether the mentor will be a good fit for your career goals requires time, patience, and diligence and should not be decided hastily.

SPONSORSHIP

As you move further in your residency, you may begin to connect with people for sponsoring. A sponsor is someone who will advocate for your professional career without necessarily providing specific career guidance the way a mentor would. Sponsors are often senior individuals who are well connected in their field. You acquire sponsors the same way

TABLE 33–1.   Types of mentorship models

Model	Advantages	Disadvantages
Dyadic mentorship	• Most traditional model • 1:1 relationship (mentor-mentee) • Specific and targeted guidance • Deeper relationship that can last throughout all stages of your career	• Unable to provide support in areas in which the mentor does not have expertise • May require finding another mentor if mentor is unable to provide guidance on your specific goal
Multiple mentorship and/or co-mentorship	• Multiple mentors simultaneously guiding and supporting your growth and development • Able to nurture multiple areas of your career because each mentor has a unique contribution • Emphasizes collaboration between mentors • Increased likelihood of finding a combination of mentors with similar values and goals	• Conflicting suggestions from multiple mentors • Increased time commitment due to engaging in multiple mentoring relationships • Working on multiple career aspects at once (vs. one at a time) • Increased likelihood of feeling overwhelmed because of multiple relationships
Peer mentorship	• Removal of hierarchy • Emphasizes mutual learning and support	• Limited insight into career advancement due to being in similar career stages • Challenges of competition in the field
Functional mentorship	• Guidance on a specific task or project • Highly targeted	• Time limited • Unable to address other career aspects outside the specific goal or project
Hybrid of all models	• Able to incorporate desired features of each of the models • Able to target specific needs and career goals	• Challenges with balancing multiple mentoring relationships • Challenges with balancing various expectations and goals in each of the relationships

---

TABLE 33–2. Sample goals for mentorship

- Enhance teaching skills
- Identify career path aligned with values
- Career development
- Networking
- Problem-solve difficult conversations and situations
- Navigate work-life balance
- Address burnout
- Address impostor phenomenon

---

you acquire mentors—by reaching out and making a professional connection or by finding them through common acquaintances. Your sponsor may be someone you heard speak at a national conference, someone you learned about via social media, or someone to whom you were introduced. Someone doing similar work at another institution or with whom you collaborate on projects may also serve as a sponsor. As the relationship with your sponsor grows through collaborative work or mutual interests or projects or as you proactively reach out as needed, your sponsor may recommend you for an employment opportunity, write you a letter of recommendation, or recommend you for a collateral project with others. In contrast to a mentoring relationship, you may have only brief interactions with a sponsor. However, some of your mentors also may become your sponsors over time throughout your career. Staying connected with your mentor following graduation can lead to their sponsoring you for employment or academic opportunities along with continuing to nurture your growth and development in your career.

SPECIFIC CHALLENGES AND STRATEGIES

⌘ **I don't think my mentor is providing me guidance that is consistent with my goals.** A mentor provides guidance, but it is your decision to act on this guidance. If you feel as if your mentor is trying to make you an extension of themselves, try to discuss this openly in a respectful manner. Although the power differential between you and your mentor can make having a frank discussion challenging, reflecting back on your initial goals previously discussed with your mentor may be helpful. Ask your mentor, "Can you help me understand how your suggestion relates to my goals?" or "Can you guide me as to how I can work toward X goal by implementing the suggestion you provided?" Furthermore, consulting a trusted colleague can provide guidance in navigating challenging conversations. You may use this person to role-play discussions, solicit feedback, and/or request assistance in resolving the issue with the other mentor. Although the hope is that both you and your mentor are able to ultimately resolve the issue, it may be helpful to transition to another mentor who fits your needs better if problems continue despite constructive conversations.

⌘ **I have a unique cultural, social, racial, or ethnic background, and there is no one like me at my program.** Not all mentor-mentee pairings will share common backgrounds or identities. For example, although you may wish to seek out someone from a similar background as your own, there may not be many women or underrepresented minority faculty within your department or program. You might seek out affinity groups at your institution specifically for your desired background (e.g., women in medicine). Involvement in national organizations may also offer access to additional mentors. On the other hand, mentoring across cultural, racial, and/or gender lines can also be very helpful in providing a rich collaborative relationship in which each member brings a unique perspective and insight. Having a mentor who you feel is an ally is more important than sharing a similar background (DeCastro et al. 2014).

⌘ **My mentor is making assumptions about my background, which negatively affects me.** With differences in gender, race, and/or ethnicity in mentor-mentee pairings, a risk of experiencing microaggressions in your mentor-mentee relationship is possible. Often, the assumptions are the result of a lack of knowledge, understanding, or even awareness. If your mentor does not attend to the rupture, try to address the comments directly with them. Because the power differential in the dyad can add additional stress in being able to engage in this conversation, consider reaching out to your program director or other residency leadership for support and assistance in addressing the situation. Some institutions have both resident- and department-level committees to look at how to manage microaggressions and other acts of racism. See Chapter 39, "Handling Mistreatment and Discrimination."

⌘ **My mentor is making inappropriate sexual advances.** Just as egregious as microaggressions is sexual harassment. And similar to microaggressions, the events can vary from small slights to very direct assaults. Many who experience these types of events often are not aware of what is happening until later. You may have a sense of unease or discomfort about the interaction. You may wonder if you (the mentee) did something wrong to bring on this behavior and/or may be unsure what to do next. Other times, sexual harassment is more obvious. If that is the case, clearly state that your mentor's behavior is inappropriate, leave the situation safely, and end communication with them. Immediately notify your program leadership, who may in turn notify the institution. This may involve both a formal and an informal investigation and a referral to institutional or local law enforcement depending on the nature of the concerns. Although the inherent power differential between you and your mentor may pose a barrier to addressing the mistreatment, especially in more subtle cases, try to discuss your concerns with a peer or trusted individual (e.g., another mentor, senior faculty, program leadership) to get support and to ensure a healthy and safe work environment.

⌘ **I am not getting the credit I deserve, and my mentor is undervaluing my efforts.** Another challenge might involve a mentor appropriating your work or minimizing your role in their work. It is not uncommon for mentors to invite mentees to partner on projects together, and your contributions as a mentee should be appropriately credited. Have discussions up front about your role in your mentor's work and questions of authorship (see Chapter 31, "Publishing"). Consider documenting these discussions in email for future reference; concerns about stolen work should be brought up to program and departmental leadership.

SELF-REFLECTIVE QUESTIONS

1. In which areas of my career would I like guidance or assistance?
2. What are some qualities I have found helpful and important in a mentor?
3. If challenges do arise, how comfortable do I feel in addressing them with my mentor?
4. What resources do I have available when trying to shape my career?

RESOURCES

Websites

American Association of Directors of Psychiatric Residency Training: Mentorship Program, www.aadprt.org/training-directors/mentorship-program

American Psychiatric Association: Mentorship Program for APA/APAF Fellows, www.psychiatry.org/residents-medical-students/residents/fellowships/additional-opportunities-for-fellows/mentorship-program

Brigham and Women's Hospital Mentoring and Curriculum and Toolkit: https://bwhmentoringtoolkit.partners.org/structuring-the-mentoring-relationship-expectations-boundaries/pearls-for-mentors-and-mentees

Clinical and Translational Science Institute, University of Minnesota: Mentor training, www.ctsi.umn.edu/education-and-training/mentoring/mentor-training

Podcasts

The Medicine Mentors: https://themedicinementors.libsyn.com

Books

Donahue A, Yager J: How to approach mentorship as a mentee, in The Academic Medicine Handbook: A Guide to Achievement and Fulfillment for Academic Faculty. Edited by Roberts LW. New York, Springer, 2020, pp 157–162

Humphrey H: Mentoring in Academic Medicine. Philadelphia, PA, American College of Physicians, 2010

Maxwell JC: Mentoring 101: What Every Leader Needs to Know. Nashville, TN, HarperCollins Leadership, 2008

REFERENCES

American Psychiatric Association: Diagnostic and Statistical Manual of Mental Disorders, 5th Edition, Text Revision. Washington, DC, American Psychiatric Association, 2022

DeCastro R, Griffith KA, Ubel PA, et al: Mentoring and the career satisfaction of male and female academic medical faculty. Acad Med 89(2):301–311, 2014 24362376

Geraci SA, Thigpen SC: A review of mentoring in academic medicine. Am J Med Sci 353(2):151–157, 2017 28183416

Sambunjak D, Straus SE, Marusic A: Mentoring in academic medicine: a systematic review. JAMA 296(9):1103–1115, 2006 16954490

Sambunjak D, Straus SE, Marusic A: A systematic review of qualitative research on the meaning and characteristics of mentoring in academic medicine. J Gen Intern Med 25(1):72–78, 2010 19924490

Straus SE, Chatur F, Taylor M: Issues in the mentor-mentee relationship in academic medicine: a qualitative study. Acad Med 84(1):135–139, 2009 19116493

Straus SE, Straus C, Tzanetos K, et al: Career choice in academic medicine: systematic review. J Gen Intern Med 21(12):1222–1229, 2006 17105520

CHAPTER 34

Preparing for Your Career

Amit Parikh, M.D.

Sallie G. De Golia, M.D., M.P.H.

Anna Kerlek, M.D.

...[I]t is impossible to have a great life unless it is a meaningful life. And it is very difficult to have a meaningful life without meaningful work.

—*Jim Collins (2001, p. 210)*

Career development does not come to the forefront of most residents' minds when beginning psychiatry residency. However, as you gain experience working with patients of all ages and diagnoses across patient populations and practice settings, you may start to identify your interests. As you continue to build your portfolio of clinical and professional interests and experience, you will become a strong candidate for the job or fellowship you desire at the end of training. In this chapter you will learn about how to go about setting yourself up to obtain the job you want.

KEY POINTS

- Engage in a variety of clinical and nonclinical experiences while maintaining an up-to-date curriculum vitae (CV).

- Mentors and colleagues can help shape your future career.

- Fellowship training can provide valuable experience.

DETERMINE A DIRECTION

The first step in preparing for your career is determining how you want to use your expertise as an attending psychiatrist—your options are endless, from the clinical space to private industry. Although this may sound like a daunting task, with some thoughtful planning and solid guidance, you may find this an exciting adventure. The structure of psychiatry residency allows you to work in different areas of clinical practice for months at a time. In most residencies, you will spend the first 2 years rotating through acute psychiatric services such as the emergency department, inpatient service, and consultation-liaison service. The third year is typically a longitudinal outpatient year, and the fourth year is often a time to pursue your own interests and take on potential leadership roles. Although the primary focus remains patient care and educational experiences, remember to reflect during and after each rotation. If you find specific work particularly enjoyable, meet with those attending physicians on service to understand their role more fully. This may help you contextualize what that type of practice might look like for you.

Geographic Locations

Most residency programs are embedded within hospital systems, but the physical setting can range widely from rural to urban. Different locations bring with them varied patient populations and cultures. Although your program may expose you to only a limited geographic location (rural vs. urban), it may provide you with opportunities to experience different settings, such as academic, community, or the Veterans Administration (VA).

Work Settings

Psychiatry is a unique field in medicine because of the vast number of clinical job types that are available to you when you graduate. It is one of the few fields of medicine where true private practice is also feasible. Most practices will fall into three main categories: academic, community, and private. If you train only in an academic hospital setting, your understanding of potential work environments may be skewed. The majority of psychiatrists in the United States do not work in academic centers. There is a variety of practice settings, including hospital employee single-specialty or multispecialty groups, health maintenance organizations (e.g., Kaiser Permanente), the VA, state hospital facilities, and Federally Qualified Health Centers, as well as solo or group private practice.

Almost all residency programs are based in academic or community settings. Academic practices tend to be linked with major universities and, often, VA hospitals and have requirements of teaching and/or research. Community practices are more focused on clinical care, although some community psychiatrists continue to be involved in research, advocacy, administration, and teaching. Private practices usually are centered fully on providing clinical care. Private practitioners may still affiliate with an academic center, psychoanalytic institute, or other mental health organization to participate in research or teaching.

Types of Work

Within the three main categories of clinical practice, you will find a variety of different types of work. These include, but are not limited to, outpatient, inpatient, consultation-liaison, alcohol and drug rehabilitation, emergency or crisis, partial hospitalization program or intensive outpatient program (PHP/IOP), residential, integrative behavioral health (a psychiatrist embedded within a collaborative care model), telepsychiatry, and clinical research. Depending on patient care needs as well as innovation, new care delivery models may be developed that have an impact on where psychiatrists might work and types of jobs offered.

Practice Style

Many psychiatrists work in multiple practice settings at the same time. As such, psychiatrists may effectively work part time in completely different institutions, perform different duties within the same setting as a full- or part-time employee, or move between geographic locations (e.g., locum tenens). Locum tenens is a unique form of practice. Rather than having a full-time job, locum tenens physicians provide their services to geographic areas of need for shorter periods of time (weeks to months). Physicians choose this model for the increased flexibility in schedule, travel opportunities, extra income, or additional clinical experience. These are positions that urgently need filling to provide patients with the care they need.

Diagnostic Focus

You can also have a specific diagnostic focus within your clinical practice. These more specialized practices center on specific clinical areas such as mood disorders, psychosis, child and adolescent psychiatry, geriatric psychiatry, substance use and detox, neuropsychiatry (including intellectual disability and autism spectrum disorder), and eating disorders. These specific areas can exist in any of the different categories of practice described in the subsection "Types of Work." Some require a fellowship to fully specialize.

Beyond Clinical Work

Traditional clinical care, although important, makes up only part of the job that many psychiatrists perform. Nonclinical care can include teaching (e.g., undergraduate education, medical school, graduate medical education, supervising other mental health providers), working in administration (e.g., hospital leadership positions, department chair, residency or fellowship program director), research (e.g., basic, translational, clinical, quality improvement), or joining private industry (e.g., pharmaceutical companies, insurance companies, health care technology companies).

While in residency, you will have the opportunity to explore teaching, leadership (similar to administration), and various forms of research. Reflect on these experiences to determine if you may want to integrate this kind of work into your career. Although some of you will not have the chance to explore private industry in your training, you will graduate with a valuable skill set and clinical knowledge base that may be attractive to private industry.

WRITE A MISSION STATEMENT

Writing a mission, vision, or values statement is a great way to begin to hone your professional and personal goals (Figure 34–1). It is never too early to create one. Try to revise it every 6–12 months throughout residency as your interests evolve. Developing a mission statement helps you identify your core values, which will guide you into the practice style and setting that best fit your goals. Think about your best moments when you thought to yourself, "This is who I am meant to be; this is what I am meant to do." Then begin to draft a strategy to get there—a clear plan that describes the path by which you intend to reach your vision.

Whom do you admire? *Qualities you would like to emulate (character, values, achievements, personality, or the way they lived)*	
Ideal self *Example: As an ideal partner, I want to:*	*Partner:* *Friend:* *Parent:* *Physician:* *Colleague:* *Community contributor:*
Legacy *How do you want others to perceive you?*	*Career:* *Family:* *Community:*

FIGURE 34–1. Mission statement worksheet.

IDENTIFY A MENTOR

Throughout residency, mentors can help you to reach your professional goals (see Chapter 33, "Mentorship and Sponsorship"). Although you may find mentors in your home program, you will also have the ability to network with psychiatrists across the country. If your program provides funds to attend meetings, use them. Attending both local and state meetings of the American Psychiatric Association (APA) and meetings of local organizations is a great way to meet potential employers, learn about job openings, and obtain mentors. Attending national confer-

Write goals for each element of who you are	*Physical:* *Mental:* *Emotional:* *Spiritual:*
Clarify your strengths *Make a list of all of your personal and professional talents, skills*	*Personal* *Professional* *Talents:* *Skills:*
Define specific goals for your life (based on above)	*Short-term* *Long-term* *Relationships:* *Work:* *Hobbies:* *Other:*

MISSION STATEMENT:

Write a statement of purpose that will help drive choices you make for your career (and life) and outlines an action plan. It should define the personal, moral, and ethical guidelines within which you can most happily express and fulfill yourself.

FIGURE 34–1.   Mission statement worksheet, *(continued)*

ences, particularly those in your area of interest, may also help you land the fellowship or job you want as well as offer mentorship. Popular national conferences include the APA Annual Meeting and APA Mental Health Services Conference, the Association of Academic Psychiatry Annual Meeting, and psychiatric subspecialty annual conferences. Ask your program or department leaders for introductions to mentors, especially those you admire, who can help you. Stay organized as you meet people by maintaining a repository of information, including name, role, and area of expertise of the people you meet, as well as contact information. Creating a social media presence can be another way to stay in contact and extend your reach to others who may possess valuable resources (see Chapter 28, "Navigating Use of Social Media").

BUILD YOUR PORTFOLIO

Now that you have thought through what area of psychiatry and type of practice you might want to pursue, consider what criteria might be required for you to reach your professional goals and try to gain the required experiences and skills. For example, if you are pursuing a fellowship or applying to an academic institution, doing research within that subspecialty may benefit you.

If research is relevant to your future career, you might consider writing for publication (e.g., case reports), being part of clinical research trials, evaluating an educational intervention, or getting involved in quality improvement, depending on your specific goals. See what types of research interest you early on in training. If you do not have mentors in your area of interest at your program, attend specialty conferences to find one (see previous section). Although private employers tend to place less weight on research, it can demonstrate your expertise in areas that matter to them and future patients.

Residency is an invaluable time when you get experience working in different clinical settings. After each service you rotate on, ask yourself, "Can I imagine myself doing this in the future?" If you find an area of great interest, you might try to spend more time in the area to deepen your expertise. Locum tenens or moonlighting work (if allowed by your program) may further bolster your clinical skills while providing you with extra income. All these experiences can be added to your CV to demonstrate developing clinical expertise.

Although clinical expertise is important, many employers also appreciate nonclinical experience. As the field of medicine has evolved, being able to navigate the nonclinical workspace has become necessary and is also a way to show your leadership potential. Consider joining a hospital committee (e.g., safety, quality, wellness) or residency committee (chief resident, program evaluation, recruitment), and remember to include them on your CV.

If your interest lies in medical education, consider developing an educator portfolio. This type of document may be used in academic institutions for promotion. It provides a review of your educational activities over time and serves as a tool to highlight your teaching experiences. It can include not only lists of your experiences but also significant results of your teaching (e.g., teaching evaluations, thank you letters from internal or external departments). See the "Resources" section at the end of the chapter for more information about an educator profile.

MAINTAIN YOUR CURRICULUM VITAE

Your CV should be a brief written summary of your experiences, qualifications, and education. Many institutions are able to provide templates to help in creating your CV. Each time you complete a lecture, presentation, teaching experience, publication, or other noteworthy achievement, add it to your CV and include a brief description of what you did. It is particularly important to include any initiatives you have developed and implemented, no matter how small (e.g., book clubs, lecture for trainees or staff). Unless you maintain an up-to-date list of activities you have worked on since first year, you are unlikely to remember all the different projects you have completed and accolades you have received. A well put together CV that is tailored to the role you are applying for can be the deciding factor in getting the interview you want. Last, make sure you have several trusted people review your CV and provide feedback regarding font, level of detail, and overall length.

CONSIDER FURTHER TRAINING

An important question is whether you need to pursue a fellowship in order to practice in a subspecialty area. In some areas of the country, you may be hired without this additional board certification. However, many would argue that fellowship training is invaluable. Although year(s) of additional training do mean lost attending or practice salary (which can be significant depending on your debt burden), it is an opportunity to expand your knowledge base and obtain free supervision. It is an opportunity to develop yourself as an expert and may potentially lead to a higher salary or more job offers. Some trainees will choose to work as an attending for a few years to help reduce their educational debt prior to starting a fellowship, although this is less common. Remember, once you leave training, consultation (known as supervision within training) costs money.

Five main Accreditation Council for Graduate Medical Education (ACGME)-accredited fellowships within psychiatry are boarded within the American Board of Psychiatry and Neurology: addiction psychiatry, child and adolescent psychiatry, consultation-liaison psychiatry, forensic psychiatry, and geriatric psychiatry (see Table 6–4 in Chapter 6, "Professional and Personal Life"). Other nonpsychiatry accredited fellowships available to psychiatry graduates include addiction medicine, brain injury medicine, hospice and palliative medicine, neuropsychiatry and behavioral medicine, and sleep medicine. In addition, nonaccredited fellowships that may be of interest and provide extra specialization for psychiatry residents include perinatal and women's mental health, public and community psychiatry, institution-specific research fellowships, and psychoanalytic training.

Whether or not you pursue a fellowship, you can still specialize clinically. For example, you might spend extra time participating in clinical research or treat additional patients with obsessive-compulsive disorder, despite the lack of a fellowship. Finding a niche is a great way to distinguish yourself from others when applying for jobs and to further establish an area of clinical excellence. This may lead to creating a specialized program at an institution or being the sought-after physician for that disorder in your community.

Depending on your career goals, you may choose to pursue further academic study outside medicine, including a Master's of Public Health (M.P.H.), Master's of Business Administration (M.B.A.), Master's of Public Administration (M.P.A.), or Juris Doctor (J.D.) degree. As a physician, you are a unique candidate to any of these potential areas.

SEARCH FOR THE RIGHT JOB

Attempting to find the absolute perfect job may be setting yourself up for disappointment. According to a survey by CompHealth in 2018, only 37% of physicians stay in their position beyond the end of their contract, although this is not psychiatry specific (Saley 2018). This lower-than-expected percentage may be the result of many variables, including 1) not enough information or less than ideal preparation leading into this first position, 2) changing clinical interests, and 3) changing life circumstances as many graduates start families while also caring for aging relatives. These factors may help inform a job transition.

If you take the time to consider the nonnegotiables for your first position, the more likely you are to be content (see Chapter 35, "Steps to Securing Your First Job"). In addition to practice setting and specialization, it is important to consider such factors as the level of support (e.g. administrative, nursing), protected time for teaching, flexibility of hours, call amount, benefits, and loan repayment.

Specific Challenges and Strategies

⌘ **I like everything I've done so far—it is so hard to choose!** That is a good problem to have. This means that you will likely be content in your first position as well. You should still take the time and effort during training to speak to as many upper-level trainees, young faculty who recently went through this same process, and senior mentors (both inside and outside your institution and in different parts of the country) to learn about all the possibilities. Also, work on your mission statement to home in on what might best fit your life right now. Many people stay in their first position only a few years, which is not necessarily frowned on.

⌘ **I wonder if it will hurt my job prospects if I take time off after training.** Some people may need to take care of loved ones, need emotional space before moving into a postgraduate career, or have other reasons to take a break following training. Although this may present financial or health insurance challenges, taking a break can be enormously useful. It is advised to keep your medical license up to date and remain in contact with your previous institution(s). This may be a time to explore additional practice settings or specific patient populations to which you were not exposed during training, which can help you secure the first best position when the time is right.

⌘ **I'm worried that my struggles during training with poor evaluations or conflict with others may haunt me in getting a job posttraining.** Unless formal corrective action was taken, which may prompt your future employer to contact your training director, your issues during training should not necessarily affect your finding a new job, pending reference checks. However, those same challenges experienced during training may follow you into your new employment. Seek outside mentorship and feedback. Embrace a growth mindset to strengthen skills and work on areas that may have been problematic for you during training. Do not hesitate to identify additional supports during the initial years out of training to help you thrive in your new job.

Self-Reflective Questions

1. Which patient population is most interesting to me?
2. What do I most enjoy about my work?
3. Would a fellowship add to my skill set and increase my chances of obtaining the job I want?
4. What would be my ideal job in 10 years?

RESOURCES

Mission Statement

Forbes Coaches Council: 13 ways you can craft a strong personal mission statement. Forbes, November 7, 2017. Available at: www.forbes.com/sites/forbescoachescouncil/2017/11/07/13-ways-you-can-craft-a-strong-personal-mission-statement. Accessed October 14, 2022.

Educator Portfolio

Simpson D: How to develop an educator's portfolio, in Roberts Academic Medicine Handbook. Edited by Roberts LW. Cham, Switzerland, Springer, 2020, pp 497–507

Curriculum Vitae

Murphy B: CV writing 101: tips for medical residents entering job market. Chicago, IL, American Medical Association, January 25, 2022. Available at: www.ama-assn.org/medical-residents/transition-resident-attending/cv-writing-101-tips-medical-residents-entering-job. Accessed October 14, 2022.

Additional Career Guidance

Gih DE: Guiding psychiatry trainees on their first job search. Acad Psychiatry 41(3):423–426, 2017 27718169

Newman WJ, Hearn J, McBride A, et al: Subspecialty training in psychiatry, in Handbook of Psychiatric Education, 2nd Edition. Edited by Sudak D. Washington, DC, American Psychiatric Association Publishing, 2021, pp 221–238

REFERENCES

Collins J: Good to Great: Why Some Companies Make the Leap…and Others Don't, 1st Edition. New York, HarperCollins, 2001

Saley C: Survey report: millennial doctors still finding jobs the old-fashioned way. CompHealth Blog, April 2018. Available at: https://comphealth.com/resources/millennial-doctors-survey. Accessed October 14, 2022.

CHAPTER **35**

Steps to Securing Your First Job

Sara Baumann, M.D.

Jorien Campbell, M.D.

Ambarin Faizi, D.O.

Searching for a job post residency or fellowship can sometimes be confusing, difficult, and frustrating. In this chapter we focus on navigating the job search—discussing how to approach a job search by identifying your priorities, recognizing your value, and staying focused. It can also help you project both assertiveness and confidence and ensure that you earn your true value as you go through the negotiation process.

KEY POINTS

- Knowing your value, including your experiences in leadership, research, and advocacy, lays the groundwork for current and future job searches.

- Identifying your priorities before beginning your job search can help you target jobs that would be a good fit for you.

- Your network and contacts are good sources for researching potential employers during your job search and the interview process.

- During salary negotiations, come prepared with knowledge about who makes salary decisions and what is negotiable and let the employer make the first offer.

- The most important factor in negotiating with an employer is your interpersonal communication style; be confident and emphasize how your strengths align with the employer's mission statement.

- During negotiations, you should know your walk-away point and have a backup plan.

KNOW YOUR VALUE

Recognizing your value before beginning the job search process will greatly serve you not only when pursuing your first job but also when you are at a position to renegotiate in later stages of your career. Knowing your value can also help to organize and ground you throughout the process. You have a breadth of skills, experiences, and accomplishments unique to you, and you have traversed a particular path to get here. Take some time to reflect on what is in your skill set. You should not only consider your experience treating patients but also include your experience in leadership positions, research, advocacy, consulting, or volunteering to explain the breadth of your skills.

Once you are clear about your own value, research how your skill set could meet unmet needs in your potential workplace. What are the resources you would require to successfully meet that need? For example, if you demonstrated active leadership in a quality improvement initiative during your training, this has prepared you for a leadership role to optimize the working environment for the benefit of patients and staff at your future workplace. Identify areas where your skills would be valuable so that you can enter the job search with a clear sense of your worth and emphasize it accordingly. Be aware that employers often devote significant time and resources to candidate searches and want to come to an agreement that will ensure your success in the position.

KNOW YOUR MUST-HAVES

Writing out your priorities before you begin your job search will provide clarity and focus. A good place to start is having a list of must-haves. Consider creating a chart with three columns: must-haves, nice-to-haves, and don't-wants. Then, turn your must-have list into a target list of potential jobs that you would be interested in. Examples of priorities for a job search are provided in Table 35–1. This list is certainly not exhaustive, but it gives you an idea of how broadly you can and should think beyond salary alone.

TABLE 35–1.   Aspects to consider and prioritize in your job search

---

Salary and benefits

    Salary structures (set salary or based on relative value units?)

    Signing bonus

    Relocation bonus or expenses covered

    Health benefits

    Parental leave

    Retirement savings options (e.g., contribution match)

Schedule

    Time allocation (including administrative, research, teaching, inpatient vs. outpatient)

    Teaching requirements

    Vacation and sick leave

    Professional development time off and/or funds, including for travel

    Call schedule

    Control over schedule and flexibility

Resources

    Office space and location

    Start-up funds

    Research equipment and materials, laboratory access

People

    Mentorship

    Future colleagues

    Company retention rates and morale

Other factors

    Patient population and volume

    Opportunities for growth and leadership development

    Title

    Tail coverage insurance

    Parking

Don't allow your eagerness to secure employment take precedence over your need to find a job that checks the most important boxes on your must-have list. In the long run, this will save you time and help you avoid accepting a position that is not a good fit.

DO YOUR RESEARCH

To get a sense of what jobs are out there, a good place to start would be to check posted or advertised job listings at local or national conferences or in academic journals. However, many jobs are not formally posted until late in the process, and you might miss out to candidates who have already been identified through word of mouth or other informal contacts. For that reason, it is important to make a list of people in your network you feel comfortable approaching—such as residency supervisors, mentors from medical school, or recent graduates from your program—and let them know you are looking for a job. This can be a helpful way of hearing about relevant opportunities. Participating in career development opportunities through organizations such as the American Psychiatric Association or reaching out to a recruiter can also help with your search, especially when you are looking for jobs far from where you completed your training.

Networking during the interviewing process can help you identify people you have something in common with as you are learning more about the position. Leverage any contacts you have as you research a potential job and employer. Finding friendly or communicative insiders is invaluable; they can potentially provide information on the workplace environment, the employer's needs and wants in a candidate, and what is negotiable in the contract, among other helpful insights. Mentors, colleagues, and friends in similar jobs may also be able to weigh in and help guide you. You can also find helpful data, such as average salary information for your specialty and geographic area, from online sources (e.g., Salary.com, Glassdoor, Medscape Salary Explorer) to get a sense of your market value.

PREPARE FOR CONTRACT NEGOTIATION

Generally, the negotiation process begins after your potential employer sends you a contract or an offer letter. Sometimes, the offer is presented verbally after the interview. If you feel pressured to negotiate or name your terms prior to receiving a formal offer, it is generally considered reasonable to request the offer in writing so that you can review it first.

So you have the job offer—now what? Be gracious, express enthusiasm for the role, and thank the employer for their effort. Then schedule time to negotiate the offer or initiate an email thread. Negotiating via email can be helpful if you do not feel confident that you can negotiate as effectively in person. The purpose of negotiation is to match your compensation to your value. Some early career psychiatrists may consider salary negotiations to be quite daunting. Asking for more money makes most people feel uncomfortable. However, contract negotiation is a consequential endeavor. It has the potential to have major impacts on your career, salary, and more. Missing out on even one negotiation can have a cumulative impact, as illustrated by Babcock et al. (2006):

> Suppose that a man and a woman begin work at age 25 for the same employer at the same salary and their employer offers both of them 2% raise every year. If the woman accepts the raise but the man negotiates his raise to receive a 3% increase every year, then after 40 years on the job, the woman will be earning 67.7% as much as the man. (p. 240)

As highlighted in this example, women are less likely than men to initiate negotiations. Such phenomena as the gender wage gap and the glass ceiling have been attributed to women's tendency to negotiate less often and less successfully than men (Babcock et al. 2006). Negotiation disparities have also been found to occur along racial lines. Hernandez and colleagues (2019) found that Black job seekers are expected to negotiate less than their white counterparts and are penalized in negotiations with lower salary outcomes when this expectation is violated (especially when negotiating with a more racially biased evaluator). Although the onus in proactively targeting and overcoming these gender and racial disparities lands firmly with employers, it can be helpful for women and underrepresented minorities in medicine to prepare for negotiation in advance by going through the steps outlined in this chapter, preparing and practicing with trusted attending physicians or mentors, using online resources (e.g., LeanIn.org, which offers videos and discussion guides to help women improve their negotiation skills), and understanding the costs of not negotiating.

Avoid expressing your feelings or thoughts about the offer itself until you have reviewed the contract and consulted with an attorney. Generally, showing your cards to your potential employer early in the process is a losing proposition. When you meet to negotiate the terms, let the employer make the first offer and then negotiate everything from there. It is important to be knowledgeable about your potential future employer to understand the relationship between the person you will be negotiating with and the person who makes the decisions about salary and benefits. For example, in academic psychiatry, negotiations are usually conducted with the direct supervisor of the position or the director of the program. In small group practices, the person who is negotiating may have the ability to affect benefits and salary, but in institutional settings such as an academic center or state hospital, salary and benefits are likely determined by the larger institution. Use your network to talk to psychiatrists who work in similar jobs to gather this type of information and to get a sense of what is negotiable. It is also appropriate to ask your potential employers to connect you with other psychiatrists in their organization to help you get a sense of the organizational culture regarding compensation.

If you value the financial outcome of the contract the most, you can make the first offer to anchor the negotiation in your favor. However, if you volunteer a salary amount first, you risk being uninformed of the true salary potential, and you may second-guess whether you could have negotiated a higher amount. It is best to let the employer state a number first because it is possible that the employer would be willing to make a higher salary offer than the one you propose. If the number is lower than what you expected, you can always make a counteroffer. If it is still short of your expectations, you can continue the negotiation process until an agreeable number is reached.

If the salary associated with your potential job is not negotiable, it may be worth considering in advance what nonsalary aspects of the job might be important to negotiate. Some nonsalary examples to consider include vacation days, sign-on bonus, relocation costs, administrative time, leadership title, and professional development time. Such requests may not cost the organization much, but they can render you opportunities for additional recognition and increased autonomy with regard to your time. Consider the whole package without becoming fixated on the money alone.

Position Yourself Well During the Negotiation Process

Negotiating your first contract is just that, a negotiation. It is a give-and-take process in which both parties must be willing to make concessions in order to get them in return. Label and define the concessions you are willing to make. To ensure that your concession is not undervalued, communicate why and how the concession affects you and emphasize the benefits to the other side. Doing so will trigger your potential employer to reciprocate. Reciprocity is an underlying fundamental principle in negotiations. To increase the likelihood that your potential employer will reciprocate your concession, tactfully incorporate your expectation when you communicate the concession you are willing to make. Consider that interests and constraints change over time, and what is nonnegotiable today may be negotiable tomorrow. Making concessions and reciprocating the potential employer's concessions demonstrates goodwill and goes a long way in establishing trust.

Don't panic if you hear a "no" from your potential employer. Use the opportunity to ask focused questions, gain information about the constraints that underlie the denial, and understand why your request was denied. This will provide a window into their rationale and aid you in constructing a counteroffer. If you launch into a counterargument without an understanding of the other side, you risk putting the employer on the defensive and shutting down additional conversation. If you find yourself in a difficult situation during the negotiation process and are pressed on deciding certain terms, remember that you do not have to provide a definitive answer in the moment. You can ask for time to think about it and offer to respond in a reasonable time frame. Do more research and seek consultation from your peers and mentors to help you consider all aspects and form your response.

Remember that the most important factor in negotiating with an employer is your interpersonal communication style. Politeness and professionalism aside, an employer is more likely to be flexible with their offer if they like interacting with you. Be confident yet practical with your requests and help the employer understand why you deserve what you are requesting. Highlight your strengths and connect your requests to the qualities that set you apart. Emphasize how your strengths align with the employer's mission statement and can further their vision. You will be more successful with negotiating your terms if your options satisfy both parties and speak to the interests of the employer. Be prepared and present your requests simultaneously to the employer, not serially. Present your requests in a way that demonstrates the value you will add to the organization. For example, if you ask for additional conference days, you can emphasize how your staying current in the field enhances patient care and allows you to share knowledge with the team.

Certain statements, such as giving ultimatums to an employer, decrease a candidate's appeal. Even if negotiations are delayed because you have not reached an agreeable offer, maintain your professionalism until the end. Both parties should treat each other with respect and utmost consideration. The world of psychiatry is small, and it is possible that you will encounter this employer in the future in other circumstances. Your professionalism during the entire process will leave a lasting impression even if you do not sign on the dotted line.

Prepare to Walk Away

When a potential employer is unable to meet your salary requirements or you have concerns about certain aspects of the job, it may be best to walk away from the offer. One way to be confident in your position is to know your walk-away point and have a backup plan in case your desired outcome is not reached. This will increase your protection against both accepting an agreement you should reject and rejecting an agreement you should accept.

Effective negotiation requires both parties to be flexible to achieve a mutually satisfactory outcome. An employer's approach to negotiating can be very telling of the organization's culture. For example, if you get penalized for negotiating, you may be facing potential bias by your prospective employer. This should be carefully considered along with other aspects of the position. Be comfortable with saying no thanks and declining a position if it is not the best fit for you. Negotiation is a skill, and you will get better at getting what you are worth with experience and practice. Use these tips to craft the kind of job that gives you satisfaction and maintains balance in your life.

Consider Having an Attorney Review Your Contract

Do not sign a contract without understanding the responsibilities, the salary, and the legal jargon. The provisions of your contract, and the exact language in which it is expressed, will control your obligations, responsibilities, and rights in your new job, as well as your employer's obligations and responsibilities to you. Consider hiring an attorney to review your contract. Find an attorney who has experience with physician contracts early in your job search, so when you receive a contract you can move quickly. Your attorney should know the pitfalls, loopholes, and specific state laws that apply, such as noncompete clauses.

SPECIFIC CHALLENGES AND STRATEGIES

✻ **I'm not worthy of a higher salary.** This cannot be stressed enough: Know your worth! You have dedicated years to your profession, and your knowledge, skills, and training are in high demand. Your personal strengths and experiences will add value to an organization. Review your curriculum vitae, assess your qualities and accomplishments objectively, be your own advocate, and imagine you are negotiating on behalf of your best friend.

✻ **Negotiating a higher salary will make me appear greedy.** On the contrary, negotiating a higher salary indicates that you have done your research and understand the demand for your skill set. Be confident yet reasonable with your negotiation expectations. Negotiating a salary offer is about more than money—it sets the stage for future earnings and career opportunities.

⌘ **The salary is nonnegotiable and seems fine, so I don't need to engage in negotiation.** Several aspects of the job are worth negotiating, such as your schedule, time off for professional development, conferences, and office space. An organization might be unable to offer a higher salary, but they may be able to offer a flexible schedule, competitive benefits, additional paid time off, or remote work opportunities. Your salary is just one piece of your compensation. Consider the whole package in your final decision.

SELF-REFLECTIVE QUESTIONS

1. What do I need to thrive day to day in this job? What do I need and want in order to grow? Is there a path forward for me here?
2. What value will I add to my future workplace? What do they have to learn and gain from me?
3. What is my number one priority for my first job?

RESOURCES

CNN Money: Cost of living: how far will my salary go in another city? Atlanta, GA, CNN, January 2021. Available at: https://money.cnn.com/calculator/pf/cost-of-living. Accessed August 25, 2021.

Fisher R, Ury W, Patton B: Getting to YES: Negotiating Agreement Without Giving In, 3rd Edition. New York, Penguin, 2011

Lean In: Negotiation advice for women. Palo Alto, CA, Lean In Foundation, 2021. Available at: https://leanin.org/negotiation. Accessed August 25, 2021.

Malhotra D: Four strategies for making concessions. Cambridge, MA, Harvard Business School, March 6, 2006. Available at: https://hbswk.hbs.edu/item/four-strategies-for-making-concessions. Accessed August 25, 2021.

Medscape: Medscape salary explorer. Medscape, 2021. Available at: www.medscape.com/physician-salary-explorer. Accessed August 25, 2021.

Medscape: Medscape physician compensation report 2020. Medscape, 2021. Available at: www.medscape.com/sites/public/physician-comp/2020. Accessed August 25, 2021.

Shonk K: Negotiation advice: when to make the first offer in negotiation. Cambridge, MA, Program on Negotiation Daily Blog, Harvard Law School, July 26, 2022. Available at: www.pon.harvard.edu/daily/negotiation-skills-daily/when-to-make-the-first-offer-in-negotiation. Accessed October 3, 2022.

REFERENCES

Babcock L, Gelfand M, Small D, et al: Gender differences in the propensity to initiate negotiations, in Social Psychology and Economics. Edited by Cremer DD, Zeelenberg M, Murnighan JK. New York, Routledge, 2006, pp 239–259

Hernandez M, Avery DR, Volpone SD, Kaiser CR: Bargaining while Black: the role of race in salary negotiations. J Appl Psychol 104(4):581–592, 2019 30335407

CHAPTER 36

Beyond Training

Board Certification and Continuing Medical Education

Ashley E. Walker, M.D.
Tessa L. Manning, M.D.

The completion of residency training is a monumental achievement that should be celebrated. It also represents an early milestone in what should be a physician's lifelong journey toward learning and honing their craft. Because many learning activities in residency are prescribed and supplied by others, it can be daunting for an early-career physician to access and curate the wide array of postresidency educational opportunities. Additionally, it is important for senior residents to plan to obtain board certification just after graduation. This can be an overwhelming process during a time when you will likely also be starting your first job out of residency or a new fellowship program. In this chapter we provide a guide to navigating the self-directed learning required after residency training and a clear understanding of the board certification process.

KEY POINTS

- Psychiatry residents should register and begin preparing for initial board certification early in their senior year.

- After obtaining initial board certification, psychiatrists must then devise a plan to fulfill all of the requirements in the maintenance of certification program.

- Continuing medical education and other opportunities ensure physicians engage in the practice of lifelong learning.

INITIAL BOARD CERTIFICATION

Board certification is an extra step that most physicians choose to complete after residency. Traditionally, being board certified indicates a physician is an expert in their specialty, meets the highest standards, and works continually to improve the quality of care they deliver to their patients. Practically, most physicians are also compelled to complete this process to meet requirements of insurance panels and employers.

Psychiatrists in the United States become board certified through the American Board of Psychiatry and Neurology (ABPN), a member board of the American Board of Medical Specialties (ABMS). In order to apply for initial certification, an applicant must have a license to practice medicine in at least one U.S. state or Canadian province. Additionally, applicants must have successfully completed an Accreditation Council for Graduate Medical Education–accredited or ABPN-approved residency training program in the United States or Canada or be on track to finish training before taking the examination. If you will be graduating residency off-cycle, check the ABPN website (www.abpn.com) to see whether you meet requirements to take that year's exam. You must obtain initial certification in an ABPN primary specialty prior to obtaining subspecialty certification if you plan to complete a fellowship. Also, the examination for board certification must occur within 7 years following completion of your residency program. You may take the exam as many times as available during the 7-year period.

All details about the exam, including information about registration, test dates, scoring, reporting, examination procedures, and special accommodations for nursing mothers and applicants with disabilities, can be found at the ABPN website. The exam is typically administered annually in September, but dates are subject to change. Make sure to register for and schedule your exam early so that you can get a spot at the testing center of your choice. Registration generally opens the November before you take the exam, with the deadline for initial registration and payment in February. Results are typically available in 8–10 weeks. The pass rate for first-time exam takers from 2016 to 2020 was 88% (American Board of Psychiatry and Neurology 2021b).

Several published texts and comprehensive programs are available for purchase to help you prepare for the certification examination. A list of popular materials is provided in the "Resources" section at the end of this chapter. You are encouraged to select study methods (books, question banks, groups, courses) on the basis of how you learn best. It is also important to devise a scheduled study plan prior to taking your examination. After obtaining your materials, estimate how much time you will need per week to complete your review prior to taking the exam and then schedule specific time blocks in your day to devote to study only. Cramming for this type of exam likely will not yield satisfactory results. You are also advised to review the APBN website regarding the details of the exam (which are subject to change), such as the number of questions and amount of time allotted for test taking and breaks. The website will also have demonstration exams and sample screens you can review to familiarize yourself with the format.

MAINTENANCE OF CERTIFICATION

Once a psychiatrist completes the initial ABPN board certification requirements and passes the exam, they are designated a diplomate of the ABPN and enrolled in the Continuous Maintenance of Certification (C-MOC) Program. Documentation of completion of all requirements will be via the online ABPN Physician Folios (American Board of Psychiatry and Neurology 2021a) website, which includes a list of all approved products for each component of C-MOC. Currently, the requirements must be fulfilled and attested in 3-year blocks and generally include the following:

- Maintenance of an active, full, unrestricted medical license in the United States or Canada
- Completion of a specified number and type of continuing medical education (CME) credits
- Completion of improvement in medical practice activities
- Regular evaluation of knowledge (through recertification exams or a journal-based reading and assessment program)

In order to maintain active certification, you must also pay a yearly fee through the ABPN Physician Folios account. If you are employed, you might receive a budget to cover CME credits and your board certification fees.

Generally, you will receive a certificate of completion for CME courses. It is wise to have an organized digital or paper file to keep these certificates so that you have proof of your completion of requirements in case you are ever audited by the ABPN. It is not recommended that you attempt to complete all of your C-MOC requirements in the months just before each 3-year block is ending. Having a plan to slowly accumulate regular credits will ensure that you do not make this mistake. This is also more likely to keep you up to date in the field and continuing to improve your clinical practice.

Multiple Board Certifications

Physicians who hold multiple board and subspecialty certifications must participate in maintenance of certification requirements separately for each program. However, CME credits earned can be applied to the requirements for multiple programs.

Alternative Board Certification

Increasingly, some physicians are choosing not to renew certification with the ABMS programs, expressing frustration that the C-MOC requirements are overly time-consuming, burdensome, and costly. In reaction to this controversy, an alternative board, the National Board of Physicians and Surgeons (NBPAS; https://nbpas.org) was formed. Diplomates who are initially certified by any ABMS program (including ABPN) are eligible to apply for board certification through the NBPAS. Requirements include only a valid medical license in at least one U.S. state and submission of CME credits (50 hours every 24 months). However, you are encouraged to discuss this option with your employer before pursuing this route because many insurance companies and hospital credentialing committees do not recognize this certification.

CONTINUING MEDICAL EDUCATION

CME includes educational activities designed to develop, increase, or maintain medical knowledge, skills, and attitudes on an ongoing basis after training (during training, scheduled didactic activities ensure residents are up to date in these areas). In addition to obtaining CME credits to meet licensure and board certification requirements, you also may obtain CME to meet specific practice needs (e.g., new billing and coding guidelines). Hopefully, the desire to engage in lifelong learning and genuine interest in your field also motivate you to engage in CME.

Each U.S. state medical board has its own requirements for CME credits to maintain your medical license. Although states' requirements are different, it is typical that ABPN MOC requirements will meet most if not all of your state's requirements. Some common exceptions are specific extra credits for opioid prescribing safety or medical ethics. Physicians licensed through an osteopathic board are subject to CME requirements that must be American Osteopathic Association accredited. Your state's osteopathic medical board will have additional information about CME credits that will qualify. You are encouraged to look at the specific requirements of your state and certifying boards. Most medical boards will randomly select a number of licensees to audit each year to verify that CME requirements are being met. Again, make sure you are keeping records of your certificates of completion for this purpose.

There are many opportunities for CME in varied formats, including journals, conferences, and podcasts (see "Resources"). If you stay in an academic setting after graduation, you will likely have easy and free access to ongoing learning through grand rounds, faculty development workshops, and institutional access to journals. These may also be available (and sometimes paid for) if you are in larger hospital or other practice settings, whereas if you are in a smaller, private practice setting, you likely will need to seek out and pay for these opportunities on your own. If you have any interest in teaching but do not want a full-time academic position, it may be worth volunteering with a local medical school or residency training program because volunteer faculty appointments often provide access to institutional libraries and opportunities to collaborate. Publishing papers and precepting medical students may also earn you CME credits.

Conferences, whether in person or virtual, have long been a traditional form of acquiring annual CME credits. In addition to primary specialty organization (e.g., American Psychiatric Association) and subspecialty or niche organization (e.g., American Association for Geriatric Psychiatry, American College of Neuropsychopharmacology) conferences, your state medical association and state branch of the American Psychiatric Association likely have annual or ongoing CME events, which also offer opportunities for local networking. Industry-sponsored CME events also abound, although they carry increased risk of bias that may unduly influence treatment decisions and may be proscribed for individuals working in academic settings.

PROFESSIONAL GROWTH BEYOND CME

The transition from residency to independent practice is often a time of tremendous professional growth. It is not uncommon for a first-year attending physician to find that they were leaning more heavily on supervision than they realized. For this reason, purposefully seeking and asking for mentorship is encouraged. You may seek this from someone more tenured within your organization or someone you respect in the field with whom you have formed a trusting relationship. Simply asking is typically all that is necessary. However, many early-career psychiatrists also pay for supervision for improving both general clinical practice and psychotherapy skills. These resources are best found through professional networking. Networking events at state and national organization meetings are a good place to meet others from whom you can seek assistance, especially if you are working in a specialized field. These relationships can also serve as a way to seek consultations for complicated cases. It will also be helpful to make an intentional effort to network with other clinicians in your community to better understand local resources for your patients and support for your practice.

Opportunities abound for professional growth after residency beyond the basic expectations of meeting CME requirements. Consider joining or forming an in-person or virtual supervision group with colleagues from residency or in your community that meets regularly. This allows you to draw on the expertise and experience of others in the field, as well as cultivate support in a career that can be emotionally and cognitively challenging. Joining a book or journal club that focuses on psychiatric practice or professional development is also a common way to foster growth.

Other forms of non-CME venues for continuing professional growth include seeking your own individual therapy, attending retreats or leadership trainings (often offered through your employer), obtaining additional certifications, participating in clinical research, publishing articles, joining social media professional groups, and teaching others. Multiple prospects for teaching are available even if you are not a member of an academic organization. Consider becoming a volunteer faculty member at your local medical school or residency program. This will also help you form relationships with other physicians as they transition into independent practice. Who knows? They may ask you to be a mentor one day.

SPECIFIC CHALLENGES AND STRATEGIES

⌘ **I'm not sure I need to pursue board certification.** Not all physicians choose to become board certified in their specialty. Some may later decide not to renew. Although this choice can be made for a number of reasons, it can lead to limitations in your ability to practice and deserves careful consideration. For example, many hospital and academic medical systems require board certification for you to receive privileges to practice. It is also possible for insurance plans and third-party payers to refuse to add a physician to their panel or to offer different reimbursement of professional fees on the basis of board certification status. Patients and employers may also equate board certification with a higher-quality physician, leading to a lack of competitiveness in certain markets. Make sure that you understand the full ramifications of your current and future employment prior to making a decision about obtaining or maintaining board certification.

⌘ **I'm having difficulty budgeting my time and finances for CME.** Finding and scheduling the amount of time you will need to complete CME requirements should be considered on a yearly basis. Typically, it takes an hour to complete a 1-hour CME credit. Most physicians need a minimum of 20–30 hours of CME per year to maintain their certifications. Many conferences, journals, newsletters, and other forms of CME require fees. Many employers provide CME funds that can be used for these purposes. If you work in a private practice or do not have access to employer funds, you will need to budget money each year for this purpose. However, there are a number of ways to obtain CME credits free of charge. These are easily accessed if you are part of an academic institution or work as volunteer faculty for a medical school. You also have the option to obtain free CME credits from local and national psychiatric associations if you pay for a yearly membership.

⌘ **I'm lacking motivation to keep up with all these requirements.** After exiting the structured learning environment of training and being faced with the demands of clinical practice, you may find it difficult to maintain the individual momentum to sustain lifelong learning. Prioritize topics that are interesting to you and will keep you fresh in your practice, such as new neuromodulation techniques or addressing racial inequities in patient care. There is no reason ongoing education has to be done alone. The recent explosion of virtual learning options has introduced more ways than ever to maintain old connections and form new ones. Your residency classmates will likely take the initial board certification exam and complete maintenance of certification requirements at the same time. Consider forming a group that meets regularly once a month (or more, before the initial exam) in person or via videoconferencing. The added benefit of maintaining social connections is that it can boost your well-being. This group might also provide peer support regarding challenging clinical cases or issues related to practical or business management concerns.

SELF-REFLECTIVE QUESTIONS

1. What will be my study plan for board certification? What resources do I need? How much time will I need?
2. What knowledge and skills do I need to develop to become a more expert psychiatrist?
3. How will I budget my time for lifelong learning while also working?

RESOURCES

Selected Board Certification Study Resources

American College of Psychiatrists: Purchase old PRITES. Chicago, IL, American College of Psychiatrists, 2002. Available at: www.acpsych.org/prite/purchase-old-prites. Accessed October 8, 2022.

American Psychiatric Association: Psychiatry review and exam prep for psychiatrists. Washington, DC, American Psychiatric Association, 2022. Available at: www.psychiatry.org/psychiatrists/education/apa-learning-center/psychiatry-review-and-exam-prep. Accessed October 8, 2022.

Beat the Boards!: Psychiatry certification board review. Westmont, IL, American Physician Institute, 2022. Available at: www.beattheboards.com/psychiatry-board-review-certification. Accessed October 8, 2022.

BoardVitals: Psychiatry board review questions and practice tests. New York, BoardVitals, 2022. Available at: www.boardvitals.com/psychiatry-board-review. Accessed October 8, 2022.

Muskin PR, Dickerman AL: Study Guide for the Psychiatry Board Examination. Arlington, VA, American Psychiatric Association Publishing, 2016

Sadock BJ, Ruiz P, Sadock VA: Kaplan and Sadock's Study Guide and Self Examination Review in Psychiatry, 9th Edition. Philadelphia, PA, Lippincott, Williams & Wilkins, 2011

Spiegel JC, Kenny JM: Psychiatry Test Preparation and Review Manual, 4th Edition. New York, Elsevier, 2020

Stern TA, Herman JB, Rubin DH: The Massachusetts General Hospital Psychiatry Update and Board Preparation, 4th Edition. Boston, Massachusetts General Hospital Psychiatry Academy, 2017

TrueLearn: Psychiatry certification practice questions: ABPN certification test prep. TrueLearn, 2022. Available at: www.truelearn.com/psychiatry/psychiatry-abpn-board-exam. Accessed October 8, 2022.

Selected CME and Lifelong Learning Resources

AudioDigest—www.audio-digest.org: CME credits and Board review through high-quality audio files

Carlat Psychiatry Report—www.thecarlatreport.com: a CME newsletter subscription offered for general psychiatry, child and adolescent psychiatry, hospital psychiatry, and addiction treatment themes

Clinical Care Options—www.clinicaloptions.com: numerous free virtual webcasts and simulcasts, although they may have industry funding

Focus: The Journal of Lifelong Learning in Psychiatry—https://focus. psychiatryonline.org: a journal published by the American Psychiatric Association that offers clinical reviews and original research for practicing psychiatrists to keep abreast of significant advances in the field

MasterPsych CME to go—www.masterpsych.com/psychiatry-cme-to-go: all necessary yearly ABPN credits in audio format

National Neuroscience Curriculum Initiative—www.nncionline.org: a comprehensive set of shared resources to train psychiatrists and other mental health professionals to integrate a modern neuroscience perspective into every facet of their clinical work

Psychopharmacology Institute—https://psychopharmacologyinstitute. com: paid membership for access to video lectures, podcast episodes, and a newsletter

Simple and Practical Mental Health—https://simpleandpractical.com: monthly subscription service that provides regular email topic updates and access to website resources for mental health clinicians

UpToDate—www.wolterskluwer.com/en/solutions/uptodate: subscribers can use time spent researching clinical information toward CME requirements

Social Media Physician Groups

Psychiatry Network— www.facebook.com/groups/psychnetwork: Facebook group that periodically hosts live webinars and journal clubs

Women's Psychiatry Group—www.facebook.com/groups/womens psychiatrygroup: Facebook group for women in psychiatry for support, learning, and networking

Podcasts

Carlat Psychiatry Podcast: www.thecarlatreport.com/podcast

Neuroscience Education Institute (NEI) Podcast: https://podcasts. apple.com/us/podcast/nei-podcast/id288425495

Psychiatry and Psychotherapy Podcast: www.psychiatrypodcast.com

Forums and Blogs

APA Blogs: www.psychiatry.org/news-room/apa-blogs
Reddit Psychiatry: www.reddit.com/r/Psychiatry

Medical News Websites

Doximity: www.doximity.com/newsfeed
Medscape: www.medscape.com
MindSiteNews: https://mindsitenews.org
Science Daily: www.sciencedaily.com/news/mind_brain/mental_health

Selected High-Quality Journals

See Table A–1 in the Appendix, "Self-Directed Learning."

REFERENCES

American Board of Psychiatry and Neurology: ABPN physician folios. Deerfield, IL, American Board of Psychiatry and Neurology, 2021a. Available at: https://apps.abpn.com/physicianportal/folios.aspx. Accessed September 9, 2021.

American Board of Psychiatry and Neurology: Pass rates for first-time takers. Deerfield, IL, American Board of Psychiatry and Neurology, May 10, 2021b. Available at: www.abpn.com/wp-content/uploads/2022/02/ABPN-Pass-Rates-First-time-Taker-5-year-2021.pdf. Accessed September 9, 2021.

PART 6

Maintaining a
Professional and
Personal Life

CHAPTER 37

Work-Life Integration

Accomplishing Your Professional and Personal Goals

Elizabeth E. Hathaway, M.D.
Jessica L.W. Mayer, M.D.
You Na P. Kheir, M.D.
Joanna Chambers, M.D.
Raziya S. Wang, M.D.

Residency is a momentous time in any physician's career. It is a period of significant personal growth filled with both triumphs and challenges as you evolve into a competent and autonomous physician. The intensity of the experience contributes to its transformative effect but also brings great stress because life outside residency does not stop. Beyond meeting self-care needs, residents also may face weighty personal obligations and challenges. Reflecting on your professional and personal priorities while securing workplace and personal support is fundamental to accomplishing your goals and maintaining a sense of balance.

KEY POINTS

- Anticipating the full range of life stressors during residency training will help you be intentional about identifying your priorities and your supports.

- Reflecting on your personal and professional priorities as you start residency and then revising them as you progress through training will help you make choices that align with your values.

- Accessing structured workplace supports, which are common across programs, can be essential to work-life balance.

- Leaning on your personal support system will nourish both your professional and your personal activities and help you meet challenges.

ANTICIPATING POTENTIAL STRESSORS

As a resident, you may experience a broad range of stressors during training, including personal stressors, work stressors, and, at times, community and societal stressors (Figure 37–1).

Personal life events and experiences enrich our lives, but they may also bring additional difficulty. Some examples include relationships, caregiving, loss and grief, physical or mental health issues, sleep deprivation, immigration status, minoritized identity, and religious questioning. Furthermore, residency falls during a time in life when you may desire to bring children into your family. Unfortunately, infertility in physicians has been documented at higher rates than in the general population, with as many as a quarter of female physicians being diagnosed with infertility (Stentz et al. 2016). Compounding the issue is the exorbitant cost of fertility treatments (often out of pocket on a tight resident salary), particularly given their relatively low success rates. Similarly, the financial, emotional, and time commitments related to gestational surrogacy, fostering, or adoption also can take their toll. These reproductive traumas affect all domains of life and can have long-term effects such as increased depressive symptoms, diminished well-being, and more health problems (Becker et al. 2019; Mahlstedt 1985; Rogers et al. 2008).

Work-related stressors in residency may include interpersonal conflicts, low morale, long work hours, patient deaths or suicide, discrimination, racism, lack of program or institutional diversity, limited access to health care, and few work-life policies. Unresponsive program leadership can further magnify these issues.

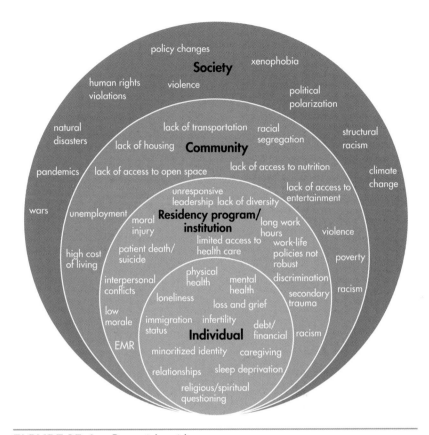

FIGURE 37–1. Potential resident stressors.

Note. EMR=electronic medical record.

Source. Adapted from Bronfenbrenner 1977, 1979.

In addition to personal and work-related stressors, community and societal stressors may also affect your work. A few examples include lack of community access to housing, nutrition, transportation, or entertainment; racism and racial segregation; and violence, poverty, natural disasters, pandemics, and wars. Although these problems require more systemic changes and interventions, it is important to recognize and acknowledge how you are personally being affected by challenges at all levels.

Psychiatry training itself may intensify and personalize life's stressors. In listening to the problems of your patients, you may find that they are similar to or relate to your own stressors; although this may stir empathy, it can also make it more challenging to help them and to manage countertransference. Similarly, you may experience secondary trauma in your work with patients in great psychological suffering, or you may experience moral injury when a systemic constraint conflicts with your personal values.

REFLECTING ON PROFESSIONAL AND PERSONAL PRIORITIES

Knowing your priorities will help you navigate the wide range of stressors throughout your psychiatry training. For example, identifying your particular interests, whether in research, psychodynamics, public psychiatry, or a particular subspecialty path, helped you make choices about the type of training program you sought as a student. Once you are in residency, you might choose certain mentors, rotations, projects, or groups that nourish these interests. However, your interests may evolve, and it will be important to reassess your priorities over time. Sometimes, your personal interests, such as your health, family considerations, or cultural factors, may be far more important priorities. It is important to reflect on all your values and priorities so that you have this scaffolding to fall back on in challenging times. Consider writing a personal mission statement or simply making a list of personal and professional goals to aid in this reflection.

WORKPLACE SUPPORTS

Each program has its own culture when it comes to structured supports, but many aspects of support are common across programs.

Faculty Mentors

Mentors may share similar professional or personal interests with you. Whether brief or long-term, connections with faculty mentors can help ease the transition to residency as well as provide guidance and emotional support in the face of challenges. Mentors may be particularly helpful in your navigation of boundaries during residency. Boundaries are useful as you seek the work-life balance that you desire and select or eliminate opportunities in line with your short- and long-term goals. With each new opportunity, think realistically about your priorities and desires and be honest about the time commitments they will bring. The time must come from somewhere; opportunities you pursue will either take away time elsewhere (frequently self-care or personal time) or push lower priorities out. Mentors may have helpful guidance as you navigate your choices and the interpersonal and professional implications that each path may hold (see Chapter 33, "Mentorship and Sponsorship").

Resident Buddy and Big Sib Programs

Buddy programs link postgraduate year 1 (PGY-1) or PGY-2 residents and senior residents together. As a new psychiatry resident, you may find that your senior residents are a repository of information unavailable anywhere else. Each program has its own culture when it comes to protecting time for professional experiences, such as didactics, psychotherapy education (including personal psychotherapy), attending national meetings, and interviewing for fellowship. In addition, each program's culture and policies affect time for personal experiences, such as family leave, part-time status, and weekend and holiday coverage. Your senior residents can give you invaluable advice ranging from which conferences to attend to how to use the program's parental leave.

Mental Health and Well-Being Resources

Most residents experience stressors and challenges during training and will have a wide range of associated emotions. Mental health and well-being resources for residents have more recently been prioritized by the Accreditation Council for Graduate Medical Education and should be available at all programs. There may be a variety of options to seek out, from burnout self-assessments to support groups. If affordable, engaging in your own personal psychotherapy may allow you to have a safe place to work through emotions while contributing to your understanding of psychotherapy practice.

Work-Life Policies

As you consider personal priorities such as your health or starting your own family, it is important to clarify your program's work-life policies, particularly because policies may vary by state (Van Niel et al. 2020) and by program (Riano et al. 2018). Although residency programs on the whole have trended toward greater support for residents requiring accommodations or family leave, formally requesting support or leave at various programs may range from a common and supported occurrence to a rare and isolating event. Talk to residents who have used the policies or to your program director, who can be helpful when policies are not clearly communicated otherwise.

Childcare

Appropriate childcare is a common logistical and financial concern for residents who have children. Whether choosing a daycare or in-home care such as a nanny or an au pair, these decisions are very personal to each parent. Some residents may find that working on a part-time basis offers the best arrangement for their family, if your residency allows it. However, even with the best-laid plans for childcare coverage, there are many contingencies to anticipate, including last-minute backup coverage in case of child or provider illness and such occurrences as doctor appointments. Having a supportive program can make a world of difference in how you feel about your ability to balance parenthood and work. Relevant program attributes may include on-site childcare, structured backup call, and a general program philosophy that is tolerant and non-shaming of last-minute needs.

Lactation Rooms

Women who wish to breastfeed may find pumping at work to be onerous. Health systems vary in their level of accommodation and the availability of lactation rooms. Navigating these accommodations with various attending physicians or practice settings can feel awkward. Advance notice, potentially including blocking time in the clinic schedule, and talking to other residents and staff who have pumped in the relevant health system may help smooth the way. Additionally, reaching out to the Graduate Medical Education office may serve as a resource if your program is not supportive.

Confidential Reporting Structures

Sometimes, residents experience harassment or discrimination during training. Workplace policies prohibit these behaviors and often include confidential reporting structures for mistreatment. It may be worthwhile to make note of the appropriate phone numbers in advance so that you can access them easily in a stressful moment (see Chapter 4, "The Underrepresented in Medicine Experience").

Moonlighting

Most residents enter training with educational debt that causes stress and may affect quality of life. In addition to using loan deferral programs, many psychiatry residents pursue moonlighting to supplement their income. Depending on the program, moonlighting (either in-house or external) may be actively encouraged, grudgingly approved, or even prohibited. Many types of moonlighting opportunities exist, from outpatient clinics to inpatient coverage, with a variety of schedules and responsibilities. Senior residents are often the most knowledgeable about moonlighting opportunities in the area. Many residents find moonlighting has other benefits, including learning about other systems of practice, exposure to different patient populations, developing self-confidence in an independent professional identity, and increasing comfort in evaluating and treating patients.

Program Administration

Although using supports may be necessary at times, it is also important to communicate with your program when you feel overwhelmed or face a personal situation that conflicts with the demands of residency. Talking to your mentors, attendings, and program director allows them to provide emotional support, direct you to appropriate resources, and collaborate with you to find helpful solutions to challenges. You cannot help others with competence and compassion if you are under duress, so be sure to honor your feelings and your need to adequately manage stressors.

PERSONAL SUPPORTS

In residency, personal time may be scarce, with inflexible or unpredictable work schedules adding to the strain of limited time. On top of clinical duties, seemingly innumerable other tasks pile up: annual trainings, didactic readings, running errands, paying bills. Fatigue may manifest in various forms, including sleep deprivation, difficulty focusing, or burnout, all of which trigger a sense of exhaustion with every patient interaction. Many of these stressors are familiar to medical students but frequently bring new intensity in residency. The optimal strategies to manage these challenges will vary by person and may require trial and error. Thoughtful self-care, using your support system, and organizational skills all may play a role in managing these challenges (see Chapter 38, "Wellness").

Self-Care

Self-care is extremely personal to you, so keep in mind that what may feel like self-care to one person can often be a stressor for another. Be honest about your own needs at any given time, and find what works for you.

Your Support System

Your support system may include loved ones and friends outside work as well as coresidents, mentors, and program directors from your institution. Taking time to maintain connections with your family and friends can be both meaningful and enjoyable, and it can offer a buoy when you need it most. Making friends with other residents brings a sense of camaraderie and an understanding of a demanding shared experience, and friends from outside the medical field bring pleasant reminders of life beyond the hospital and clinic.

Managing Chores

Finding time to get groceries, maintain a livable home, do laundry, and meet other demands can become daunting. Maintaining a calendar and a simple to-do list may be helpful if tasks tend to slip off the radar. An organized schedule may help fit these tasks in more efficiently, but it may be worthwhile to pay for help with these tasks. Paying for a house cleaner, laundry service, or grocery pickup can feel extravagant, especially when facing debt from training, but it may be worth the extra free time and associated mental health benefits.

SPECIFIC CHALLENGES AND STRATEGIES

⌘ **I feel like I'm working all the time, and it's overwhelming.** Maintaining a life outside work is helpful for de-stressing and keeping perspective on challenges on the job. You may find it helpful to schedule time for hobbies, or you may find it more pleasant to see where unstructured time takes you. Either way, you are encouraged to make time for enjoyable activities. You may prefer compartmentalizing, focusing solely on work-related tasks during defined parts of the day, or you may enjoy mixing in leisure activities while catching up on lingering tasks outside work. It may take some time to figure out how to balance your time in a way that feels most comfortable for you.

⌘ **I'm afraid to let my program know that I'm struggling.** It's understandable to be concerned about sharing difficulties with a supervisor or program director who has an evaluative role in your training. Consider initially connecting with your personal support system and with coresidents, mentors, or the chief resident for advice and support within your program. However, it is important to remember your responsibility to patient care. If you are not well, your patient care will likely also suffer. Ultimately, you may need to speak with your program director to request accommodations or even take a leave of absence. Physicians who care for themselves well care for their patients well (see Chapter 40, "Physician Impairment").

SELF-REFLECTIVE QUESTIONS

1. What are my professional and personal values? Do my goals align with my values? How have these goals evolved over the course of my educational, personal, and professional life?
2. Have I had past experiences in which I balanced personal and professional obligations particularly well or particularly poorly? What factors might have led to each?
3. What workplace and personal supports might be available to me during my residency training?

RESOURCES

General Residency Resources

American Psychiatric Association: Resources for residents: www.psychiatry.org/residents-medical-students/residents
American Psychoanalytic Association: https://apsa.org

Family-Related Resources

Birth Injury Guide: A comprehensive resource for families coping with birth injuries. Houston, TX, Birth Injury Guide, 2021. Available at: www.birthinjuryguide.org. Accessed October 7, 2022.
The Compassionate Friends: www.compassionatefriends.org—support for family after a child dies
First Candle: https://firstcandle.org—support for families experiencing sleep-related infant deaths.
HealGrief: https://healgrief.org—social support network for individuals grieving people or pets.
RESOLVE: The National Infertility Association: https://resolve.org

REFERENCES

Becker MA, Chandy A, Mayer JLW, et al: Resource document on psychiatric aspects of infertility. APA Resource Document. Washington,DC, American Psychiatric Association, February 2019. Available at: www.psychiatry.org/File%20Library/Psychiatrists/Directories/Library-and-Archive/resource_documents/Resource-Document-2019-Psychiatric-Aspects-of-Infertility.pdf. Accessed August 1, 2020.
Bronfenbrenner U: Toward an experimental ecology of human development. Am Psychol 32(7):513–531, 1977
Bronfenbrenner U: The Ecology of Human Development: Experiments in Nature and Design. Cambridge, MA, Harvard University Press, 1979

Mahlstedt PP: The psychological component of infertility. Fertil Steril 43(3):335–346, 1985 3979571

Riano NS, Linos E, Accurso EC, et al: Paid family and childbearing leave policies at top US medical schools. JAMA 319(6):611–614, 2018 29450516

Rogers CH, Floyd FJ, Seltzer MM, et al: Long-term effects of the death of a child on parents' adjustment in midlife. J Fam Psychol 22(2):203–211, 2008 18410207

Stentz NC, Griffith KA, Perkins E, et al: Fertility and childbearing among American female physicians. J Womens Health (Larchmt) 25(10):1059–1065, 2016 27347614

Van Niel MS, Bhatia R, Riano NS, et al: The impact of paid maternity leave on the mental and physical health of mothers and children: a review of the literature and policy implications. Harv Rev Psychiatry 28(2):113–126, 2020 32134836

CHAPTER 38

Wellness

Am I Well or Am I Burned Out?

Kristen Kim, M.D.
Rashi Aggarwal, M.D.

Psychiatry residency training is undoubtedly a challenging experience. As a resident, you spend 4 years with little control over your daily schedule and often face seemingly insurmountable demands and expectations within an imperfect health system. Maintaining wellness as you go through this process can be difficult. Stress is normal, expected, and even adaptive, but burnout is problematic and requires attention. Unsurprisingly, residents are more likely to experience burnout compared with the general population (Dyrbye et al. 2014). The first step in enhancing wellness and combating burnout is to ask yourself, *Am I well, or am I burned out?*

KEY POINTS

- Wellness is more than the absence of burnout.

- Stress is normal, but burnout is not and is important to address.

- Burnout is a systemic problem that requires systemic solutions.

- Individual strategies to enhance well-being can also be helpful.

WELLNESS AND RESILIENCE

Case Vignette: Taylor

Taylor is a psychiatry resident. After taking a nap and eating a healthy dinner, she drives to the hospital for a Saturday night call shift. As she interviews a suicidal patient in the emergency department, Taylor grows concerned and takes care to conduct a thorough suicide risk assessment. After determining that the patient is at a low acute risk for suicide, Taylor reviews safety plans with the patient and discusses return precautions before discharging him. During morning sign-out, the day team questions Taylor's decision to discharge the patient. Taylor is initially flustered but then explains her clinical reasoning behind the decision and gracefully accepts feedback.

Is Taylor well or burned out? Do you identify with any of Taylor's thoughts, emotions, or behaviors? Are you well or burned out?

Myth: *Wellness is the absence of burnout.*

Fact: Just as health is not defined as the absence of disease, wellness is not simply the absence of burnout. Rather, it is the presence of frequent positive affect and high life satisfaction. It means being well in all aspects of your life, including physical, mental, and emotional. Resilience is a related concept that is defined as the ability to adapt to and bounce back from the stress of the clinical environment. Resilience allows a resident to recover from the unavoidable stresses of residency training without lasting negative consequences.

Myth: *It is impossible to be well during residency training.*

Fact: Despite the barriers, it is possible to be well during residency training. Both organizational and individual interventions for enhancing wellness have been shown to be effective (Panagioti et al. 2017; Shanafelt and Noseworthy 2017). Burnout is fundamentally a systemic problem and thus requires systemic changes, which likely are beyond an individual resident's control. However, there are ways that you can approach your training to optimize your chances of maintaining wellness, as we discuss later in this chapter.

Case Vignette: Taylor *(continued)*

Taylor seems stressed but is able to engage in her work and express empathy toward her patient. Even when under pressure, Taylor is able to explain her clinical reasoning and accept feedback as part of the training process. In short, Taylor is appropriately dealing with stress and is not burned out.

BURNOUT AND MORAL INJURY

Case Vignette: Sam

Sam is a psychiatry resident. He dreads driving to the hospital for a Saturday night call shift. As he interviews a suicidal patient in the emergency department, Sam feels apathetic and rushes through the interview to get enough information to adequately fill out a consultation note. After discharging the patient, Sam feels relieved and crosses the patient's bed number off his to-do list. During morning sign-out, the day team questions Sam's decision to discharge the patient. Sam becomes defensive and leaves the hospital feeling discouraged.

Is Sam well or burned out? Do you identify with any of Sam's thoughts, emotions, or behaviors? Are you well or burned out?

Myth: *If I am stressed, I am not well.*

Fact: Stress is normal, expected, and even adaptive during residency training. As you have likely experienced during medical school, stress can facilitate learning and motivation to grow as a clinician. On the contrary, burnout can lead to serious consequences and is important to address.

Myth: *It is my fault if I am burned out.*

Fact: Burnout is an individual's response to excessive work-related stress characterized by emotional exhaustion, depersonalization, and a diminished sense of personal accomplishment (Maslach and Jackson 1981). An individual resident experiences burnout, but the root cause of burnout lies within the greater system—that is, the residency training program, the institution, and the health system at large—and not within the individual trainee. Moral injury, a related concept, captures the distress that one experiences as a result of the clash between one's moral values and a health system that makes it impossible to act according to those values. As a resident, you sacrifice your time, energy, finances, and youth to training because you want to help patients. Furthermore, you were likely attracted to psychiatry because you value spending time with and getting to know your patients on a deeper level. However, as a resident, you may find yourself having to spend more time documenting in the electronic health record than talking to your patients. You may be forced to discharge homeless patients to the streets because no alternative disposition options are available. You may be asked to discharge patients from the inpatient setting sooner than you think is clinically appropriate because of pressures from their insurance company. These are just a few examples of how residents may experience moral injury on a day-to-day basis. In short, burnout and moral injury are signs of a broken system that needs to be fixed.

Myth: *Psychiatrists specialize in mental health, so they do not struggle with burnout or depression.*

Fact: Despite our expertise in mental health topics, psychiatrists are human and not immune to burnout or its consequences, including mental illness. In a recent study, 78% of psychiatrists scored ≥35 on the Oldenburg Burnout Inventory, suggesting high levels of burnout, and 16% scored ≥10 on the Patient Health Questionnaire–9 (PHQ-9), suggesting a diagnosis of major depression (Summers et al. 2020). Of participants who rated themselves as moderately or severely depressed, 98% also had significant burnout. Notably, resident or early-career participants tended to have higher PHQ-9 scores. Another meta-analysis estimated that the prevalence of depression or depressive symptoms among residents was 29% (Mata et al. 2015). Furthermore, residents who are burned out are more likely to experience suicidal thoughts compared with those who are not (van der Heijden et al. 2008). Therefore, burnout is a serious, potentially life-threatening problem and requires prompt attention.

Myth: *The patient's preferences or needs always come before mine.*

Fact: Residents who experience discrimination, abuse, or harassment from patients are more likely to endorse symptoms of burnout and suicidal thoughts (Hu et al. 2019). Workplace discrimination occurs when others treat you less favorably because of your race, color, religion, sex, sexual orientation, gender identity, national origin, disability, status as a protected veteran, or other characteristics. It can range from more subtle forms, such as microaggressions, to more blatant forms, and it can certainly be damaging to wellness. You have the right to work in a safe environment that is free of workplace mistreatment. If you experience workplace mistreatment, use the reporting mechanisms in place at your institution, which may include speaking confidentially with an ombudsperson, and/or reach out to the Accreditation Council for Graduate Medical Education at www.acgme.org/Residents-and-Fellows/Report-an-Issue. See Chapter 4, "The Underrepresented in Medicine Experience," and Chapter 5, "Gender and Sexual Identity."

Case Vignette: Sam *(continued)*

Sam has reached the point of dreading work, treating patients as tasks rather than as people, and feeling cynical. He is likely at a point of burnout and needs to take active steps to address this. Be aware that some rotations might predispose you to feel burned out.

ORGANIZATIONAL INTERVENTIONS TO PROMOTE WELLNESS

As the alarming prevalence of physician burnout gained national attention, burnout shifted from being viewed as an individual issue to being viewed as a systemic one that requires systemic solutions. Organizational interventions to promote wellness have the strongest evidence for effectiveness (Panagioti et al. 2017; Shanafelt and Noseworthy 2017). Many interventions can be cost-effective and easy to implement (Aggarwal et al. 2019). Although there is no one-size-fits-all solution for all residency training programs or institutions, multiple guidelines have been established to assist leaders in improving wellness within their organizations. For instance, the American Psychiatric Association's Work Group on Psychiatrist Wellbeing and Burnout developed a step-by-step model for organizational interventions (American Psychiatric Association 2022). Your residency training program and the larger health system are responsible for implementing these interventions.

INDIVIDUAL INTERVENTIONS TO PROMOTE WELLNESS

Burnout is a systemic problem that requires systemic interventions, but individual interventions are also encouraged and necessary. Furthermore, they are simpler, easier, and faster to implement. Although it may seem contradictory to suggest individual interventions in light of the fact that burnout is a systemic problem, the following tips may help you remain healthy so that you can optimize your chance of being well. Remember, it can be difficult to incorporate the following on a regular basis, especially during busier rotations, and it is important to approach each intervention with self-compassion.

Practice Patient-Centered Care

The most stressful moments in residency are often due to the barriers you face as you try to help your patients. These barriers (e.g., hospital protocols, limitations of treatment options and resources) result in your inability to provide high-quality, empathetic care for your patients. Although it is important to recognize one's limitations, it is equally important to resist allowing them to lead to a sense of futility and cynicism. Whenever you are able, advocate for your patients and brainstorm creative ways to help them. For example, patients suffering from severe mental illness may find it difficult to navigate outpatient medical services on their own. As their inpatient psychiatrist, you can refer them to case management services or advocate for them to receive outpatient care while in the hospital to ensure access and compliance. Such actions may lead not only to improved care for the patient but also to a greater sense of fulfillment for you.

Search for Meaning and Purpose

Finding meaning and purpose in your work can contribute to greater fulfillment and happiness. At work, allow yourself to be fully present and actively listen to your patients. As described in the previous subsection, keep your patients at the center of your care. Get involved in other areas of psychiatry that excite you, such as advocacy, community outreach, scholarly activities, education, and mentorship. If you identify areas for improvement in your residency training program, get involved and promote the changes you would like to see. Although these activities may require additional time and energy, you may find that they rejuvenate rather than drain you.

Embrace Community

Enhancing your sense of belonging both at home and at work can improve your wellness. Stay in touch with your roots and make time for your friends and family back home. For example, set a specific time every week to call your loved ones. Because you will be spending many hours at work, build community at the hospital or clinic. Get to know your coresidents, attending physicians, nurses, social workers, and security guards. The interdisciplinary nature of psychiatry requires teamwork and coordination, so developing good relationships with your coworkers will not only make work more enjoyable but also help you accomplish your work more efficiently and effectively.

Set Boundaries

Although it is likely you became a doctor to help others, it is important to set appropriate boundaries and make time for your own needs. Set boundaries with others and learn to say no to inappropriate requests or demands. Make an agreement with your coresidents to see new patients only until a certain hour and normalize signing out unseen consultations to the incoming resident. Turn off your pager when you are off duty. Avoid taking work home, and set timers for yourself to limit the time you spend on documenting in the electronic medical record.

Maintain Balance

The phrase *work-life balance* creates undue stress for most people because it implies that one must juggle work and life tasks and try to keep as many tasks in the air as possible. This concept presents work and life as a dichotomy and pits them against each other. It may be more helpful to recognize that we all have multiple identities: we are parents, siblings, spouses, children, students, psychiatrists, athletes, violinists, and so on. In order to be fully realized human beings, we must embrace all the identities that are meaningful to us. The key is to recognize that at different life stages, different identities may be more important to attend to. If you are a parent to a newborn baby, your identity as a parent is important. If you are in college, your identity as a student is important. When you start residency, your identity as a resident is important. At each stage, we must recognize the identities that are most meaningful to us and invest more of our time and energy in them. It is the balance of how much we cultivate each identity over time that matters. See Chapter 37, "Work-Life Integration."

Seek Positivity

Day-to-day stresses can lead to focusing on things that are not going well. Taking a couple of minutes every day to focus on things that are going well can have an impact on your ability to deal with stress. Neuroscience studies show that people who tend to be happy have greater amygdala reactivity to positive stimuli. Practicing gratitude or optimism-based exercises can improve your overall well-being. For example, try downloading the Three Good Things phone app and input three things that went well for you every night before you go to bed. This exercise can promote your well-being and resilience (Rippstein-Leuenberger et al. 2017).

Reframe

Incorporation of cognitive-behavioral principles or therapy can have positive impacts on sleep, fatigue, depression, and work engagement (Melnyk et al. 2020). Consider applying the cognitive-behavioral skills you teach your patients or working through a manual such as MINDSTRONG, a cognitive-behavioral skill-building program that has been associated with decreases in depression and anxiety as well as healthier lifestyle behaviors (Melnyk et al. 2022).

Breathe

When we are stressed, our stress response system leads to activation of the sympathetic nervous system, leading to tachycardia and hypertension. Paying attention to your breath for a few minutes can disengage your sympathetic nervous system and activate parasympathetic response. A simple way to do this is to practice diaphragmatic breathing. Set a 1-minute timer, sit comfortably, take a deep breath in, let your belly expand, and then exhale, paying attention to your belly going in and out.

Be Mindful

If diaphragmatic breathing is not your cup of tea, plenty of other mindfulness exercises are available to help you reduce stress, anxiety, and depression (Melnyk et al. 2020). Some other examples of mindfulness activities include keeping a gratitude journal or visualization exercises during which you imagine yourself in a relaxing, safe space. Download an app such as Insight Timer, Calm, or Headspace for guided meditations.

Don't Forget the Basics

If your schedule permits, go back to the basics but without guilt because, again, it is not your fault that you are burned out. Eat healthy when you can and make sure you squeeze in time for at least a snack during busy shifts. Exercise as much as you can; for example, take the stairs when possible. Prioritize sleep as you are able and get blackout curtains or eye masks for postcall days. And always be safe—do not drive to and from work when sleepy.

SPECIFIC CHALLENGES AND STRATEGIES

⌘ **I am still not sure whether I am well or burned out.** Additional resources for self-assessment of stress, sleepiness, burnout, well-being, depression, and anxiety are available in the "Resources" section. However, these tools are limited, and sometimes self-assessment can be inaccurate. If you are concerned that you may be burned out, reach out to your colleagues, mentors, and training directors for support and/or seek professional help.

⌘ **I am burned out, but I am afraid of seeking help because of potential professional repercussions.** Many residents avoid reaching out for help for similar reasons. This is a valid concern because some states require physicians to report their mental health history on licensing applications. Nevertheless, burnout is crucial to address because it can have far-reaching consequences for the individual resident and the patients they care for (e.g., an increase in medical errors) (Tawfik et al. 2018). Ultimately, systemic changes are needed to create a safer environment for physicians to seek help. In the meantime, consider reaching out to someone you trust or search for confidential and low-cost mental health services that are outside your grading and evaluation pathways within your institution, in the community, or online.

⌘ **I experienced an adverse event at work.** As a psychiatry trainee, you are more likely to face adverse events, such as patient suicide or violence. Such events can be extremely distressing, demoralizing, and isolating. Prioritize your wellness after an adverse event by taking time away from work to allow yourself to experience and process your emotions in a way that is most helpful for you (e.g., talking to loved ones, writing about the experience, engaging in hobbies). Early in your training, identify the protocols that exist in cases of patient suicide or violence so you know whom to reach out to if needed.

SELF-REFLECTIVE QUESTIONS

1. What does wellness mean to me?
2. How can I enhance my own wellness and prevent burnout?
3. Do I know how and whom to approach for support in my training program and/or institution?

RESOURCES

Websites

American Medical Association: www.ama-assn.org/topics/physician-burnout

American Medical Association STEPS Forward: https://edhub.ama-assn.org/steps-forward

American Psychiatric Association: https://psychiatry.org/psychiatrists/practice/well-being-and-burnout

Screening Tools

Epworth Sleepiness Scale: www.cdc.gov/niosh/emres/longhours training/scale.html

GAD-7 Anxiety Screening: www.mdcalc.com/calc/1727/gad7-general-anxiety-disorder7

Mental Health America Stress Screener: www.mhanational.org/get-involved/stress-screener

988 Suicide & Crisis Lifeline: https://988lifeline.org

Oldenburg Burnout Inventory: https://www.mdapp.co/oldenburg-burnout-inventory-olbi-calculator-606/

PHQ-9 Depression Screening: www.mdcalc.com/calc/1725/phq9-patient-health-questionnaire9

Phone Apps (Available on iOS and Android)

Calm
Headspace
Insight Timer
Sleep Cycle
Three Good Things

REFERENCES

Aggarwal R, Kim K, O'Donohoe J, et al: Implementing organizational strategies for resident well-being: practical tips. Acad Psychiatry 43(4):400–404, 2019 30805860

American Psychiatric Association: Well-being and burnout. Washington, DC, American Psychiatric Association, 2022. Available at: https://psychiatry.org/psychiatrists/practice/well-being-and-burnout. Accessed October 4, 2022.

Dyrbye LN, West CP, Satele D, et al: Burnout among U.S. medical students, residents, and early career physicians relative to the general U.S. population. Acad Med 89(3):443–451, 2014 24448053

Hu YY, Ellis RJ, Hewitt DB, et al: Discrimination, abuse, harassment, and burnout in surgical residency training. N Engl J Med 381(18):1741–1752, 2019 31657887

Maslach C, Jackson SE: The measurement of experienced burnout. J Organ Behav 2(2):99–113, 1981

Mata DA, Ramos MA, Bansal N, et al: Prevalence of depression and depressive symptoms among resident physicians: a systematic review and meta-analysis. JAMA 314(22):2373–2383, 2015 26647259

Melnyk BM, Kelly SA, Stephens J, et al: Interventions to improve mental health, well-being, physical health, and lifestyle behaviors in physicians and nurses: a systematic review. Am J Health Promot 34(8):929–941, 2020 32338522

Melnyk BM, Hoying J, Tan A: Effects of the MINDSTRONG© CBT-based program on depression, anxiety and healthy lifestyle behaviors in graduate health sciences students. J Am Coll Health 70(4):1001–1009, 2022 32672515

Panagioti M, Panagopoulou E, Bower P, et al: Controlled interventions to reduce burnout in physicians: a systematic review and meta-analysis. JAMA Intern Med 177(2):195–205, 2017 27918798

Rippstein-Leuenberger K, Mauthner O, Bryan Sexton J, et al: A qualitative analysis of the Three Good Things intervention in healthcare workers. BMJ Open 7(5):e015826, 2017 28611090

Shanafelt TD, Noseworthy JH: Executive leadership and physician well-being: nine organizational strategies to promote engagement and reduce burnout. Mayo Clin Proc 92(1):129–146, 2017 27871627

Summers RF, Gorrindo T, Hwang S, et al: Well-being, burnout, and depression among North American psychiatrists: the state of our profession. Am J Psychiatry 177(10):955–964, 2020 32660300

Tawfik DS, Profit J, Morgenthaler TI, et al: Physician burnout, well-being, and work unit safety grades in relationship to reported medical errors. Mayo Clin Proc 93(11):1571–1580, 2018 30001832

van der Heijden F, Dillingh G, Bakker A, et al: Suicidal thoughts among medical residents with burnout. Arch Suicide Res 12(4):344–346, 2008 18828037

CHAPTER 39

Handling Mistreatment and Discrimination

Jessica Isom, M.D., M.P.H.

Aekta Malhotra, M.D., M.S.

J. Corey Williams, M.D., M.A.

Handling mistreatment and discrimination, although often neglected in formal orientation or didactic sessions, is essential for resident well-being. We define mistreatment as speech or behavior that shows disrespect for the dignity of others and significantly disrupts the learning process in an educational context. We define discrimination as the unjust or prejudicial treatment of different categories of people, especially on the grounds of social identities (e.g., race, age, sex). This includes any behavior that denigrates or disparages the person or seeks to associate the person with negative stereotypes. Although discrimination represents but one form of mistreatment, we use the terms discrimination and mistreatment interchangeably.

In this chapter we address discrimination and mistreatment that fall into three categories: 1) from patients (including their guests and families), 2) from colleagues (e.g., nurses, physicians, administration staff), and 3) from institutions (i.e., policies, norms, and practices). Each of these categories represents an important source of discrimination and mistreatment throughout residency, with personal and professional impacts well beyond residency.

We also discuss how mistreatment can be entangled in group dynamics in residency programs. This is a particularly concerning aspect of discrimination and mistreatment because of the psychological impact of marginalization from a group. Regardless of the source of mistreatment, you should be proactive about cultivating systems of support, including peers, program chiefs, and program leadership. Even in moments of relative normality, these support systems need to be in place to prevent incidents and address incidents that do occur.

KEY POINTS

- Mistreatment and discrimination are unfortunately very common and are never acceptable.

- Practicing structured or scripted responses to patient hate speech allows for preparedness and effective redirection in real time.

- Being proactive in establishing a support network of advocates and mentors at each institutional level can be helpful.

- Collective organizing is the most powerful way residents can advocate for themselves.

FORMS OF MISTREATMENT AND DISCRIMINATION

Mistreatment and discrimination can take many forms, ranging from subtle nuances of language to very explicit actions (Table 39–1). Explicit discrimination can be described as a conscious, intentional act, detectable by most observers, whereas implicit discrimination is more subtle and the result of unconscious attitudes or beliefs. To be clear, in the real world these can be difficult to distinguish. In terms of addressing the transgression, distinguishing between differences of explicit and implicit discrimination is less relevant when considering the impact of these behaviors on the target person. For example, racist hate speech is a form of explicit discrimination that is unambiguous, but racial microaggressions (e.g., a white nurse who addresses a Black resident by their first name while referring to their white colleague as "Dr.") can sometimes be difficult to detect by both perpetrators and targets. However, both types of discrimination can be very harmful.

TABLE 39–1. Examples of mistreatment and discrimination

Explicit and overt

Threatening or abusive language or profanity or language that can be perceived as rude, threatening, demeaning, sarcastic, loud, or offensive

Belittling or humiliating comments

Threats of physical harm, such as hitting, slapping, and kicking

Offensive sexist remarks or names

Racist or ethnically offensive remarks or names

Implicit and more subtle

Staff undermining the authority of the resident

Staff not referring to the resident as doctor or being overly familiar with the resident

Neglect or exclusion from communications

Source. Adapted from UTRGV School of Medicine 2021.

DISCRIMINATION IN RESIDENCY

You may have already experienced an incident of discrimination prior to residency. Issues of discrimination are all too common for residents. A national survey of 1,773 residents revealed that one-quarter had at least one experience of racial or ethnic discrimination during their first year of training, and nearly half reported that the incident came from a patient (Baldwin et al. 1994). In a survey of 823 physicians, two-thirds reported experiencing bias from patients based on a personal characteristic (Cajigal and Scudder 2017) (Figure 39–1).

In addition to understanding these statistics, we encourage you to have explicit conversations with your colleagues in your program about such incidents and listen carefully to understand and empathize, especially if you are a white-identified person and have not come across any discrimination thus far in your training.

Each of us possesses a number of social identities that represent distinguishing characteristics that may be easily observed (e.g., racial phenotype, gender-nonconforming appearance) or more hidden unless explicitly disclosed (e.g., sexual orientation, religion, socioeconomic status). In discussions of mistreatment and discrimination, it is important to identify majority (privileged) statuses and minority (marginalized) statuses. Targets of discriminatory behaviors are typically those possessing minority statuses, whereas agents are those engaging in the behavior (Table 39–2).

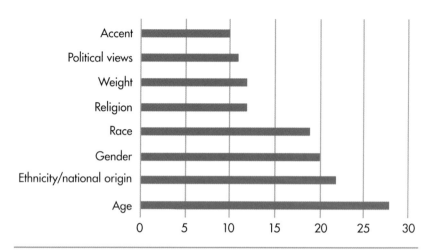

FIGURE 39–1.   Most commonly reported types of bias.
Source.   Adapted from Cajigal and Scudder 2017.

DISCRIMINATION AND MISTREATMENT FROM PATIENTS, FAMILIES, AND GUESTS

Discrimination and mistreatment from patients present a specific challenge to residents, attending physicians, and medical centers due to the complex interactions of medicolegal statutes and cultural norms within institutions. These behaviors have increased recently in relation to a broader social climate in which a proliferation of hate speech and hate groups has been observed in connection with encouragement from prominent public officials (Potok 2017). Implicit forms of discrimination from patients might include a patient assuming that the racially minoritized physician is a nonphysician staff member, addressing minoritized physicians more informally (e.g., not addressing them as "Dr."), or speaking only to the white members of the medical team. More explicit forms of discrimination might include using racist or threatening hate speech, requesting white-only or male-only care, using racial stereotypes in jokes, assuming a staff member is an immigrant or a foreigner, or asking whether staff speak English or whether they are American.

First and foremost, you should never feel that experiencing discrimination by patients, their families, or guests is acceptable. Discrimination from patients denigrates you, corrupts your learning environment, and creates an atmosphere of toxic otherness that can impair the functioning of the clinical team and undermine patient safety.

TABLE 39–2. Social identity of agent and targets within the United States

Social identity category	Agent identity (possesses structural power)	Target identity
Age	Adults (18–64 years)	Children, adolescents, elders
Disability	Able persons	Persons with developmental or acquired disability
Religion and spiritual orientation	Cultural Christians, agnostics, and atheists	Jews, Muslims, and members of all other non-Christian religions
Race/ethnicity	White European Americans	People of color
Social class culture	Middle- and owning-class persons	Poor and working-class persons
Sexual orientation	Heterosexuals	Lesbian, gay, bisexual, trans, queer/questioning, and other persons (LGBTQ+)
Indigenous heritage	Non-Native persons	Native persons
National origin	U.S.-born individuals	Immigrants and refugees
Gender	Cisgender men	Intersex persons, transgender persons, cisgender women, gender-nonbinary persons, gender-questioning persons

Source. Adapted from Hays 2001.

Furthermore, discrimination in the workplace is *unlawful*. In particular, when patients make race-based requests for certain providers, this presents a medical liability to the hospital system (even though hospital systems typically grant these requests). In one large survey, almost half of the physicians had a patient request an alternative clinician on the basis of personal characteristics; the request was granted 83% of the time (Cajigal and Scudder 2017). In general, patients have the right to refuse care, and hospitals are obligated to provide care in emergency situations. However, the patient's rights do not supersede the employee's right to be free from discrimination in the workplace. In fact, relevant case law supports Black employees who are subjected to racist requests. In 2010, the U.S. 7th Circuit Court of Appeals ruled in favor of a Black employee who sued a nursing home for violations of Title VII of the 1964 Civil Rights Act, citing that acceptance of the patient's preference created a hostile work environment (Moore 2012).

You should feel empowered to redirect discriminatory speech or behavior from patients, employing a personal zero-tolerance policy even if the institution lacks one. At the moment of the encounter, finding the right words can be difficult. When in doubt, you always have the right to end an encounter and walk away to seek out additional guidance from team members. Be sure to check in with your physical, mental, and emotional reactions to the encounter because these behaviors can evoke a trauma response. This trauma reaction and need for space to process may be misconstrued by supervisors and colleagues as a dereliction of duties and unprofessional behavior if they do not understand your internal experience, which is often the case. If possible, articulate your needs to your supervisor (e.g., "I need a moment to gather myself"). If this is not possible, consider writing (e.g., email) a well-thought out message of your concerns and proposed next steps.

There are a number of communication frameworks a resident can use when presented with a challenging situation. The ERASE framework, originally designed to guide faculty in supporting trainees, includes principles that can help trainees as well (Wilkins et al. 2019). ERASE represents the following principles: 1) **E**xpect that mistreatment will happen. 2) **R**ecognize when mistreatment occurs. 3) **A**ddress the situation in real time. 4) **S**upport the trainee after the event. 5) **E**stablish a positive culture. See Table 39–3 for sample language you can use to address discrimination in real time.

Obtaining support can be challenging, especially when a supervisor is complicit in discrimination by neglecting their duty to support their trainee. Understanding the roles and responsibilities of the supervisor is imperative for residents to effectively advocate for themselves from a well-informed perspective. Ideally, a supervisor should debrief with you and other witnesses following the mistreatment. Supervisors should check in to assess whether you have any immediate needs. Any supervisor who suggests that you should not take the discrimination "personally" or that you should "get used to it" is being neglectful of an important, primary responsibility—supporting and protecting their resident from avoidable harm (Williams and Rohrbaugh 2019). Do not hesitate to report the behavior of the patient and that of the supervisor by using the established hospital reporting system or reporting directly to hospital leadership. If you fear retaliation, seek out a program director or other training leadership, an ombudsperson, a trusted colleague, or a mentor for additional guidance.

TABLE 39–3. Communication problems and interventions

Problem	Intervention	Example	Sample language
Overt derogatory language	Set clear limits	Patient uses a racial slur in reference to a student participating in their care	"This clinic/unit/ department is an area where we treat each other with mutual respect. We cannot tolerate that kind of language."
		Angry patient yells misogynistic term at female resident	"Mr. Y, we do not use that kind of language here. We are only trying to help you, which is harder to do when you talk like that."
Microaggressions	Educate/ explain	Patient addresses female trainee as "Nurse"	"As Dr. Z explained, she is a resident physician who is caring for you. Nurses in the hospital wear blue scrubs and will introduce themselves as your nurse."
		Family member asks Latinx trainee to serve as interpreter	"Mr. V, this is not the interpreter. This is J, one of the medical students on our team. Have you met?"
Compliments	Redirect/ reframe	Patient comments on student's attractive appearance	"I know you mean well, but we are more concerned about our students' skills and abilities than their looks."
		Patient associates resident's ethnicity with superior intelligence	"Mrs. U, Dr. W is an intelligent physician, but that has nothing to do with his ethnicity."

Source. Adapted from Wilkins et al. 2019.

Ultimately, the institution should be held accountable for protecting its trainees. Institutional preparedness is essential, especially given the regular occurrence of incidents of discrimination and maltreatment. Every medical center should have 1) a zero-tolerance policy that forbids all forms of hate speech and discrimination, 2) a system of reporting incidents that respects anonymity and protects reporters from fears of retaliation, and 3) a committee and/or officer who has the authority to review incident reports and issue sanctions, if necessary. A sanction might include the patient receiving a letter to reinforce code of conduct, a conversation with a committee representative, discharge, or transfer of care. If these structures are not in place, residents can consider organizing collectively to advocate for institutional accountability.

DISCRIMINATION AND MISTREATMENT FROM COLLEAGUES

Handling discrimination from colleagues, including faculty, staff, peers, and other employees, can also prove challenging because these situations often involve entrenched workplace norms, institutional politics, and power hierarchies. Similar to cases of patient behaviors, mistreatment from colleagues can come in explicit forms such as hate speech, derogatory comments, and physical and sexual assault, as well as implicit forms such as not referring to the resident by name, compelling the resident to work longer hours than others, holding the resident to a different standard than other residents, or neglecting the resident's educational experience.

Critically, whether discrimination is explicit or implicit, what matters is the impact of the discrimination, not the intention of the perpetrator. Appeals to intentions often undermine the issue of accountability and fail to address the impact of the behaviors on the trainee. Each incident needs to be addressed within its context and impacts, regardless of intentions. In addition, the intentions of the perpetrator should not dictate the institutional response or level of support the trainee should receive. What must be centered in the response is the behavior's impact on the trainee and the trainee's subsequent needs.

Therefore, you must empower yourself with information about institutional and program requirements in order to advocate effectively for yourself. The Accreditation Council for Graduate Medical Education (ACGME) institutional requirements are clear that sponsoring institutions must cultivate a learning environment that is respectful, equitable, civil, and free of discrimination or coercion of residents. Furthermore, programs must have procedures and policies to handle resident or fellow grievances at the program and institutional levels that minimize conflicts of interest (Accreditation Council for Graduate Medical Education 2018). Power dynamics can represent a form of coercion; therefore, it is also imperative in such cases that the inherent power differential between the parties be kept at the center of all inquiries to prevent further oppression of minoritized residents.

If you find that conflicts of interest and power differentials are being ignored and your due process rights are being violated, you should first and foremost raise this concern with the Graduate Medical Education (GME) office and your program leadership. If you fail to find recourse, you must consider formally elevating the issue to the ACGME. It would be worthwhile to consult with a trusted mentor outside the institution or the school's ombudsperson to guide you through this process. Consider seeking legal advice from an employment attorney well versed in residency and higher education issues. If you suspect that the program and the GME office are already flouting the ACGME guidelines, they are unlikely to change course without direct advocacy or intervention. As such, consider all avenues to protect your residency position and prevent any further detrimental course of action, including disciplinary action, before it is too late.

As in the case of mistreatment from patients, you should feel empowered to redress mistreatment and discrimination from colleagues. Of course, this is easier said than done. Redressing discrimination from colleagues often entails a complex calculation of different considerations: Is this worth the emotional taxation it will entail? Will I be retaliated against? Will this besmirch my reputation in the program? This calculus can be draining in and of itself. However, these are questions you must reconcile for yourself when seeking to act in response to discrimination from colleagues. Research shows that minoritized persons who mention experiences of discrimination can suffer experiences of further marginalization and stigmatization (Miller and Kaiser 2001). In our experience, having quality supportive relationships with program leadership or other senior faculty can mitigate the psychological toll that results from these mental calculations. Supportive relationships with leadership can provide some reassurance of your good standing in the program and give you a sense that you have backup in times when you feel it is necessary to address mistreatment.

In some cases, where mistreatment seems nuanced or may be a result of miscommunication, having an open dialogue with the colleague is the first step. To create a productive space for dialogue, consider the following approach: be direct, be specific, plan out the conversation, use "I" language, offer a solution, pay attention to your emotions, and be empathetic. However, in some circumstances, a one-on-one conversation is not viable because of power dynamics, a strained relationship, fears of retribution, or fears of violence. In these cases, you should lean on your support network and mentors in navigating the complex ecosystem of a department or hospital. The conversation with your support network should result in an action plan, which may entail a formal report made on your behalf, a meeting with a member of leadership, and/ or an ad hoc huddle on the clinical team. The action plan should be highly specific to the nature of the incident, institutional procedures, and politics.

DISCRIMINATION AND MISTREATMENT AT THE INSTITUTIONAL LEVEL

When discrimination occurs at an institutional level, be proactive about seeking out systems of support, which can be found in each level of the institution, including peers, program leadership, departmental leadership, hospital-wide leadership, and on a national level (e.g., organized psychiatry, social media networks). This can be challenging for minoritized persons, such as racial-ethnic minorities, religious minorities, and international medical graduates, who are often represented in small numbers within institutions. In cultures such as medicine that value conformity or adherence to dominant norms, a person speaking uncomfortable truths can be labeled as "disruptive" or "unprofessional" and be subject to workplace bullying, especially from supervising physicians (Leisy and Ahmad 2016). Speaking about equity, diversity, and discrimination can be discordant with the institution and leaders' self-image and can be met with denial and defensiveness. It is advisable to use anonymous reporting channels in such circumstances and instead focus on cultivating a professional career within a nurturing and inclusive environment.

Coalition building is particularly important to ensure strength in numbers whenever possible, which also helps to diffuse concerns about retribution. When starting a training program, you should begin to take meetings with potential allies and mentors to introduce yourself and your interests. These connections will act as an advocacy and support network not only for your career goals but also in times of need. In addition, it can be prudent to seek mentorship and support outside the institution when they are unavailable in the local milieu. Although organizations can be complicated and replete with inequalities, state psychiatric societies, national organized psychiatry, and local physicians groups can be avenues where you find a supportive community.

When an issue of mistreatment or discrimination has arisen, the chief resident is often the first line for support and guidance. Chief residents are advanced-level trainees who are closest to your experience and ideally can empathize with your circumstances. Assistant program directors can be the second line of support because they often work the closest with trainees among the program leadership. However, it is important to note that depending on the institutional culture, the chief residents and assistant program directors may have been chosen for their positions specifically to maintain alliance with the program and the institution rather than to advocate for the residents. If you are uncomfortable reaching out to program leadership, the staff within the department who have leadership positions related to diversity, equity, and inclusion, if present, can be sources of support. If there is no such officer in the department, then a hospital-wide and/or school of medicine–wide diversity officer should be available. It is unacceptable for you to fear retribution when reporting incidents of discrimination. If there is a culture of fear of retribution, this represents a failure of program leadership to establish an organizational climate of trust, psychological safety, and transparency.

Be sure to find opportunities for collective organizing in residency. Often, it may feel as if the trainees (and students) are the populations that are the most vulnerable to mistreatment, and this is often true. On the other hand, there is tremendous power in the collective student and trainee body. Having GME training programs and trainee rotators is central to the mission of the hospital, and this labor is critical for the institution's prestige, reputation, and funding. Leverage this cultural and economic capital to advocate for better working conditions and support for trainees who have experienced mistreatment. Existing data suggest that residencies that have formal associations tend to have better working conditions (Sklar et al. 2011). The National Labor Relations Board has ruled that residents at private hospitals are employees—with the same right to unionize as residents at public hospitals. However, collective organizing does not always have to be in the form of a formalized union and can also come from informal or ad hoc resident work groups that are focused on a particular issue.

It is critical for you to find out about access to mental health resources for residents. Taking time for your mental health and well-being is a crucial component of handling discrimination and mistreatment. Although there is a push among some programs to normalize residents being in therapy, in other programs stigma is still associated with open and honest dialogue about residents seeking mental health treatment. Call your insurance company and ask about in-network mental health resources. If benefits are lacking, this can be an opportunity for collective organizing and advocacy. Programs are mandated by the ACGME to allow residents to take time off during regular hours to attend medical and mental health appointments (Accreditation Council for Graduate Medical Education 2020). Collective organizing can also help with establishing an institutional climate that normalizes taking time for regular mental health help.

Last, be proactive about understanding your rights and responsibilities as a trainee. Go over your contract closely, especially if you are considering taking a leave of absence or if the program is seeking to terminate your contract prematurely. In some scenarios, residents have sought legal assistance for abuse allegations or for the program's unlawful termination of their contract. In these cases, legal outcomes have not been favorable for trainees, and the court has overwhelmingly sided with programs. This is partly a result of legal precedent of the courts largely deferring to the training program's professional judgment (Brown et al. 1994). However, these cases are very rare. Programs must also have an ombudsperson who is outside the department and can advocate for the trainee. It should be noted, however, that in institutions where resident mistreatment and discrimination are rampant, the mechanisms for reporting and investigation may exist on paper, but in reality, the policies can be purposefully vague to give the advantage to the institution.

Furthermore, ombudspersons and Offices of Diversity, Equity, and Inclusion may not be given any investigative power so as to further obfuscate the process for the resident or fellow and to tip the scales against the resident trying to obtain a fair and impartial process. If you find yourself the subject of a complaint, corrective action plan, or investigation that can potentially have legal implications, it is imperative to seek help from an employment attorney who specializes in higher education and academia as soon as possible. These processes can have far-reaching consequences for your entire career, and the longer you wait to seek legal help, the worse the outcome tends to be.

SPECIFIC CHALLENGES AND STRATEGIES

⌘ **When the patient called me a racial slur, I was not sure if I should respond or if I was allowed to respond.** Mistreatment and discrimination represent significant barriers to resident well-being, and efforts to address these occurrences should be central to any educational setting. It can be challenging to navigate power dynamics within a work environment, especially because of fear of retribution. Understand that you have the right to not be discriminated against in the workplace (as per the Civil Rights Act of 1964), and you should not normalize or accept such behavior. Be prepared with a set of verbal scripts that serve to disarm or halt discriminatory incidents.

⌘ **I am not sure how I would respond to racist hate speech from a patient.** Be empowered to redirect discriminatory speech or behavior from patients by employing a personal zero-tolerance policy even if the institution does not have one. Clinical supervisors are expected to be supportive of you in such instances. If they are not, this constitutes negligence on their part and may be worthy of report to program leadership. Hold your institution accountable for having a zero-tolerance policy that forbids all forms of hate speech and discrimination, a system of reporting incidents, and a committee and/or officer who has the authority to review incident reports and issue sanctions, if necessary.

⌘ **I am worried that if I report my supervisor, I will get a bad reputation in the program and eventually be removed from the program.** Proactively and intentionally seeking out allyship and mentorship is critical to building psychological safety if the program leadership or the organization lacks commitment or self-awareness regarding an oppressive learning environment.

⌘ **I am thinking about leaving my program because of discrimination, and I am unsure of my rights.** Closely examine contract details on roles, rights, and responsibilities and options for terminating your employment contract because of abuse. If you are facing disciplinary action or have been subjected to retaliation for reporting abuse, engage an employment attorney specializing in higher education and residency issues as soon as possible. The attorney can empower you with information and carefully guide you about the next steps, which may include an ACGME complaint, an Equal Opportunity Employment Commission complaint, a request for your residency file, and other steps to protect your education and career. The consequences of GME action on your record can be career altering. It would also be worthwhile to consult with the school's ombudsperson or a trusted mentor outside the institution to guide you through this challenging process. When faced with such a situation, seek out your employee assistance program (EAP) or your therapist and prioritize your mental health.

SELF-REFLECTIVE QUESTIONS

1. If a patient is threatening or uses hate speech targeted at me, what will I say? What will I do?
2. Whom among my colleagues do I trust? Whom will I reach out to in times of need?
3. What opportunities for collective organizing exist at my institution?

RESOURCES

Goldenberg MN, Cyrus KD, Wilkins KM: ERASE: a new framework for faculty to manage patient mistreatment of trainees. Acad Psychiatry 43(4): 396–399, 2019

Rice T: Medical residents and academic due process: know your rights. Medpage Today's KevinMD.com, May 20, 2018. Available at: www.kevinmd.com/blog/2018/05/medical-residents-and-academic-due-process-know-your-rights.html. Accessed August 7, 2021.

Rice T: Understand your resident contract: what you don't know may hurt you. Medpage Today's KevinMD.com, June 17, 2020. Available at: www.kevinmd.com/blog/2020/06/understand-your-resident-contract-what-you-dont-know-may-hurt-you.html. Accessed July 21, 2021.

REFERENCES

Accreditation Council for Graduate Medical Education: ACGME institutional requirements. Chicago, IL, Accreditation Council for Graduate Medical Education, February 4, 2018. Available at: www.acgme.org/Portals/0/PFAssets/ProgramRequirements/800_InstitutionalRequirements_2021.pdf?ver=2021-02-19-090632-820. Accessed March 14 2021.

Accreditation Council for Graduate Medical Education: ACGME program requirements for graduate medical education in psychiatry. Chicago, IL, Accreditation Council for Graduate Medical Education, February 3, 2020. Available at: www.acgme.org/Portals/0/PFAssets/ProgramRequirements/400_Psychiatry_2020.pdf?ver=2020-06-19-123110-817. Accessed March 7, 2021.

Baldwin DC Jr, Daugherty SR, Rowley BD: Racial and ethnic discrimination during residency: results of a national survey. Acad Med 69(10)(suppl):S19–S21, 1994 7916815

Brown M, Shah PV, Brody A, et al: Litigation in residency training programs and suggested due process guidelines for "residents in trouble." Acad Psychiatry 18(3):119–128, 1994 24442464

Cajigal S, Scudder L: Patient prejudice survey: when credentials aren't enough. Medscape, October 18, 2017. Available at www.medscape.com/slideshow/2017-patient-prejudice-report-6009134. Accessed on March 7, 2021.

Hays PA: Addressing Cultural Complexities in Practice: Assessment, Diagnosis, and Therapy. Washington, DC, American Psychological Association, 2001

Leisy HB, Ahmad M: Altering workplace attitudes for resident education (A.W.A.R.E.): discovering solutions for medical resident bullying through literature review. BMC Med Educ 16:127, 2016 27117063

Miller CT, Kaiser CR: A theoretical perspective on coping with stigma. J Soc Issues 57(1):73–92, 2001

Moore S: The continued reign of Title VII: racial discrimination trumps patient's preferences. Tennessee Journal of Race, Gender, and Social Justice 1(1):185–189, 2012

Potok M: The year in hate and extremism. Montgomery, AL, Southern Poverty Law Center, February 15, 2017. Available at: www.splcenter.org/fighting-hate/intelligence-report/2017/year-hate-and-extremism Accessed April 15, 2021.

Sklar D, Chang B, Hoffman BD: Commentary: experience with resident unions at one institution and implications for the future of practicing physicians. Acad Med 86(5):552–554, 2011 21646972

UTRGV School of Medicine: What is mistreatment? Brownsville, University of Texas Rio Grande Valley, 2021. Available at: www.utrgv.edu/som/student-affairs/student-mistreatment-learning-environment/what-is-mistreatment/index.htm. Accessed April 2, 2021.

Wilkins KM, Goldenberg MN, Cyrus KD: ERASE-ing patient mistreatment of trainees: faculty workshop. MedEdPORTAL 15:10865, 2019 32051848

Williams JC, Rohrbaugh RM: Confronting racial violence: resident, unit, and institutional responses. Acad Med 94(8):1084–1088, 2019 30681449

CHAPTER 40

Physician Impairment

Iverson Bell, M.D., DLFAPA

Paul Hill, M.D.

Allison Ford, M.D.

Hugh Caldwell, M.D.

Jeffrey Hunt, M.D.

Raziya S. Wang, M.D.

Clinical training is a time of new activity, learning, and responsibility. The experience can be a source of great achievement and growth, yet this period can also be very challenging. Residents experience a variety of stressors, and some may experience significant health and wellness issues and even impairment. Physician impairment is defined as the inability of a physician to practice safely as result of a mental disorder, a physical illness or condition, or a substance use disorder. Although some agencies conflate illness with impairment, the Federation of State Medical Boards (2008) notes that

> Physician illness and impairment exist on a continuum with illness typically predating impairment, often by many years. This is a critically important distinction. Illness is the existence of a disease. Impairment is a functional classification and implies the inability of the person affected by disease to perform specific activities" (p. 1)

In this chapter we review how to recognize the potential for impairment in ourselves, our peers, or those in supervisory positions and discuss ways to seek treatment and support recovery.

KEY POINTS

- Anticipating common stressors during residency training can prevent future impairment.

- You should learn to recognize the signs of potential impairment in yourself as well as in coresidents and attending physicians.

- Seeking treatment early for yourself or supporting others seeking treatment promotes recovery from impairment.

ANTICIPATING STRESSORS AND PREVENTING IMPAIRMENT

One author estimates the rate of physician impairment as about 15% over a professional career, similar to other professions (Boisaubin 2009), but the exact scope of the problem is largely unknown because of the confidential nature of reporting. Residency training can be a time of stress, making residents more vulnerable to mental health issues (including substance use), physical health issues, and burnout. Untreated illness may result in impairment over time. Common potential causes of stress among new psychiatry residents include navigating the transition from medical school to residency and adjusting to a new city, institution, and training cohort. Once in residency, professional stressors may include fatigue from long shifts and experiences with patient suffering, negative outcomes, or clinical acuity. Personal stressors may include limited time for self-care, leisure, or social connections (Swensen and Shanafelt 2020). A more detailed list of stressors can be found in Chapter 37, "Work-Life Integration."

These stressors can be very impactful. A study of more than 15,000 internal medicine residents showed that more than 50% experienced burnout (West et al. 2011). Another study noted that minority medical students were almost five times more likely than nonminorities to report that their race had a negative impact on their training because of discrimination, prejudice, or isolation. The students were also more likely to experience burnout and depression (Dyrbye et al. 2007). Another study reported that 58.2% of participating medical students, 50.8% of residents and fellows, and 40% of early-career physicians screened positive for depression (Dyrbye et al. 2014). Although individuals can experience stress, depression, or burnout without becoming impaired, there is increasing acknowledgment that when left untreated, these conditions may result in physician impairment (Broquet and Rockey 2004; Brown et al. 2009). Substance use among residents may also be a source of impairment. Although estimations of substance use among physicians vary, an older study found that psychiatry and emergency medicine residents had higher rates of substance use than did residents in other specialties (Hughes et al. 1992).

However, all is not lost. By anticipating these residency-related stressors and addressing mental illness, physical conditions, and burnout, you can work to prevent impairment during your residency training. The Accreditation Council for Graduate Medical Education (ACGME) requires that your institution actively participate in wellness initiatives and provide you with the support and care you need. Check out the American Psychiatric Association's well-being resources listed in the "Resources" at the end of the chapter and review your institution's policy on resident wellness. Proactively connecting to personal supports (friends; family; and religious, cultural, and community organizations), prioritizing personal health (sleep, exercise, and nutrition), as well as seeking treatment for any psychiatric or medical conditions will all help prevent impairment (see Chapter 38, "Wellness: Am I Well or Am I Burned Out?"). If you need treatment, consider self-referring to a psychologist and/or psychiatrist, as appropriate. Often, residency programs keep a list of available and confidential resources, perhaps through a university health clinic or the Graduate Medical Education office at your institution. Word of mouth or asking a trusted colleague or training director may be another option for finding referrals.

Finally, feeling a sense of community in your program can be helpful. Reach out for support from your coresidents, chief residents, and program director when you are struggling or notice a colleague or supervisor who may need assistance. Advocate for increased awareness of discrimination and racism in your program because challenging inequities is a critical part of ensuring your and your colleagues' own wellness as well as appropriate care for your patients (see Chapter 39, "Handling Mistreatment and Discrimination").

RECOGNIZING IMPAIRMENT

In spite of your best efforts to manage stressors or access treatment, you might continue to feel unwell. In this situation, it is important to learn how to monitor yourself for signs of impairment. Have you been struggling with significant personal or professional stressors? Have you been experiencing depression, burnout, substance use, or a medical condition? Do these experiences make it hard to keep up with clinical responsibilities such as reading for didactics or charting for clinic? Do you find yourself unable to contain anger at work or find yourself more easily engaged in conflicts? Starting with an online burnout self-assessment or meeting with a mental health provider for an evaluation can be helpful. Even if your symptoms are not yet having an impact on your capacity to function as a resident, it is important to seek help to avoid potential future impairment.

Impaired Resident Colleagues

In addition to taking care of ourselves, watching for impairment in coresidents can support their recovery as well as protect patient care. Apparent intoxication at work, the scent of alcohol on the breath, and a disheveled appearance are clear signs of a coresident's impairment. More commonly, you may notice personality changes, tardiness or missed shifts, or mistakes that your colleague would not usually make. Pay attention to changes in your coresident's dependability or a decline in the quality of their work. Watch for errors and alert your coresident or the treatment team if necessary. Most importantly, listen to your coresidents. Notice increasing cynicism and irritability; be concerned about withdrawn or isolating behavior, self-criticism, or low self-worth; and take seriously any speech or messaging relating to suicide.

If you are worried about your peer, consider sharing your observations and concern with them, probing gently and refraining from judgment. Offer resources and/or connect them to other supports, such as your chief resident or program director. Your coresident might deny that anything is wrong or may feel that you are the first person willing to listen. If your peer is not ready for assistance, you can only continue to make yourself available as a support. Ultimately, however, if patient safety is at risk, you have a duty to report this to your program director. By informing your program director before a patient is harmed, you may save your coresident's career.

Peer Suicide

Among residents, suicide is the leading cause of death in male residents and the second-leading cause for female residents, with the majority of deaths occurring in the first and second years of training (Yaghmour et al. 2017). Compounding this situation is the fact that physicians may be reluctant to discuss and seek help for suicidal thoughts (Brooks 2017).

Job problems around the time of death are more common in physicians who die from suicide than in others who die from suicide (Langballe et al. 2011). These problems especially include disciplinary actions and other potentially humiliating events such as failure on examinations or in rotations. The aftermath of a patient suicide, including litigation, is another high-risk period. These risk factors are in addition to untreated depression and other mood disorders and particularly substance abuse.

Given the very high stakes with regard to missing the cues of a colleague in distress, it is important to look out for the risk factors for physician suicide and to maintain open conversations with peers. A culture of openness can be facilitated through structured modules available from the Suicide Prevention Section of the WELL Toolkit (University of Pittsburgh Medical Center 2021). One particularly helpful exercise is "seize the awkward," which enables residents to practice having difficult or awkward conversations about a peer's mental health concerns (Seize the Awkward 2020). These conversations can be incredibly helpful in facilitating engagement and intervention during times of deep despair.

Impaired Attending Psychiatrists

You may be concerned about impairment in a supervisory or attending physician. Understandably, you may feel a sense of loyalty or deference toward your attending that makes it hard to broach the subject. In addition, the existing power dynamic might cause you to hesitate to report the attending for fear of retaliation or worries about shaming them. Seeking support and guidance from your chief resident and/or program director may be useful. Most, but not all, states require that health care professionals report colleagues who are impaired. In some states, reporting requirements are met if a referral is made to the state physician health program (American Society of Addiction Medicine 2020). No one wants to be in the position of reporting their attending for concerning behavior, but it could be the move that saves a patient, the attending's career—or even the attending's life.

SEEKING HELP

Similar to reporting impairment in others, it is not uncommon for impaired residents to fear repercussions from seeking help for themselves. However, if you are impaired and do not access resources, the consequences for yourself and your patients could be grave. As mentioned in the section "Anticipating Stressors and Preventing Impairment," the ACGME requires that your program provide you access to affordable care, including an emergent mental health assessment. Review your institution's resources for guidance on how to seek help and how to report a concern. Your institution's priority—in addition to ensuring patient safety—is to provide you with the care you need.

In addition to institutional resources, most states have established physician health programs (PHPs) that operate under the auspices of the Federation of State Physician Health Programs (2018). PHPs are tasked with overseeing the care of physicians struggling with substance use disorders. Self-referral or mandated treatment can be an alternative to corrective action when a physician is reported for concerning behavior. PHPs provide evaluation and diagnosis, develop an agreement with the physician for treatment and monitoring, assist with coordinating treatment, and implement monitoring with regular drug screening, usually for 5 years. In a study of 16 PHPs, 78.7% of physicians engaged in the programs were licensed and working after 5 years (McLellan et al. 2008). This positive outcome makes engagement in PHPs a hopeful opportunity for recovery and return to practice. The American Society of Addiction Medicine recommends that impaired physicians be referred to PHPs rather than receive punitive action (American Society of Addiction Medicine 2020).

Physicians should be granted the same protections and care as patients as determined by the Americans with Disabilities Act (ADA). Although some state medical boards continue to ask questions regarding physician mental illness, the American Psychiatric Association recommends that the boards not inquire about mental illness (American Psychiatric Association 2018). Furthermore, such questions are increasingly challenged as unlawful under the ADA (Jones et al. 2018). Fortunately, many state physician advocacy programs support and speak for recovered and recovering physicians. These programs facilitate the needs of the practicing physician, but the rules and effectiveness of these programs vary by state.

SPECIFIC CHALLENGES AND STRATEGIES

⌘ **I'm afraid to tell anyone that I'm feeling burned out, and I am getting further and further behind in my clinic charting.** Fear that disclosure could lead to academic or professional repercussions often makes it hard to ask for help or access care. In addition, some states require reporting of mental health treatment for licensure. However, burnout and most psychiatric issues worsen if left untreated, sometimes with devastating consequences. Although the pile of delinquent notes may seem daunting, and burnout makes it hard to take any action, consider taking the single initial step of reaching out to a trusted colleague, friend, or family member. Or consider accessing the emergency health care services that your institution is required to provide for you.

⌘ **I noticed that my attending smelled like alcohol during rounds on the inpatient consultation-liaison service this morning, but her clinical care seemed fine.** When a colleague or attending shows evidence of substance intoxication in the workplace, it is not your responsibility to determine their level of impairment. In addition, because you are a resident, the evaluative role of the attending and her power in the medical hierarchy likely preclude your being able to discuss your concerns with her directly. Any intoxication in the workplace is inappropriate and should be reported. If you are not sure how to do this, program leadership and chief residents should be able to assist. Remember that reporting will ultimately benefit patient care and the provider as well.

⌘ **I confronted my coresident about his missing rounds, showing up late, and delaying discharge orders on his patient, but he just brushed me off.** Taking a nonjudgmental, curious, and kind approach can go a long way when you want to discuss concerns about a peer's workplace behavior. An invitation to talk more or a gentle inquiry about how things are going, rather than a confrontation, might demonstrate your genuine concern and build enough trust for your coresident to confide in you. Normalizing workplace struggles, stress, and burnout can help destigmatize his experience, and reminders about mental health resources may decrease barriers to seeking his own care. However, if he continues to dismiss your concern, you may need to just remain available in case he changes his mind at a later time. Consider elevating the issue to program leadership if your concerns persist or patient safety is an issue.

SELF-REFLECTIVE QUESTIONS

1. What stressors can I anticipate in my next rotation? How can I promote my own self-care?
2. Am I having difficulty meeting my professional responsibilities? Am I showing signs of impairment?
3. Do I know what my institution's resources are for mental health or substance use treatment?

RESOURCES

Accreditation Council for Graduate Medical Education: ACGME common program requirements section VI with background and intent. Chicago, IL, Accreditation Council for Graduate Medical Education, February 2017. Available at: www.acgme.org/globalassets/PFAssets/ProgramRequirements/CPRs_Section-VI_with-Background-and-Intent_2017-01.pdf. Accessed March 13, 2021.

AMA Council on Mental Health: The sick physician: impairment by psychiatric disorders, including alcoholism and drug dependence. JAMA 223(6):684–687, 1973 4739202

American Psychiatric Association: Well being resources. Washington, DC, American Psychiatric Association, 2022. Available at: www.psychiatry.org/psychiatrists/practice/well-being-and-burnout/well-being-resources. Accessed March 13, 2021.

Chisolm M, Lyketsos C: The Systematic Psychiatric Evaluation: A Step-by-Step Guide to Applying the Perspectives of Psychiatry. Baltimore, MD, Johns Hopkins University Press, 2012

Federation of State Physician Health Programs: www.fsphp.org/state-programs

McGugh P, Slavney P: The Perspectives of Psychiatry, 2nd Edition. Baltimore, MD, Johns Hopkins University Press, 1998

Mossman D: Physician impairment: when should you report? Current Psychiatry 10(9):67–71, 2011

Tokarz JP, Bremer W, Peters K: Beyond Survival: A Book Prepared by and for Resident Physicians to Meet the Challenge of the Impaired Physician and to Promote Well-Being Through Medical Education. The Challenge of the Impaired Student Workgroup on Physician Well-Being, Resident Physicians Section. Chicago, IL, American Medical Association, 1979

Wible P: Human Rights Violations in Medicine: A-to-Z Action Guide. Self-published, 2019

REFERENCES

American Psychiatric Association: Position statement on inquiries about diagnosis and treatment of mental disorders in connection with professional credentialing and licensing. Washington, DC, American Psychiatric Association, July 2018. Available at: www.psychiatry.org/File%20Library/About-APA/Organization-Documents-Policies/Policies/Position-2018-Inquiries-about-Diagnosis-and-Treatment-of-Mental-Disorders-in-Connection-with-Professional-Credentialing-and-Licensing.pdf. Accessed July 30, 2021.

American Society of Addiction Medicine: Public policy statement on physicians and other healthcare professionals with addiction. February 2020. Available at: www.asam.org/docs/default-source/public-policy-statements/2020-public-policy-statement-on-physicians-and-other-healthcare-professionals-with-addiction_final.pdf?sfvrsn=5ed51c2_0. Accessed July 30, 2021.

Boisaubin EV: Causes and treatment of impairment and burnout in physicians: the epidemic within, in Faculty Health in Academic Medicine. Edited by Cole TR, Goodrich TJ, Gritz ER. Totowa, NJ, Humana Press, 2009, pp 29–38

Brooks E: Preventing physician distress and suicide. Chicago, IL, American Medical Association, 2017. Available at: https://edhub.ama-assn.org/steps-forward/module/2702599. Accessed September 25, 2021.

Broquet KE, Rockey PH: Teaching residents and program directors about physician impairment. Acad Psychiatry 28(3):221–225, 2004 15507558

Brown SD, Goske MJ, Johnson CM: Beyond substance abuse: stress, burnout, and depression as causes of physician impairment and disruptive behavior. J Am Coll Radiol 6(7):479–485, 2009 19560063

Dyrbye LN, Thomas MR, Eacker A, et al: Race, ethnicity, and medical student well-being in the United States. Arch Intern Med 167(19):2103–2109, 2007 17954805

Dyrbye LN, West CP, Satele D, et al: Burnout among U.S. medical students, residents, and early career physicians relative to the general U.S. population. Acad Med 89(3):443–451, 2014 24448053

Federation of State Medical Boards: Public policy statement: physician illness vs impairment. Chicago IL, Federation of State Physician Health Programs, July 30, 2008. Available at www.fsphp.org/assets/docs/illness_vs_impairment.pdf. Accessed September 29, 2022.

Federation of State Physician Health Programs: State Programs: Chicago, IL, Federation of State Physician Health Programs, 2018. Available at: https://www.fsphp.org/state-programs#:~:text=A%20Physician%20Health%20Program%20(PHP,or%20other%20potentially%20impairing%20conditions. Accessed September 29, 2022.

Hughes PH, Baldwin DC Jr, Sheehan DV, et al: Resident physician substance use, by specialty. Am J Psychiatry 149(10):1348–1354, 1992 1530071

Jones JTR, North CS, Vogel-Scibilia S, et al: Medical licensure questions about mental illness and compliance with the Americans With Disabilities Act. J Am Acad Psychiatry Law 46(4):458–471, 2018 30593476

Langballe EM, Innstrand ST, Aasland OG, et al: The predictive value of individual factors, work-related factors, and work–home interaction on burnout in female and male physicians: a longitudinal study. Stress Health 27(1):73–87, 2011

McLellan AT, Skipper GS, Campbell M, et al: Five year outcomes in a cohort study of physicians treated for substance use disorders in the United States. BMJ 337:a2038, 2008 18984632

Seize the Awkward: Starting the conversation. New York, Jed Foundation, 2020. Available at: https://seizetheawkward.org/conversation/starting-the-conversation. Accessed August 23, 2021.

Swensen S, Shanafelt T: Applying the action sets to address the unique needs of medical students, residents and fellows, in Mayo Clinic Strategies to Reduce Burnout: 12 Actions to Create the Ideal Workplace. New York, Mayo Clinic Scientific Press, 2020, pp 259–260

University of Pittsburgh Medical Center: Suicide resources. Pittsburgh, PA, University of Pittsburgh Medical Center, June 28, 2021. Available at: https://gmewellness.upmc.com/Resources/Index?topicID=6. Accessed August 23, 2021.

West CP, Shanafelt TD, Kolars JC: Quality of life, burnout, educational debt, and medical knowledge among internal medicine residents. JAMA 306(9):952–960, 2011 21900135

Yaghmour NA, Brigham TP, Richter T, et al: Causes of death of residents in ACGME-accredited programs 2000 through 2014: implications for the learning environment. Acad Med 92(7):976–983, 2017 28514230

CHAPTER 41

Practical Finances

Creating a Budget and Beginning Investing

Timothy Ando, M.D.
James Kahn, M.D.

The lack of education around managing finances in medical school and residency curricula (Ahmad et al. 2017), combined with lack of time to manage finances, leaves many residents relatively unprepared for financial wellness. In this chapter you will learn basic principles of budgeting, investing, and debt management as a foundation for financial wellness that begins in, and extends beyond, residency. This chapter is meant to be informational, and you will want to consult a certified financial adviser or tax professional for advice specific to your financial situation.

KEY POINTS

- Most residents begin their careers with substantial debt, and it is important to consider starting to make loan payments and to understand options for loan consolidation, refinancing, and forgiveness.

- Budgeting is a key skill that will help you track your finances, understand your spending habits, reduce debts, and begin saving.

- In the short term, emergency savings should be your priority, followed by saving for large purchases and major life events by investing to grow your savings.

- In the long term, investing in the U.S. stock market, index funds in particular, is considered safe, stable, and profitable.

- Residency is a great time to start saving for retirement, thanks to compounding interest, potential employer retirement fund matching, and Roth IRA eligibility.

DEBTS

Most people enter residency with a significant amount of interest-accruing debt, such as from undergraduate and medical school, credit cards, and automobile loans. The Association of American Medical Colleges has published a free comprehensive guide to loan repayment titled *Education Debt Manager for Matriculating and Graduating Medical School Students* (see "Resources" section at the end of the chapter). You are highly encouraged to read through this guide when you start residency as part of establishing a financial wellness plan.

Strongly consider starting to pay back loans as soon as residency begins. Incorporating loan payments, no matter how small, into your residency budget could gradually and methodically reduce the principal, leading to a significant impact in the total loan repayment amount. In addition, consider options for loan consolidation, refinancing, and forgiveness. Loan consolidation and refinancing can help simplify payments and lower interest rates but can also alter benefits and protections of federal student loans such as forbearance and loan forgiveness eligibility. Public service loan forgiveness (PSLF) is available to all medical school graduates who commit to working full-time in public service and making monthly loan repayments for 10 years (see "Resources"). If you are pursuing PSLF and have verified that your residency program is an eligible employer, start making the required monthly payments at the beginning of residency. The National Institutes of Health (NIH) Loan Repayment Program also offers grants that will directly pay off loans for physician scientists who are conducting funded research, carry significant educational debt, and agree to a research commitment at either the NIH or a university (see "Resources").

BUDGETING

Budgeting is the process of creating and maintaining an intentional financial plan that allocates income toward expenses, debts, and investments. Why budget? You won't know where your money goes if you don't pay attention to it. Without budgeting, you will not be nearly as effective in managing your finances, and you will be at much greater risk of financial trouble.

A popular method of budgeting allocates income into needs, wants, and investments or savings. Needs represent the necessities of life: rent, car insurance, groceries, and utilities, to name a few. Childcare expenses, loan repayments, and money you send home to your family would be considered needs, too. Wants include any expenses that are not life necessities but are still important to you, such as eating out, watching movies, buying nice clothes, or upgrading your TV. Savings and investments are set aside for future expenses, such as a new car, a house, or retirement. A common rule of thumb for allocating your finances is the 50/30/20 formula: 50% toward needs, 30% toward wants, and 20% toward savings and investments. You may need to adjust these percentages because of cost of living or life circumstances, but most importantly, be specific, deliberate, and realistic with your budget. Allocate limits for each of these needs, wants, and investments, and stick to them, If you find yourself going over budget, consider lifestyle modifications. Incremental reductions in expenses can add up in the long run.

So, how do you create a budget? Online templates and software are available for free. Paid subscription software is also available, but save your money and try the free online programs first (see "Resources"). Remember that no matter how you go about it, budgeting is an active, not passive, effort and requires regular monitoring and maintenance.

BASICS OF INVESTING

Why invest? If you don't invest, your money will slowly depreciate over time because of inflation. Through investment, your money will instead be positioned to grow over time. One of the most popular and accessible venues of investing is the stock market. The stock market has a few categories of investments: stocks, bonds, mutual funds, and index funds. Stocks are pieces of individual companies, and the value of the stock reflects the company's performance. Stocks are considered to be high risk and high reward. Bonds are loans to government or business entities, and they are considered a safe investment with low risk and low reward. Mutual funds are a collection of stocks, bonds, or other assets that are usually hand selected and actively managed by professional investment managers. Last, for simplicity's sake, we refer to index funds and exchange-traded funds interchangeably. These funds are baskets of market assets structurally similar to mutual funds but usually passively managed, automatically following a predetermined market index. Ex-

TABLE 41–1.   Mutual and index funds

Mutual funds	Index funds
Actively managed	Passively managed
High expense ratios (0.5%–1%)	Low expense ratios (0%–0.2%)
Rarely outperform market; often underperform market	Reliably track market

amples of index funds include S&P 500 index funds, health care index funds, bond index funds, and "green" (environmentally friendly) index funds. Actively managed funds rarely outperform passively managed funds over the long term (Rompotis 2020) and incur much higher fees. For this reason, and because of the reliable growth of the overall U.S. economy over time, index funds are an increasingly popular choice for residents as they begin their investment career. When selecting index funds, pay attention to the expense ratio, which is the cost of owning the index fund and can vary widely. A comparison of mutual funds and index funds is provided in Table 41–1.

An important investment strategy is diversification, finance's version of "don't put all your eggs in one basket." Diversification means making a variety of investments so that your overall risk is spread out and a downtrend in one industry sector will not be a disaster to your total investments. Index funds are by definition diversified because they comprise a large number of different assets. However, index funds are still subject to overall market volatility, so you should consider also investing in some bonds to offset risk. Don't lose hope when there is a down year in which you may actually lose value in your investments; over the long run, market growth has consistently overcome downturns.

INVESTMENTS

There are a few reasons to start investing during residency. At the same time, even after careful budgeting, you may find that your expenses and debts leave you with little bandwidth for saving. Indeed, it is generally not a good idea to invest heavily in lieu of paying off large debts. In that case, this section on investing can still serve as useful information for when you are able to start investing.

Before investing, save for an emergency fund in case of a sudden and unexpected financial obligation or loss of income stream. One common rule of thumb is to build and maintain an emergency fund of 3 months' worth of living expenses. Keep these funds readily available in a basic checking or savings account.

Short-Term Investments

For any anticipated large purchases or major life events, you should save and invest accordingly. For the short term, investing in index funds carries some risk that the stock market will experience a downturn when you need the money. To mitigate risk, you may want to consider making investments outside the stock market. As an example, see if any banks or credit unions nearby offer interest-earning high-yield savings or money market accounts, where you can set aside some money for both your emergency fund and upcoming financial obligations. Also consider a certificate of deposit (CD). A CD has a term (length of time) for which you must not withdraw any funds or you will be penalized and an annual percentage yield (APY) or interest rate that is promised for the duration of the CD. Interest rates on CDs tend to be slightly higher than for a high-yield savings or money market account. Last, you can still invest in index funds, but you might want to invest in a significant proportion of bond index funds because bonds are much less prone to fluctuate when the stock market is unstable and will provide a relatively stable, albeit modest, rate of return.

Long-Term Investments

Retirement savings are an important form of long-term investments. Pensions are uncommon, social security benefits are meager, and you must build for your retirement by allocating a proportion of your income during your working years toward retirement savings. Why save for retirement now when it is so far away? Thanks to compounding interest, saving for retirement now is wise *because* it is so far away. Figure 41–1 compares the trajectories of a $6,000 investment at age 30 versus age 35, assuming 7% yearly growth. As you can see, growth is exponential, not linear, and the total value at the retirement age of 65 is about $19,000 greater if the initial investment was made at age 30 instead of 35.

Retirement accounts come in two broad categories: pretax accounts and after-tax accounts. With a pretax retirement account, the money you put in the retirement account is not taxed in the present but will be taxed when withdrawn in retirement; with an after-tax retirement account, on the other hand, you contribute money to the retirement account after paying income tax and withdraw the money in retirement tax-free. Generally, you can have and contribute to both types of retirement accounts, but you should be aware of income limits and yearly contribution limits.

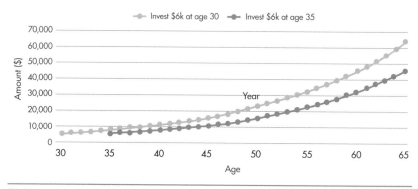

FIGURE 41–1. Compounding interest.

You should have access to an employer-sponsored pretax retirement account, typically a 401(k), 403(b), or 457(b). See if you are eligible for employer matching funds. If so, your employer will match your retirement contributions up to a certain limit or percentage. This is free money that you do not want to leave on the table. Make sure to look into the investment options within employer-sponsored retirement accounts, which usually consist of a selection of index funds. When you leave residency, you will have the option to take this account with you.

You should also strongly consider a Roth individual retirement account (IRA), an after-tax retirement account. The money you contribute to and invest in a Roth IRA will grow steadily over time, and in retirement, distributions on the entire amount, including all investment gains, are tax-free (U.S. Department of the Treasury 2022). This is a key difference from pretax retirement accounts, for which you must eventually pay income tax on your contributions as well as on investment gains. Roth IRA contributions are not allowed above a certain income limit, which resident incomes are well within (unless you have substantial additional income), making residency a perfect time to contribute to a Roth IRA.

SPECIFIC STRATEGIES AND CHALLENGES

⌘ **I'm not used to talking about finances, and I don't know whom to talk to.** You can talk to your coresidents, for one. After all, you are likely to be in similar financial situations, having attended medical school, earning the same salary now, and anticipating similar salaries in the future. Also talk to attending physicians, family, significant others, and anyone else whom you trust. Finances can seem especially daunting if nobody is talking about them, and at the same time, it is very likely that many people around you have, or once had, the exact same questions and uncertainties as you.

⌘ **I don't know how to start to invest in the stock market.** In order to start investing in the stock market and index funds, you will need to open a brokerage account. A brokerage account is similar to the checking account that you probably already have, in that it can be easily opened online, comes with a routing number and account number, and can initiate and accept transfers to and from other bank accounts. The primary difference is that a brokerage account also comes with an interface for making and tracking investments, so once you have some money in the account, you will be able to purchase stocks, bonds, and index funds with it. Some common large brokerage firms include Vanguard, Fidelity, Teachers Insurance and Annuity Association of America–College Retirement Equities Fund (TIAA-CREF), TD Ameritrade, and Schwab. Opening a Roth IRA can be done at the same brokerage firms and involves an equally simple online process.

⌘ **I'm not sure I can do this myself or whether I should hire a financial adviser.** A financial adviser can provide investment expertise as well as peace of mind and additional financial advice around loan repayment, home ownership, and estate planning. Some of the online brokerage businesses provide free investment advice, too. Make sure to understand the fee structures of a financial planner before hiring one, especially because expenses can add up over time; your residency or Graduate Medical Education office may also work with financial planners who offer free consultation to residents. It is also important to remember that active investing (buying and selling assets to try to beat the market) generally falls short of passive investing (purchasing and holding on to reliable long-term investments such as index funds).

⌘ **I've often wondered if credit cards are safe.** Credit cards have significant benefits and drawbacks. The benefits include earning rewards on purchases, easily contesting fraudulent charges (simply call your credit card issuer), and building your credit score so that you can secure better future loans. However, drawbacks include ease of spending leading to unnecessary expenditures and the potential to enter credit card debt. If you are worried about going over budget or losing track of expenses, consider using a debit card or cash instead; carrying an outstanding balance from a partial or minimum credit card payment comes with extremely high interest rates and should be avoided at all costs. You should pay off any balance as aggressively as possible.

⌘ **I can't decide whether to pay back loans or save for future expenses or retirement.** Consider doing both. As mentioned in the section "Debts," you should strongly consider starting to pay back loans in residency to reduce the principal or maintain PSLF eligibility. At the same time, you should not pass up certain benefits of saving for retirement during residency, such as employer matching or Roth IRA eligibility. Make a concerted effort toward financial wellness by both reducing debts and building future savings.

SELF-REFLECTIVE QUESTIONS

1. What are my debts, and how can I incorporate debt repayments into my overall budget?
2. Do I have an emergency fund, and if not, can I prioritize making one?
3. Do I have people in my community with whom I can discuss finances, such as friends and family, coresidents and attendings, or financial advisers through my residency or bank?

RESOURCES

Association of American Medical Colleges: Education Debt Manager for Matriculating and Graduating Medical School Students. Washington, DC, Association of American Medical Colleges, 2021. Available at: https://store.aamc.org/education-debt-manager-for-matriculating-and-graduating-medical-school-students.html. October 15, 2022.

Budgeting resources: Mint (https://mint.intuit.com, free); YNAB (www.youneedabudget.com, paid)

NIH Loan Repayment Programs: www.lrp.nih.gov/eligibility-programs

Public Service Loan Forgiveness: https://studentaid.gov/manage-loans/forgiveness-cancellation/public-service

White Coat Investor: www.whitecoatinvestor.com (popular physician finance blog)

REFERENCES

Ahmad FA, White AJ, Hiller KM, et al: An assessment of residents' and fellows' personal finance literacy: an unmet medical education need. Int J Med Educ 8:192–204, 2017 28557777

Rompotis GG: Actively versus passively managed equity ETFs: new empirical insights. International Journal of Banking, Account, and Finance 11(1):95–135, 2020

U.S. Department of the Treasury: Publication 590-B (2021): distributions from individual retirement arrangements (IRAs). Washington, DC, Internal Revenue Service, May 2, 2022. Available at: www.irs.gov/publications/p590b. Accessed October 15, 2022.

Self-Directed Learning

Jon Sole, M.D.

Bronwyn Lane Scott, M.D.

Karen Li, M.D.

JOURNALS

Many of the journals in Table A–1 represent the top 20 journals in psychiatry according to impact factor, grouped by general area of interest, in addition to education-focused journals.

TABLE A–1.   Journals grouped by area of interest

Area	Journal	Impact factor
Biological psychiatry	*Biological Psychiatry*	7.04
	Lancet Psychiatry	4.88
	Molecular Autism	6.87
	Molecular Psychiatry	10.23
	Translational Psychiatry	5.69
Child and adolescent psychiatry	*Developmental Review*	7.68
	Journal of Child Psychology and Psychiatry and Allied Disciplines	6.47
Clinical psychology	*Annual Review of Clinical Psychology*	16.47
	Clinical Psychology Review	11.48

TABLE A–1.   Journals grouped by area of interest *(continued)*

Area	Journal	Impact factor
	Depression and Anxiety	5.88
	Journal of Abnormal Psychology	5.83
Dementia	*Alzheimer's and Dementia*	13.68
General psychiatry	*Academic Psychiatry*	3.29
	American Journal of Psychiatry	6.91
	British Journal of Psychiatry	3.43
	JAMA Psychiatry	8.16
	World Psychiatry	9.57
Neurology	*Journal of Neurology, Neurosurgery and Psychiatry*	5.58
Psychopharmacology	*Neuropsychopharmacology*	5.66
Psychosis	*Schizophrenia Bulletin*	5.04
Teaching and education	*Academic Medicine*	6.89
	Academic Psychiatry	3.29
	Clinical Supervisor	2.19
	MedEdPORTAL: The Journal of Teaching and Learning Resources (open access)	0.85
	Medical Education	6.25
	Medical Teacher	2.71

SEMINAL ARTICLES

Seminal studies are those that were first to present an idea or paradigm of great importance or influence within a discipline, often stirring subsequent research or altering current understanding. Determining what study fulfills *seminal* criteria is a point of discussion. The studies included in Table A–2 were selected for their significant influence and were cross-referenced with numerous publicly available seminal lists. This list is in no way exhaustive and is meant to serve as a starting point for psychiatric academic literature.

PODCASTS AND WEBSITES

With expanding technological innovation and greater use of online interfacing in mental health, learning and treatment happen through a variety of forums, including podcasts and websites (Tables A–3 and A–4).

Although some of these podcasts and websites may become outdated in the influx of rapidly developing e-resources, residents have found them to be useful for their own learning.

TABLE A–2. Seminal articles in psychiatry

Topic	Article
Addiction	Anton RF, O'Malley SS, Ciraulo DA, et al: Combined pharmacotherapies and behavioral interventions for alcohol dependence: the COMBINE study: a randomized controlled trial. JAMA 295(17):2003–2017, 2006 16670409
	Johnson RE, Chutuape MA, Strain EC, et al: A comparison of levomethadyl acetate, buprenorphine, and methadone for opioid dependence. N Engl J Med 343(18):1290–1297, 2000 11058673
	Jones HE, Kaltenbach K, Heil SH, et al: Neonatal abstinence syndrome after methadone or buprenorphine exposure. N Engl J Med 363(24):2320–2331, 2010 21142534
	McKetin R, Lubman DI, Baker AL, et al: Dose-related psychotic symptoms in chronic methamphetamine users: evidence from a prospective longitudinal study. JAMA Psychiatry 70(3):319–324, 2013 23303471
	Sees KL, Delucchi KL, Masson C, et al: Methadone maintenance vs 180-day psychosocially enriched detoxification for treatment of opioid dependence: a randomized controlled trial. JAMA 283(10):1303–1310, 2000 10714729
Bipolar disorder	BALANCE investigators and collaborators; Geddes JR, Goodwin GM, Rendell J, et al: Lithium plus valproate combination therapy versus monotherapy for relapse prevention in bipolar I disorder (BALANCE): a randomised open-label trial. Lancet 375(9712):385–395, 2010 20092882
	Cipriani A, Barbui C, Salanti G, et al: Comparative efficacy and acceptability of antimanic drugs in acute mania: a multiple-treatments meta-analysis. Lancet 378(9799):1306–1315, 2011 21851976
	Goodwin FK, Fireman B, Simon GE, et al: Suicide risk in bipolar disorder during treatment with lithium and divalproex. JAMA 290(11):1467–1473, 2003 13129986
	Judd LL, Akiskal HS, Schettler PJ, et al: The long-term natural history of the weekly symptomatic status of bipolar I disorder. Arch Gen Psychiatry 59(6):530–537, 2002 12044195

Topic	Article
	Sachs GS, Nierenberg AA, Calabrese JR, et al: Effectiveness of adjunctive antidepressant treatment for bipolar depression. N Engl J Med 356(17):1711–1722, 2007 17392295
Borderline personality disorder	Clarkin JF, Levy KN, Lenzenweger MF, et al: Evaluating three treatments for borderline personality disorder: a multiwave study. Am J Psychiatry 164(6):922–928, 2007 17541052
	Gunderson JG, Stout RL, McGlashan TH, et al: Ten-year course of borderline personality disorder: psychopathology and function from the Collaborative Longitudinal Personality Disorders study. Arch Gen Psychiatry 68(8):827–837, 2011 21464343
	Linehan MM, Comtois KA, Murray AM, et al: Two-year randomized controlled trial and follow-up of dialectical behavior therapy vs therapy by experts for suicidal behaviors and borderline personality disorder. Arch Gen Psychiatry 63(7):757–766, 2006 16818865
Child psychiatry	Bass C, Halligan P: Factitious disorders and malingering: challenges for clinical assessment and management. Lancet 383(9926):1422–1432, 2014 24612861
	Bloch MH, McGuire J, Landeros-Weisenberger A, et al: Meta-analysis of the dose-response relationship of SSRI in obsessive-compulsive disorder. Mol Psychiatry 15(8):850–855, 2010 19468281
	Brent D, Emslie G, Clarke G, et al: Switching to another SSRI or to venlafaxine with or without cognitive behavioral therapy for adolescents with SSRI-resistant depression: the TORDIA randomized controlled trial. JAMA 299(8):901–913, 2008 18314433
	Brent DA, Greenhill LL, Compton S, et al: The Treatment of Adolescent Suicide Attempters study (TASA): predictors of suicidal events in an open treatment trial. J Am Acad Child Adolesc Psychiatry 48(10):987–996, 2009 19730274
	Cortese S, Adamo N, Del Giovane C, et al: Comparative efficacy and tolerability of medications for attention-deficit hyperactivity disorder in children, adolescents, and adults: a systematic review and network meta-analysis. Lancet Psychiatry 5(9):727–738, 2018 30097390

TABLE A–2. Seminal articles in psychiatry *(continued)*

TABLE A–2. Seminal articles in psychiatry *(continued)*

Topic	Article
	Geller B, Luby JL, Joshi P, et al: A randomized controlled trial of risperidone, lithium, or divalproex sodium for initial treatment of bipolar I disorder, manic or mixed phase, in children and adolescents. Arch Gen Psychiatry 69(5):515–528, 2012 22213771
	Hammad TA, Laughren T, Racoosin J: Suicidality in pediatric patients treated with antidepressant drugs. Arch Gen Psychiatry 63(3):332–339, 2006 16520440
	Jensen PS: A 14-month randomized clinical trial of treatment strategies for attention-deficit/hyperactivity disorder: The MTA Cooperative Group Multimodal Treatment Study of Children with PTSD. Arch Gen Psychiatry 56(12):1073–1086, 1999 10591283
	March JS: Cognitive-behavior therapy, sertraline, and their combination for children and adolescents with obsessive-compulsive disorder: the pediatric OCD treatment study (POTS) randomized controlled trial. JAMA 292(16):1969–1976, 2004 15507582
	March JS, Silva S, Petrycki S, et al: The Treatment for Adolescents with Depression Study (TADS): long-term effectiveness and safety outcomes. Arch Gen Psychiatry 64(10):1132–1143. 2007 17909125
	Walkup JT, Albano AM, Piacentini J, et al: Cognitive behavioral therapy, sertraline, or a combination in childhood anxiety. N Engl J Med 359(26):2753–2766, 2008 18974308
Consultation-liaison psychiatry	Appelbaum PS: Assessment of patients' competence to consent to treatment. N Engl J Med 357(25):1834–1840, 2007 17978292
	Barsky AJ, Saintfort R, Rogers MP, et al: Nonspecific medication side effects and the nocebo phenomenon. JAMA 287(5):622–627, 2002 11829702
	Bass C, Halligan P: Factitious disorders and malingering: challenges for clinical assessment and management. Lancet 383(9926):1422–1432, 2014 24612861
	Beach SR, Celano CM, Noseworthy PA, et al: QTc prolongation, torsades de pointes, and psychotropic medications. Psychosomatics 54(1):1–13, 2013 23295003
	Boyer EW, Shannon M: The serotonin syndrome. N Engl J Med 352(11):1112–1120, 2005 15784664

TABLE A–2.	Seminal articles in psychiatry *(continued)*
Topic	**Article**
	Kayser MS, Kohler CG, Dalmau J: Psychiatric manifestations of paraneoplastic disorders. Am J Psychiatry 167(9):1039–1050, 2010 20439389
	Levenson JL: Neuroleptic malignant syndrome. Am J Psychiatry 142(10):1137–1145, 1985
	Maldonado JR: Delirium pathophysiology: an updated hypothesis of the etiology of acute brain failure. Int J Geriatr Psychiatry 33(11):1428–1457, 2018 29278283
	Stone J, Carson A, Sharpe M: Functional symptoms and signs in neurology: assessment and diagnosis. J Neurol Neurosurg Psychiatry 76(suppl 1):i2–i12, 2005 15718217
Depression	DeRubeis RJ, Hollon SD, Amsterdam JD, et al: Cognitive therapy vs medications in the treatment of moderate to severe depression. Arch Gen Psychiatry 62(4):409–416, 2005 15809408
	Elkin I, Shea MT, Watkins JT, et al: National Institute of Mental Health Treatment of Depression Collaborative Research Program: general effectiveness of treatments. Arch Gen Psychiatry 46(11):971–982, 1989 2684085
	Gaynes BN, Rush AJ, Trivedi MH, et al: The STAR*D study: treating depression in the real world. Cleve Clin J Med 75(1):57–66, 2008 18236731
	Kirsch I, Deacon BJ, Huedo-Medina TB, et al: Initial severity and antidepressant benefits: a meta-analysis of data submitted to the Food and Drug Administration. PLoS Med 5(2):e45, 2008 18303940
	Lespérance F, Frasure-Smith N, Koszycki D, et al: Effects of citalopram and interpersonal psychotherapy on depression in patients with coronary artery disease: the Canadian Cardiac Randomized Evaluation of Antidepressant and Psychotherapy Efficacy (CREATE) trial. JAMA 297(4):367–379, 2007 17244833
	Nunes EV, Levin FR: Treatment of depression in patients with alcohol or other drug dependence: a meta-analysis. JAMA 291(15):1887–1896, 2004 15100209
Diversity, equity, and inclusion	Metzl JM, Hansen H: Structural competency: theorizing a new medical engagement with stigma and inequality. Soc Sci Med 103:126–133, 2014 24507917
Eating disorders	Treasure J, Claudino AM, Zucker N: Eating disorders. Lancet 375(9714):583–593, 2010 19931176
	Yager J, Andersen AE: Clinical practice: anorexia nervosa. N Engl J Med 353(14):1481–1488, 2005 16207850

Topic	Article
Electroconvulsive therapy	Geddes J, Carney S, Cowen P, et al: Efficacy and safety of electroconvulsive therapy in depressive disorders: a systematic review and meta-analysis. Lancet 361(9360):799–808, 2003 12642045
	Kellner CH, Fink M, Knapp R, et al: Relief of expressed suicidal intent by ECT: a consortium for research in ECT study. Am J Psychiatry 162(5):977–982, 2005 15863801
	Rose D, Wykes T, Leese M, et al: Patients' perspectives on electroconvulsive therapy: systematic review. BMJ 326(7403):1363, 2003 12816822
	Tess AV, Smetana GW: Medical evaluation of patients undergoing electroconvulsive therapy. N Engl J Med 360(14):1437–1444, 2009 19339723
Epidemiology	Kessler RC, Wai TC, Demler O, et al: Prevalence, severity, and comorbidity of 12-month DSM-IV disorders in the National Comorbidity Survey Replication. Arch Gen Psychiatry 62(6):617–627, 2005 15939839
	Whiteford HA, Degenhardt L, Rehm J, et al: Global burden of disease attributable to mental and substance use disorders: findings from the Global Burden of Disease Study 2010. Lancet 382(9904):1575–1586, 2013 23993280
Gerontology	Morin CM, Colecchi C, Stone J, et al: Behavioral and pharmacological therapies for late-life insomnia: a randomized controlled trial. JAMA 281(11):991–999, 1999 10086433
	Schneider LS, Dagerman KS, Insel P: Risk of death with atypical antipsychotic drug treatment for dementia: meta-analysis of randomized placebo-controlled trials. JAMA 294(15):1934–1943, 2005 16234500
	Schneider LS, Tariot PN, Dagerman KS, et al: Effectiveness of atypical antipsychotic drugs in patients with Alzheimer's disease. N Engl J Med 355(15):1525–1538, 2006 17764624
	Tariot PN, Farlow MR, Grossberg GT, et al: Memantine treatment in patients with moderate to severe Alzheimer disease already receiving donepezil: a randomized controlled trial. JAMA 291(3):317–324, 2004 14734594
Obsessive-compulsive disorder	Abramowitz JS, Taylor S, McKay D: Obsessive-compulsive disorder. Lancet 374(9688):491–499, 2009 19665647

TABLE A–2. Seminal articles in psychiatry *(continued)*

TABLE A–2.   Seminal articles in psychiatry *(continued)*

Topic	Article
	Bloch MH, McGuire J, Landeros-Weisenberger A, et al: Meta-analysis of the dose-response relationship of SSRI in obsessive-compulsive disorder. Mol Psychiatry 15(8):850–855, 2010 19468281
	Foa EB, Liebowitz MR, Kozak MJ, et al: Randomized, placebo-controlled trial of exposure and ritual prevention, clomipramine, and their combination in the treatment of obsessive-compulsive disorder. Am J Psychiatry 162(1):151–161, 2005 15625214
Panic disorder	Barlow DH, Gorman JM, Shear MK, et al: Cognitive-behavioral therapy, imipramine, or their combination for panic disorder: a randomized controlled trial. JAMA 283(19):2529–2536, 2000 10815116
Professionalism	Carrese JA, Malek J, Watson K, et al: The essential role of medical ethics education in achieving professionalism: the Romanell Report. Acad Med 90(6):744–752, 2015 25881647
	Doukas DJ, Volpe R: Why pull the arrow when you cannot see the target? Framing professionalism goals in medical education. Acad Med 93(11):1610–1612, 2018 29697430
	Hickson GB, Pichert JW, Webb LE, et al: A complementary approach to promoting professionalism: identifying, measuring, and addressing unprofessional behaviors. Acad Med 82(11):1040–1048, 2007 17971689
	Ludwig S: Domain of competence: professionalism. Acad Pediatr 14(2 suppl):566–569, 2014 24602656
	Swick HM: Viewpoint: professionalism and humanism beyond the academic health center. Acad Med 82(11):1022–1028, 2007 17971685
Psychosis	Cannon TD, Cadenhead K, Cornblatt B, et al: Prediction of psychosis in youth at high clinical risk: a multisite longitudinal study in North America. Arch Gen Psychiatry 65(1):28–37, 2008 18180426
	Jones PB, Barnes TRE, Davies L, et al: Randomized controlled trial of the effect on quality of life of second- vs first-generation antipsychotic drugs in schizophrenia: Cost Utility of the Latest Antipsychotic Drugs in Schizophrenia Study (CUtLASS 1). Arch Gen Psychiatry 63(10):1079–1087, 2006 17015810
	Kane J, Honigfeld G, Singer J, et al: Clozapine for the treatment-resistant schizophrenic: a double-blind comparison with chlorpromazine. Arch Gen Psychiatry 45(9):789–796, 1988 3046553

TABLE A–2.	Seminal articles in psychiatry *(continued)*
Topic	**Article**
	Lieberman JA, Stroup TS, McEvoy JP, et al: Effectiveness of antipsychotic drugs in patients with chronic schizophrenia. N Engl J Med 353(12):1209–1223, 2005 16172203
	McEvoy J: Effectiveness of clozapine versus olanzapine, quetiapine, and risperidone in patients with chronic schizophrenia who did not respond to prior atypical antipsychotic treatment. Am J Psychiatry 163(4):600–610, 2006 16585434
	Meltzer HY, Alphs L, Green AI, et al: Clozapine treatment for suicidality in schizophrenia: International Suicide Prevention Trial (InterSePT). Arch Gen Psychiatry 60(1):82–91, 2003 12511175
	Ray WA, Chung CP, Murray KT, et al: Atypical antipsychotic drugs and the risk of sudden cardiac death. N Engl J Med 360(3):225–235, 2009 19144938
	Reilly JG, Ayis SA, Ferrier IN, et al: QTc-interval abnormalities and psychotropic drug therapy in psychiatric patients. Lancet 355(9209):1048–1052, 2000 10744090
	Stroup TS, McEvoy JP, Ring KD, et al: A randomized trial examining the effectiveness of switching from olanzapine, quetiapine, or risperidone to aripiprazole to reduce metabolic risk: Comparison of Antipsychotics for Metabolic Problems (CAMP). Am J Psychiatry 168(9):947–956, 2011 21768610
	Tiihonen J, Haukka J, Taylor M, et al: A nationwide cohort study of oral and depot antipsychotics after first hospitalization for schizophrenia. Am J Psychiatry 168(6):603–609, 2011 21362741
	Woods SW, Morgenstern H, Saksa JR, et al: Incidence of tardive dyskinesia with atypical versus conventional antipsychotic medications: a prospective cohort study. J Clin Psychiatry 71(4):463–474, 2010 20156410
PTSD	Ehlers A, Clark DM: A cognitive model of posttraumatic stress disorder. Behav Res Ther 38(4):319–345, 2000 10761279
	Hoge CW, McGurk D, Thomas JL, et al: Mild traumatic brain injury in U.S. soldiers returning from Iraq. N Engl J Med 358(5):453–463, 2008 18491417
	Summerfield D: The invention of post-traumatic stress disorder and the social usefulness of a psychiatric category. Br Med J 322(7278):95–98, 2001 11154627

Topic	Article
	TABLE A–2. Seminal articles in psychiatry *(continued)*
Social phobia	Davidson JRT, Foa EB, Huppert JD, et al: Fluoxetine, comprehensive cognitive behavioral therapy, and placebo in generalized social phobia. Arch Gen Psychiatry 61(10):1005–1013, 2004 15466674
Suicide	Cipriani A, Hawton K, Stockton S, et al: Lithium in the prevention of suicide in mood disorders: updated systematic review and meta-analysis. BMJ 346:f3646, 2013 23814104
	Harris EC, Barraclough B: Suicide as an outcome for mental disorders: a meta-analysis. Br J Psychiatry 170:205–228, 1997 9229027
	Mann JJ, Apter A, Bertolote J, et al: Suicide prevention strategies: a systematic review. JAMA 294(16):2064–2074, 2005 16249421
	Stone M, Laughren T, Jones ML, et al: Risk of suicidality in clinical trials of antidepressants in adults: analysis of proprietary data submitted to US Food and Drug Administration. BMJ 339:431–434, 2009 19671933
Tic disorders	Kurlan R: Clinical practice: Tourette's syndrome. N Engl J Med 363(24):2332–2338, 2010 21142535

TABLE A–3. Psychiatry podcasts

Topic	Podcast	Link	Description
Child psychiatry	*Journal of Child and Adolescent Psychiatry* Podcast Program	www.jaacap.org/content/podcast	Interview with the author of a selected article from JAACAP in which the author shares aspects of their science
	Shrinking It Down: Mental Health Made Simple	www.mghclaycenter.org/multimedia/podcasts	Shines light on the fact that mental health is anything but simple while helping parents and caregivers navigate some tough questions. Cohosts Dr. Gene Beresin and Dr. Khadijah Booth Watkins explore and provide guidance on topics related to the mental health of children, teens, and young adults.
General psychiatry	*American Journal of Psychiatry* Podcast	https://ajp.psychiatryonline.org/audio	In-depth look at one of the articles featured in that month's issue of the *American Journal of Psychiatry*; side-ranging interviews with article authors
	The Carlat Psychiatry Podcast	www.thecarlatreport.com/podcast	Practical updates on clinical psychiatry
	Finding Our Voice	https://psychiatryonline.org/finding-our-voice	A production of APA Publishing and Psychiatric News, this podcast brings viewpoints and opinions of the next generation of psychiatrists—including residents, fellows, and early-career psychiatrists—to the forefront. Each episode focuses on systemic racism within a racial, ethnic, or minority group.

TABLE A–3. Psychiatry podcasts (continued)

Topic	Podcast	Link	Description
	Hidden Brain	https://hiddenbrain.org	NPR's Shankar Vedantam uses science and storytelling to reveal the unconscious patterns that drive human behavior, shape our choices, and direct our relationships.
	JAMA Psychiatry Author Interviews	https://jamanetwork.com/journals/jamapsychiatry/pages/jama-psychiatry-author-interviews	Editors and authors discuss articles published in *JAMA Psychiatry*.
	The Journal of Clinical Psychiatry Publisher's Podcast	www.psychiatrist.com/jcp-podcast	Includes monthly audio updates of the features in each issue of JCP, plus special features added from time to time
	Psychcast	www.mdedge.com/podcasts/psychcast	Hosted by Editor-in-Chief Lorenzo Norris, M.D., Psychcast features mental health care professionals discussing the issues that most affect psychiatry.
	PsychEd	www.psychedpodcast.org	Mental health educational podcast by a team of psychiatry residents based out of the University of Toronto catering to a resident training level; features resident interviews with faculty and experts on common psychiatric conditions
	Psych Essentials	https://psychessentials.org	Psychiatry education podcast for students and learners

TABLE A–3. Psychiatry podcasts *(continued)*

Topic	Podcast	Link	Description
	Psychiatric Services Podcast	https://ps.psychiatryonline.org/podcast	*Psychiatric Services* Editor and Podcast Editor discuss key aspects of research recently published by *Psychiatric Services*.
	Psychiatry and Psychotherapy Podcast	www.psychiatrypodcast.com	Drawing on wisdom from mentors, research, in-session therapy, and psychiatry experience, David Puder, M.D., explores topics that affect mental health professionals and psychology enthusiasts.
	Psychiatry Unbound	https://psychiatryonline.org/psychiatry-unbound	APA Publishing's books authors discuss their scholarship and its impact in clinical settings throughout the world.
Innovations in mental health	The Medical Mind Podcast	www.psychiatry.org/psychiatrists/education/podcasts/the-medical-mind-podcast	Interviews with APA members and other health care professionals about new initiatives in psychiatry from the APA Division of Education
Mental health crisis	Mentally Healthy Nation	https://apafdn.org/news-events/mentally-healthy-nation-podcast	Candid conversations from the American Psychiatric Association Foundation focusing on educating the public and providing tangible solutions to our mental health crisis
Patient-oriented psychiatry	Ask Lisa: The Psychology of Parenting	https://drlisadamour.com/resources/podcast	*New York Times* columnist and author Dr. Lisa Damour provides a timely and practical perspective to parenting questions.

TABLE A–3. Psychiatry podcasts (continued)

Topic	Podcast	Link	Description
	Feeling Good Podcast	https://feelinggood.com/category/podcast	Dr. David Burns, author of *Feeling Good: The New Mood Therapy*, explores TEAM-CBT.
	NPR Life Kit	www.npr.org/lifekit	Explores various topics from sleep to finances to parenting, including a lot of mental health–oriented content
	NPR Life Kit: Parenting	www.npr.org/tags/797069332/life-kit-parenting	Explores parenting-related topics
	Respectful Parenting Podcasts: Janet Lansbury Unruffled	www.janetlansbury.com/2015/08/respectful-parenting-podcasts-janet-lansbury-unruffled	Podcast on parenting
Psychopharmacology	Psychopharmacology and Psychiatry Updates	https://psychopharmacology.libsyn.com	Practical psychopharmacology updates for mental health clinicians, with expert interviews and soundbites from CME presentations
	Psychopharmacology Institute	https://psychopharmacologyinstitute.com	Unbiased and practical psychopharmacology updates for prescribers
	NEI Podcast	https://neiglobal.libsyn.com	High-quality, visually engaging, evidence-based activities to enhance the competence of health care professionals in the diagnosis and treatment of patients with mental illness

TABLE A–3. Psychotherapy podcasts *(continued)*

Topic	Podcast	Link	Description
Psychotherapy	Psychiatry and Psychotherapy Podcast	www.psychiatrypodcast.com	Drawing on wisdom from mentors, research, in-session therapy, and psychiatry experience, David Puder, M.D., explores topics that affect mental health professionals and psychology enthusiasts.

Note. APA=American Psychiatric Association; CBT=cognitive-behavioral therapy; CME=continuing medical education; NPR=National Public Radio; TEAM=testing, empathy, agenda setting, methods.

TABLE A–4.   Psychiatry websites

Topic	Website	Link	Description
General psychiatry	Bullet Psych	www.bulletpsych.com	Free online curriculum with short lessons on the basics of psychiatry for psychiatry residents or medical students
	American Psychological Association	www.apa.org/about/awards	Information about external funding opportunities for research and clinical fellowships, as well as awards
	One Mind PsyberGuide	https://onemindpsyberguide.org	Nonprofit project that aims to help people use technology to live a mentally healthier life by reviewing apps against rating criteria developed by experts in the field
	Epocrates	www.epocrates.com	Clinical database
Neuroanatomy	Radiopaedia	https://radiopaedia.org/?lang=us	Annotated MRI with associated brain areas
Patient-centered websites	Parents Helping Parents	www.php.com	A trusted source of information for helping parents, caregivers, and children with special needs.
	Atlas of Emotions	http://atlasofemotions.org	Interactive tool that builds your vocabulary of emotions and illuminates your emotional world
Psychopharmacology	Psychopharmacopeia	https://psychopharmacopeia.com	Psychotropic database
	Psychopharmacology Algorithms	https://psychopharm.mobi/algo_live	Psychopharmacology algorithms for common indications

TABLE A–4. Psychiatry websites *(continued)*

Topic	Website	Link	Description
Research	Visualmed	www.visualmed.org	Visual guides to landmark studies in medicine
Serious mental illness	SMI Adviser	https://smiadviser.org	SAMHSA-funded and APA-administered website that provides access to in-depth mental health courses, vetted resources, consultations, and more for free

Note. APA=American Psychiatric Association; SAMHSA=Substance Abuse and Mental Health Services Administration; SMI=serious mental illness.

Index

*Page numbers printed in **boldface** type refer to figures, tables, or tools.*